MEDICAL EDUCATION IN OKLAHOMA
VOLUME III

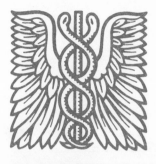

MEDICAL EDUCATION IN OKLAHOMA VOLUME III

The University of Oklahoma
College of Medicine and
Health Sciences Center 1964–1996

Mark Allen Everett
Howard Dean Everett

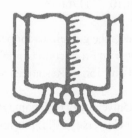

Norman • University of Oklahoma Press

This book is published with the generous assistance of the Wallace C. Thompson Endowment Fund, University of Oklahoma Foundation, the Arthur C. Curtis Fund, and the Herzog Foundation.

Library of Congress Cataloging in Publication Data

Everett, Mark Reuben, 1899–1981
    Medical education in Oklahoma.
    ISBN 0-8061-3268-X
    Includes bibliographical references and index.
    1. Oklahoma.   University.   School of Medicine—
History.   2. Oklahoma.   University.   Medical Center,
Oklahoma City—History.   I. Everett, Alice Allen,
joint author.   II. Title.   III. Everett, Mark Allen and Howard
Dean, joint authors.
R747.067E82   610'.7'1176638   70-177333

The paper in this book meets the guidelines for permanence and durability of the Committee on Production Guidelines for Book Longevity of the Council on Library Resources.∞

1 2 3 4 5 6 7 8 9 10

This book is inscribed in memoriam to
Kathleen Everett Upshaw
and Lloyd Rader

Contents

	List of Illustrations	ix
	List of Tables	xiii
	Acknowledgments	xv
	Authors' Note and Abbreviations	xvii
	Prologue	3
Chapter I	Passing the Torch: The Everett Legacy, 1964	7
Chapter II	Expansion and Struggle: The Dennis Years, 1965–1969	21
Chapter III	Strife in the Executive Suites, 1970–1975	61
Chapter IV	The Provost Governs, 1975–1979	138
Chapter V	Storms in the Sea of Tranquility, 1980–1992	196
Chapter VI	The New CEOs: Academe Lost, 1992–1996	305
	Epilogue	343
	Appendices	347
	Notes	393
	Index of Persons	401
	General Index	407

Illustrations

Mark R. Everett   52
E. T. Dunlap, with William Banowsky   53
The University of Oklahoma Board of Regents
   with President George Lynn Cross   53
John Schilling   54
The old Children's Hospital and the new
   Basic Science Education Building   55
James Dennis   56
Robert M. Bird and James M. Merrill   56
Stewart G. Wolf   57
Dean A. McGee   57
George Lynn Cross at the presentation of Mark R. Everett's portrait   58
Herbert A. Hollomon   59
The Dermatology Clinic   59
The Oklahoma City Clinic   60
Leonard P. Eliel   60
Mark Allen Everett   129
Paul Sharp   129
Lloyd Rader   130
Gordon Deckert   130
The old Children's Hospital   131
A ward in the old Children's Hospital, ca. 1945   132
Oklahoma Memorial Hospital and Clinics, Everett Tower   133
G. Rainey Williams   133
The Child Study Center, 1973   134
Donald Halverstadt   135
Thomas N. Lynn, Jr.   135
The new Presbyterian Hospital   136

Stanton Young   137
William G. Thurman   190
The University of Oklahoma Health Sciences Center campus, 1975   191
Dee Replogle   192
Nancy Davies   192
The Dean A. McGee Eye Institute   193
The Oklahoma Asthma and Allergy Clinic   194
Don H. O'Donoghue   194
William Thurman   195
Clayton Rich   195
The University of Oklahoma College of Medicine, Tulsa Branch   294
The Health Sciences Center's
    Oklahoma Medical Research Foundation   294
The Health Sciences Center's College of Nursing   295
The Health Sciences Center's
    Colleges of Allied Health and Public Health   295
The Health Sciences Center's College of Pharmacy   296
The Health Sciences Center's Robert M. Bird Library   296
Charles B. McCall   297
A Medi-Flight helicopter on landing pad of
    Children's Memorial Hospital   297
Lloyd Rader with his assistant Vera Alder   298
William Banowsky   298
University of Oklahoma Board of Regents and their
    executive secretary, with President Banowsky   299
Joseph Kopta   300
Lloyd Rader and Ralph Hudgins with the infamous wrecking ball   300
Patrick A. McKee   301
The University of Oklahoma Health Sciences Center
    and downtown Oklahoma City, 1985   301
George Garrison   302
Donald G. Kassebaum   302
Lloyd Rader   303
William E. Brown   303
Edward N. Brandt, Jr.   304
Hans Brisch   304
Donald B. Halverstadt, Douglas Voth, and Jay Stein   338
R. Timothy Coussons   338

David Boren	339
The Family Medicine building	340
The Alfred P. Murrah Federal Building after the bombing, 1995	340
Joseph Ferretti	341
Jerry Vannatta	341
The University of Oklahoma Health Sciences Center campus, 1998	342

Photographs are from the collection of Alice Allen Everett (AAE) or are courtesy of the Oklahoma Department of Human Services (DHS), the photography service of the University of Oklahoma Health Sciences Center (OUHSC), and the University of Oklahoma Division of Public Affairs (OUPA).

Tables

1. College of Medicine Budget, 1973–1978   161
2. Salaries of Instructional Staff, Health Sciences Center, 1980   199
3. Salary Ranges, Health Sciences Center, 1981   210
4. College of Medicine Budget, 1985–1986   238
5. Agency Special Accounts for Professional Practice Plans   256
6. Evening of Excellence Honorees, 1985–1995   310

CHART

University of Oklahoma Health Sciences Center
    Timeline, 1964–1996   xix

Acknowledgments

The authors wish to thank the following individuals for their kindness in responding to our often intrusive questioning with good humor, tolerance, and insight: University of Oklahoma President Emeritus Paul Sharp, Dr. Stewart Wolf, Dr. "Monty" DuVal, Professor Patrick McKee, Professor Gordon Deckert, Professor Emeritus James Merrill, Dr. Harris D. Riley, former Provost William G. Thurman, Dr. Thomas N. Lynn, Jr., Dr. Donald Halverstadt, Dr. Timothy Coussons, Dr. Oscar Parsons, Dr. Ronald Elkins, Dr. Joseph Kopta, Mrs. Mark R. Everett, Regent Julian Rothbaum, Vice-chancellor of Higher Education Gary Smith, Ms. Vera Alder (assistant to Lloyd Rader), and the late Professor G. Rainey Williams, who shared not only his observations but also many of his last precious hours in friendship with the authors. To each of these we are most grateful.

We also wish to acknowledge the guidance and suggestions of our editors, Kim Wiar and Karen Couch Wieder, as well as the generous assistance of Ruby Humphrey, Patty L. Lawson, Barbara Sappenfield, Joann Taylor, Dr. Loy Markland, and Leland Alexander and his staff at the Tulsa Medical School. We also appreciate the assistance of the following individuals in assembling photographs for this publication: Kyle Noble of the Department of Human Services; Lanay J. David, Teri Jennings, and Terry Stover of the University of Oklahoma Health Sciences Center Photographic Service; and Katherine Bishop and Jerri Culpepper of the University of Oklahoma Office of Public Affairs.

Last on our list but not in our gratitude are Dean Douglas Voth for his persistent encouragement to write this history, and to Dr. Chris Purcell, Executive Secretary of the University of Oklahoma Board of Regents, and her hard-working staff, and Dean Sul Lee of the Bizzell Memorial Library.

Without their generous assistance and resources, this book could not have been written.

In addition to the contributions of the individuals cited above, the authors relied on several major print resources in compiling this history: (1) The multivolume *Minutes of the Board of Regents of the University of Oklahoma, 1964–1998*. These volumes, which are official state documents on file at the Norman offices of the University of Oklahoma Board of Regents, were the source of much factual information regarding personnel appointments, terms of service, salaries, contracts, dates, cost and construction of buildings, political disputes, medical programs, relations with other government agencies, and every imaginable topic affecting the Health Sciences Center and its personnel. Rare is the page in this history that does not contain at least one tidbit gleaned from the *Regents Minutes*. (2) *The Daily Oklahoman* and, to a lesser extent, the *Oklahoma City Times*, the *Tulsa World*, the *Journal Record*, and the *Oklahoma Daily* (the University of Oklahoma newspaper). The *Daily Oklahoman*, which has been, with few exceptions, extremely supportive of the Health Sciences Center, also provided a great deal of information and insight into the relationships of the Center to the outside world and to Oklahoma's political establishment. If the dry bones of this history came largely from the *Regents Minutes*, much of its color and life came from the *Daily Oklahoman* and other state newspapers.

Author's Note and Abbreviations

 To conserve space and spare readers the necessity of consulting countless notes, quotations from major sources are cited in italics and brackets at the conclusion of the quoted material, as follows:

[RM, 14619]   *Regents Minutes*, p. 14619
[FBM, 3–30–94]   *Faculty Board Minutes*, Mar. 30, 1994
[DO, 6–19–82]   *Daily Oklahoman*, June 19, 1982
[JR, 9–1–88]   *Journal Record*, Sept. 1, 1988

Other less-frequently used sources are cited with their full nomenclature in italics and brackets at the end of the quoted material—e.g., *[Tulsa World, 11–4–88]*—or as numbered notes.

Careful readers may notice that several quotations are not followed by citations. When this occurs, it is the result of a request by the source to "speak off the record." We have attempted to honor all such requests.

The opinions expressed in this history, unless they appear as quoted material, are entirely those of the authors, and in no way do they purport to represent the opinions of the administration or staff of the University of Oklahoma, the Health Sciences Center, or the University of Oklahoma Press. By its very nature, a history will reflect the viewpoint (and, despite their best efforts to remain objective, the biases) of the authors who wrote it. This history, then, reflects the observations and experiences of Dr. Mark Allen Everett, who wrote much of the text from his point of view as chair of the Faculty Board during the period 1974–1990, as well as the views of Dr. Howard D. Everett, who performed most of the research and edited the book. Both Drs. Everett accept responsibility for any errors in fact readers may find, including errors in dates of individual service which were not recorded in official documents.

University of Oklahoma Health Sciences Center
Timeline 1964–1996
(New appointees appear in **bold**.)

Year	O.U. President	O.U. Board of Regents	HSC Provost	HSC Dean and Director	Governance of HSC Hospitals	HSC Hospitals Chiefs of Staff	HSC Hospitals CEOs
1964	George L. Cross	James G. Davidson, John M. Houchin, Mark R. Johnson, Quintin Little, Ira Eph Monroe, Glenn Northcutt, Julian J. Rothbaum, Reuben K. Sparks	No Provost	Mark R. Everett, Dean and Director, retired in March; **Joseph M. White**, interim **James L. Dennis** appointed Dean on September 1	University: O.U. Children's: O.U.	University and Children's: William A. Parry	Joseph M. White through August 31; James L. Dennis, September 1
1965	George L. Cross	**Horace K. Calvert**, Davidson, Houchin, Johnson, Little, Monroe, Rothbaum, Sparks	No Provost	James L. Dennis	University: O.U. Children's: O.U.	University and Children's: William A. Parry	James L. Dennis
1966	George L. Cross	Calvert, **Nancy J. Davies**, Davidson, Houchin, Johnson, Little, Rothbaum, Sparks	No Provost	James L. Dennis	University: O.U. Children's: O.U.	University and Children's: William A. Parry; James B. Snow, Jr., July 1	James L. Dennis
1967	George L. Cross	Calvert, Davies, Davidson, Houchin, **Huston Huffman**, Johnson, Little, Sparks	No Provost	James L. Dennis; title of Vice-President for Medical Center Affairs added on May 11	University: O.U. Children's: O.U.	University and Children's: James B. Snow, Jr.	James L. Dennis

Year	O.U. President	O.U. Board of Regents	HSC Provost	HSC Dean and Director	Governance of HSC Hospitals	HSC Hospitals Chiefs of Staff	HSC Hospitals CEOs
1968	George L. Cross; **John Herbert Hollomon**, July 1	Calvert, Davies, Davidson, Houchin, Huffman, Little, **Jack H. Santee,** Sparks	No Provost	James Dennis	University: O.U. Children's: O.U.	University and Children's: James B. Snow, Jr.; Ben Heller, July 1	James L. Dennis
1969	John Herbert Hollomon	Calvert, Davies, Houchin, Huffman, Little, **Walter Neustadt, Jr.,** Santee, Sparks	No Provost	James Dennis	University: O.U. Children's: O.U.	University and Children's: Ben Heller	James L. Dennis
1970	John Herbert Hollomon; **Pete Kyle McCarter,** Acting President, effective September 1	Calvert, Davies, Houchin, Huffman, **Vernon M. Lockard, Robert C. Lollar,** Neustadt, Santee, Sparks	**James L. Dennis** becomes, in effect, the first Provost with new title of Executive Vice-President for Medical Center Affairs and deletion of title of Dean; Dennis replaced by **John Colmore** in September, who dies in November; **Leonard P. Eliel** appointed Interim Executive Vice-President for Medical	James Dennis; Regents add title of Executive Vice-President for Medical Center Affairs and delete title of Dean, School of Medicine; **John P. Colmore** appointed as Interim successor to Dennis September 15; title of Associate Dean of School of Medicine added in July; then deleted in September; Colmore dies November	University: O.U. Children's: O.U.	University and Children's: Ben Heller through June 30; Gordon Deckert, July 1	James L. Dennis through August 31; John Colmore, September 1 through November 26 (death); Leonard P. Eliel, December 1

1971 McCarter, Interim; **Paul F. Sharp**, appointed in April, attends first Regents meeting in August	**Mack M. Braly, Thomas R. Brett,** Calvert, Davies, Huffman, Lockard, Neustadt, Santee	Center Affairs and Interim Director of the Medical Center effective December 1 Leonard P. Eliel made permanent Executive Vice-President for Medical Center Affairs and Director of the Medical Center	26; **Robert M. Bird** selected as Dean of School of Medicine, July 1 Robert M. Bird; title of School of Medicine changed to College of Medicine at November 11 Regents meeting; title of Univeristy of Oklahoma Medical Center changed to Oklahoma Health Sciences Center November 11	University: O.U. Children's: O.U.	University and Children's Gordon Deckert	Leonard P. Eliel
1972 Paul F. Sharp	Braly, Brett, Calvert, Davies, Huffman, **Bob G. Mitchell** Neustadt, Santee	Leonard P. Eliel	Robert M. Bird	University: O.U. Children's: O.U. DISRS agrees to provide funds for Children's Hospital rather than consolidate it with University Hospital	University and Children's: Gordon Deckert	Leonard P. Eliel
1973 Paul F. Sharp	**Kenneth Dexter Bailey,** Braly, Brett, Davies, Huffman, Mitchell, Neustadt, Santee	Leonard P. Eliel; title changed to Vice-President for Health Sciences in March; President Sharp	Robert M. Bird; Regents approve establishment of a Tulsa branch of the Medical School in	University: O.U. Children's: **Welfare Commission**; Agreement between OU and DISRS	University and Children's: Gordon Deckert through June 30; University: G. Rainey Williams, July	Leonard P. Eliel through January 11. Governance of University

Year	O.U. President	O.U. Board of Regents	HSC Provost	HSC Dean and Director	Governance of HSC Hospitals	HSC Hospitals Chiefs of Staff	HSC Hospitals CEOs
1973			recommends in May that title of Vice-President for Health Sciences be changed to Provost for the Health Sciences; Regents approve; Dr. Eliel announces resignation effective July 1; **William E. Brown**, DDS, Dean of College of Dentistry named Acting Provost of the Health Sciences Center June 1	July and begin search for Tulsa Dean	regarding Title XIX funding for Children's March 17; **University Hospital placed under control of its own Board of Trustees** (Senate Bill 325) in May; Regents transfer Hospital to Board in June; Children's: Regents transfer **Children's Hospital to Welfare Commission** in June	1; Children's: Donald B. Halverstadt July 1	and Children's split. University: Jeptha Dalston January 12; Children's: Donald B. Halverstadt
1974	Paul F. Sharp	Bailey, **Richard Allen Bell**, Braly, Brett, Huffman, Mitchell, Neustadt, Santee	William Brown (acting); **William G. Thurman** appointed November 14	Robert M. Bird resigns July 12; **Thomas N. Lynn** appointed Acting Dean, July 26	University: Board of Trustees; Children's: Welfare Commission	University: G. Rainey Williams; Children's: Donald B. Halverstadt	University: Jeptha Dalston; Children's: Donald B. Halverstadt
1975	Paul F. Sharp	Bailey, Bell, Braly, Brett, Mitchell, **Dee A. Replogle, Jr.**, Santee	William Brown, Acting Provost, attends final Regents meeting in March; William G. Thurman	Thomas N. Lynn	University: Board of Trustees; Children's: Welfare Commission	University: G. Rainey Williams through June 30; Stanley Deutsch, July 1; Children's:	University: Jeptha Dalston; Don Brown (interim)

	becomes Provost in April		Donald B. Halverstadt		University: Stanley Deutsch; Children's: Donald B. Halverstadt	University: Bruce M. Perry; Children's: Donald B. Halverstadt
1976 Paul F. Sharp	Bailey, Bell, Braly, Brett, **Charles E. Engleman**, Mitchell, Neustadt, Replogle	William G. Thurman	Thomas N. Lynn	University: Board of Trustees; Children's: Welfare Commission	University: Stanley Deutsch; Children's: Donald B. Halverstadt	University: Bruce M. Perry; Children's: Donald B. Halverstadt
1977 Paul F. Sharp	Bailey, Bell, Braly, Brett, Engleman, Mitchell, Replogle, **Ronald H. White**	William G. Thurman	Thomas N. Lynn	University: Board of Trustees; Children's: Welfare Commission	University: Stanley Deutsch through June 30; G. Rainey Williams, July 1; Children's: Donald B. Halverstadt	University: Bruce M. Perry; Children's: Donald B. Halverstadt
1978 Paul F. Sharp; **William Slater Banowsky**, August 14	Bailey, Bell, Brett, Engleman, Little, Mitchell, Replogle, White	William G. Thurman	Thomas N. Lynn	University: Board of Trustees; Children's: Welfare Commission	University: G. Rainey Williams; Children's: Donald B. Halverstadt	University: Bruce M. Perry; Children's: Donald B. Halverstadt
1979 William S. Banowsky	Bailey, Bell, Engleman, Little, Mitchell, **Julian J. Rothbaum**, Replogle, White	William G. Thurman resigns November 1 to accept OMRF presidency; **Donald B. Halverstadt**, Interim Provost	Thomas N. Lynn	University: Board of Trustees; Children's: Welfare Commission	University: G. Rainey Williams through June 30; James Merrill, July 1; Children's: Donald B. Halverstadt	University: Bruce M. Perry Children's: Donald B. Halverstadt

Year	O.U. President	O.U. Board of Regents	HSC Provost	HSC Dean and Director	Governance of HSC Hospitals	HSC Hospitals Chiefs of Staff	HSC Hospitals CEOs
1980	William S. Banowsky	Bailey, Bell, Engleman, Little, **Thomas M. McCurdy, II,** Rothbaum, Replogle, White	Donald B. Halverstadt, Interim Provost; **Clayton Rich**, June 1	Thomas N. Lynn resigns; **G. Rainey Williams** appointed Interim Dean, effective January 1	University: Board of Trustees; then to **Welfare Commission** on August 28; Children's: Welfare Commission	University: James Merrill through June 30; Mark Allen Everett, July 1; Children's: Donald B. Halverstadt	University and Children's: Donald B. Halverstadt
1981	William S. Banowsky	Bell, Engleman, **John M. Imel**, Little, McCurdy, Rothbaum, Replogle, White	Clayton Rich	G. Rainey Williams, Interim Dean	University: Welfare Commission; Children's: Welfare Commission	University: Mark Allen Everett; Children: Webb Thompson	University and Children's: Donald B. Halverstadt
1982	William S. Banowsky (resigns Sept. 1; returns Nov. 11); **J.R. Morris** Interim	Engleman, Imel, **Thomas Elwood Kemp**, Little, McCurdy, Rothbaum, Replogle, White	Clayton Rich; title changed to Provost and Vice-President for Health Sciences, December 9	G. Rainey Williams, Interim until February 1; **Charles McCall,** February 1; given additional title of Executive Dean, October 14	University: Welfare Commission; Children's: Welfare Commission	University: Mark Allen Everett; Children's: Webb Thompson	University and Children's: Donald B. Halverstadt
1983	William Banowsky	Engleman, Imel, Kemp, Little, McCurdy, Rothbaum,	Clayton Rich	Charles McCall	University: Welfare Commission; Children's: Welfare	University: Mark Allen Everett; Children's:	University and Children's:

	Charles F. Sarratt, White				Commission	Webb Thompson	Donald B. Halverstadt through June 30; Owen Rennart
1984	William S. Banowsky	Imel, Kemp, Little, McCurdy, Rothbaum, Sarratt, White	Clayton Rich	Charles McCall; on sick leave April 20 through September 21; **William Knisely** appointed Acting Dean in McCall's absence	University: Welfare Commission; Children's: Welfare Commission	University: Mark Allen Everett; Children's: Webb Thompson	University and Children's: Owen Rennart
1985	William S. Banowsky resigns February 1; **Martin C . Jischke,** Interim, to September; **Frank E. Horton,** September 10	**Sarah C. Hogan,** Imel, Kemp, Little, McCurdy, Rothbaum, Sarratt, White	Clayton Rich	Charles McCall (William Knisely); **G. Rainey Williams** appointed Interim Executive Dean and Interim Dean, College of Medicine, June 13	University: Welfare Commission; Children's: Welfare Commission	University: Mark Allen Everett through June 30; Robert McCaffree, July 1; Children's: Webb Thompson through June 30; Owen Rennert July 1	University and Children's: Owen Rennart through June 30; Antonio Padilla, July 1
1986	Frank E. Horton	Hogan, Imel, Kemp, **Sylvia A. Lewis,** McCurdy, Rothbaum, Sarratt, White	Clayton Rich	G. Rainey Williams, Interim; Donald G. Kassebaum, selected June 12, reports to duty August 1	University: Welfare Commission; Children's: Welfare Commission	University: Robert McCaffree; Children's: Owen Rennert	University and Children's: Antonio Padilla

Year	O.U. President	O.U. Board of Regents	HSC Provost	HSC Dean and Director	Governance of HSC Hospitals	HSC Hospitals Chiefs of Staff	HSC Hospitals CEOs
1987	Frank E. Horton	Hogan, Imel, Kemp, Lewis, McCurdy, **Samuel R. Noble**, Sarratt, White	Clayton Rich	Donald Kassebaum	University: Welfare Commission; Children's: Welfare Commission	University: Robert McCaffree; Children's: Andy Sullivan	University and Children's: Bobby G. Thompson
1988	Frank E. Horton resigns August 1; **David Swank**, Interim, August 1	**E. Murray Gullatt**, Hogan, Imel, Kemp, Lewis, Noble, Sarratt, White	Clayton Rich	Donald Kassebaum resigns June 30; **G. Rainey Williams** appointed Interim Executive Dean and Interim Dean, College of Medicine, July 1; **Edward N. Brandt, Jr.** selected as Executive Dean and Dean, College of Medicine, December 8	University: Welfare Commission; Children's: Welfare Commission	University: Robert McCaffree; Children's: Andy Sullivan	University and Children's: Bobby G. Thompson through June 30; Andrew A. Lasser, July 1
1989	David Swank, Interim; **Richard L. Van Horn**, July 15	Gullatt, Hogan, Kemp, Lewis, Noble, Sarratt, **J. Cooper West**, White	Clayton Rich	G. Rainey Williams, Interim through May; Edward N. Brandt, Jr. assumes post on June 1	University: Welfare Commission; Children's: Welfare Commission	University: Robert McCaffree; Children's: Andy Sullivan through June 30; John Grunow, July 1	University and Children's: Andrew A. Lasser
1990	Richard L. Van Horn	**G. T. Blankenship,** Gullatt, Hogan, Lewis,	Clayton Rich	Edward N. Brandt, Jr.	University: Welfare Commission;	University: Robert McCaffree	University and

					University/Children's	University/Children's	University/Children's
		Noble, Sarratt, West White			Children's: Welfare Commission	through June 30; Russell G. Postier, July 1; Children's: John Grunow	Children's: Andrew A. Lasser
1991	Richard L. Van Horn	Blankenship, Gullatt, Hogan, Lewis, Noble, West, White, **C. Victor Williams**	Clayton Rich	Edward N. Brandt, Jr.	University: Welfare Commission; Children's: Welfare Commission	University: Russell G. Postier; Children's: John Grunow through June 30; Joe Leonard	University and Children's: Andrew A. Lasser
1992	Richard L. Van Horn	Blankenship, **Ada Lois Sipuel Fisher**, Gullatt, **Melvin C. Hall**, Lewis, Hogan, West, Williams	Clayton Rich through June 30; **Jay H. Stein** appointed Senior Vice-President and Provost, Health Sciences Center, July 1	Edward N. Brandt, Jr. through July 31; **Douglas W. Voth** appointed Executive Dean of the College of Medicine, November 11	University: Welfare Commission; Children's: Welfare Commission	University: Russell G. Postier through June 30; M. DeWayne Andrews, July 1; Children's: Joe Leonard	University and Children's: Andrew A. Lasser
1993	Richard L. Van Horn	**Stephen F. Bentley**, Blankenship, Fisher, Gullatt, Hall, **Donald B. Halverstadt**, West	Jay H. Stein	Douglas W. Voth	University: Welfare Commission; Children's: Welfare Commission; Hospitals transferred to University Hospitals Authority July 1	University: M. DeWayne Andrews; Children's: Joe Leonard through June 30; Tom Lerher, July 1	University and Children's: Andrew A. Lasser through June 30; R. Timothy Coussons, July 1

Year	O.U. President	O.U. Board of Regents	HSC Provost	HSC Dean and Director	Governance of HSC Hospitals	HSC Hospitals Chiefs of Staff	HSC Hospitals CEOs
1994	Richard L. Van Horn, through June 5; **J. R. Morris** Interim, June 6; **David L. Boren,** November 1	Bentley, Blankenship, Gullatt, Hall, Halverstadt, **C. S. Lewis III,** West	Jay H. Stein	Douglas W. Voth	University Hospitals Authority	University: M. DeWayne Andrews through June 30; M. Alex Jaycocks, July 1; Children's: Tom Lerher	University and Children's: R. Timothy Coussons
1995	David L. Boren	Bentley, Blankenship, Gullatt, Hall, Halverstadt, Lewis, **Robin Siegfried,** West	Jay Stein resigns June 30; **Joseph Ferretti** appointed Interim Vice-President and Provost July 1	Douglas Voth resigns; **Jerry B. Vannatta** Associate Provost for Medical Affiars July 1	University Hospitals Authority	University: M. Alex Jaycocks; Children's: Tom Lerher through June 30; Curtis Gruel, July1	University and Children's: R. Timothy Coussons
1996	David L. Boren	Bentley, Blankenship, Gullatt, Hall, Halverstadt, Lewis **Mary Jane Noble,** Siegfried	Joseph Ferretti named Senior Vice-President and Provost April 25	Jerry Vannatta named Vice President for Health Affairs and Associate Provost April 25; named Interim Executive Dean July 1	University Hospitals Authority	University: M. Alex Jaycocks through June 30; Dwight Reynolds, July 1; Children's: Curtis Gruel	University and Children's: R. Timothy Coussons
1997	David L. Boren	Bentley, Blankenship	Joseph Ferretti	Jerry Vannatta	University Hospitals Authority	University: Dwight Reynolds;	University and

Year	President		Dean	Event	Provost	Interim
		(reappointed), Gullatt, Hall, Halverstadt, Lewis, Noble, Siegfried	Joseph Ferretti		Children's: Curtis Gruel through June 30; Morris Gessouroan, July 1	Children's: R. Timothy Coussons
1998	David L. Boren	Bentley (reappointed), Blankenship, **Christie Everest**, Gullatt, Halverstadt, Lewis, Noble, Siegfried	Jerry Vannatta	Merger with Columbia/HCA-Presbyterian	University: Dwight Reynolds through June 30; Ronald Elkins, July 1; Children's: Morris Gessouroan	University and Children's: R. Timothy Coussons until arrival of Gerald J. Maier

MEDICAL EDUCATION IN OKLAHOMA
VOLUME III

Prologue

The three decades between the retirement of Dean and Medical Center Director Mark R. Everett in 1964 and the ascension of Provost Joseph J. Ferretti in 1996 witnessed a sea change on the University of Oklahoma Health Sciences Center campus. A vast building program, financed by two state bond issues, abundant federal matching money, and the moral and financial support of Department of Human Services Director Lloyd Rader, dramatically transformed the physical appearance of the campus. The addition of new schools and colleges altered the educational and political scenes, diminishing the once overwhelming influence of the College of Medicine while elevating the others to near-equal status. The combination of local political pressure (primarily from Tulsa legislators and osteopaths throughout the state) and federal encouragement of medical school class expansion led to a large increase in the annual production of physicians and osteopaths, while a legislatively mandated branch medical school in Tulsa put enormous strains on the fiscal stability of the parent Center in Oklahoma City. Throughout this same period, there was a large increase in federal research grants from the National Institutes of Health (primarily in the 1960s and again in the 1990s), which fed the growth of scientific investigation and the size of departmental payrolls.

The 1965–1969 period was notable for the physical growth of the campus, the separation of the position of dean of the College of Medicine from that of Medical Center director, and the increasingly bitter struggle for power between Dean James L. Dennis and University of Oklahoma President Herbert Hollomon, which ultimately led to the departure of both.

The years 1970–1975 were characterized by campus leadership vested in the faculty and continuing fiscal crises, primarily as a result of rising health care costs, the great expense of operating new facilities in Oklahoma City and Tulsa, wage inflation, diminishing federal funds, and the unwillingness of the state legislature to provide sufficient yearly increments in appropriations to operate the expanding campus and mandated growth in its programs. Additionally, there was a constant struggle to find funds to provide medical care for Oklahoma's indigent population. There was no state program to fund unreimbursed care, and the counties, which were mandated by law to pay the teaching hospitals for the care given to their indigents, refused to honor this obligation. Oklahoma never came to grips with the problem of providing medical care to indigents, and the arrival of Medicare did little more than lessen the visibility of the problem.

The period from 1975–1980, under the strong direction of Provost William Thurman, saw a realignment of administrative power on the Oklahoma City campus. Authority and dominion moved away from the geheimrat clinical professors—who controlled the destinies of their respective medical departments and, through the Faculty Board, determined the curricula and direction of the College of Medicine—to a layered bureaucracy of administrators, their hands firmly on the finances and direction of the Center's hospitals, as well as on its growing collection of colleges: Medicine, Nursing, Health, Allied Health, and Pharmacy. And, to no one's surprise, the marginal fiscal viability of the entire operation continued throughout the period.

From 1980–1992, centralization of power and control increased more slowly and with less trauma under Provost Clayton Rich, who was both less confrontational and less aggressive as an administrator than his predecessor. This period was also characterized by a series of "revolving door" deans in the College of Medicine, which contributed to a lessened influence of the College on the campus overall.

During the 1992–1996 period, the need for increased numbers of "health care providers" in the state and nation was challenged, and liberal government funding for large medical classes was discontinued, with consequent tighter budgets and decreases in student enrollments nationwide. The advent of managed care placed great pressure on the rising costs of health care and had an especially adverse effect on academic heath centers. These factors in aggregate caused a reexamination of the fundamental basis upon which such centers were operated, leading to further dispersion of students among community hospitals, and to increased emphasis on the delivery of health care by academic faculty, which generated funds that the institutions came to depend on for daily operation. In the early 1990s, Provost Clayton Rich was succeeded by the vigorous and uncompromising Jay Stein, who completed the transformation of the Medical Center to a health delivery organization.

Throughout the thirty-plus years of this history, there were three vital constants: 1) the critical role of the Veterans Administration Hospital in providing teaching beds, resident stipends, and faculty salaries; 2) the consistent financial and administrative support of the Department of Human Services, especially under the direction of Lloyd E. Rader; and 3) the unswerving dedication of the Presbyterian Foundation to excellence in medical education. There also were thousands of changes that affected the lives of every individual connected to the University of Oklahoma Health Sciences Center. Of these changes, however, only a few were of such overriding significance that they can be labeled fundamental or even historic. Among these were: (1) The Medical School deanship, originally an office representing the faculty to the administration, became less aligned with the faculty and more primarily an administrative position, carrying out the policies of the various provosts and University presidents. (2) With the prominent expansion of enrollment in the College of Medicine (from 75 in 1951 to 184 in 1987) and the division of the third- and fourth-year students between Tulsa and Oklahoma City, the previous, often close relationships between faculty and students diminished. Students did not even always know the names of their own classmates, much less of the faculty. Lost in this growth was the collegiality and esprit de corps of earlier periods in the Center's history, a trend that persisted even when enrollments declined after 1987. (3) The increase in student numbers was accompanied by (and principally due to) an increased emphasis on the production of, and perceived need for, primary care physicians, with dispersion of medical students to numerous sites and the concomitant growth of graduate programs in Family Practice. (4) The change in concept from a "medical center" to a "health sciences center" removed the dean of the College of Medicine from the central role on the campus and placed him under the overall supervision or control of a provost or vice president. This had the effect of making the several other colleges on campus and their deans the "equals" of the College of Medicine and the medical dean, even though the budget for medicine and research exceeded that of the sum of the budgets for all the other colleges. (5) The "health sciences" concept led to both a greatly enlarged Center and to a blurring of the central role of the University Hospitals as the primary training site for medical students, as new hospitals and clinics, both on-campus (Presbyterian Hospital) and off-campus (primary care clinics), came to be utilized for medical student education. (6) Finally, after 1995 the position of dean was merged with the position of associate provost for medical affairs, further removing the dean from his former role of faculty advocate and leader, and establishing the dean's primary function as a "CEO" of managed care at the Center. This essentially relegated the College of Medicine and its hospitals to a "health provider" role, rather than what it had been historically, an enterprise dedicated to scholarship and education.

Three institutions lie at the heart of this history and all three underwent numerous changes in name, mission, governance, and effectiveness: (1) the University of Oklahoma College of Medicine, (2) the University Hospital, and (3) the Children's Hospital of Oklahoma. Their stories constitute the essence of this account.

Chapter I.
Passing the Torch:
The Everett Legacy,
1964

 Exceptional events often have unexceptional beginnings. For example, who suspected in 1914 that World War I would evolve from the assassination of an Austrian archduke by an unknown political fanatic in Sarajevo, Bosnia? On a vastly smaller scale, how many Oklahomans imagined that a 1961 trip to Washington, D.C., by University of Oklahoma Medical Center Dean Mark R. Everett would initiate a funding renaissance that would continue, albeit sporadically, far into the century and drag the Center kicking and screaming into the mainstream of U.S. medical education and patient care?

Not even Dean Everett had an inkling of the significance of his 1961 journey. For him, it was another in a long line of begging trips to acquire federal operating funds and building capital for a Medical Center[1] that was historically—and often woefully—underfunded by the Oklahoma legislature. The dean, who frequently brought with him one of the brilliant young department heads he recruited during his seventeen-year stewardship, viewed the trip as merely another salvo in the decades-long battle to mold the Medical Center into an institution without peer, public or private, in the state of Oklahoma. To paraphrase the ironic comment of longtime University of Oklahoma President George L. Cross, Dean Everett sought to build a Medical Center that "even the football team can be proud of."

In the early 1960s, according to Mark R. and Alice Everett's *Medical Education in Oklahoma*, "The School of Medicine needed about $500,000 a year [above legislative appropriations] to stabilize its operations, which leaves much in the land of limbo."[2] These funds (which equate to millions in contemporary dollars) were above and beyond the annual state appropriation for such purposes and were necessary simply to keep the doors open. In addition, the Medical Center required additional funds for research, modernization, expansion, and construction of new buildings that would allow it to increase class sizes and graduate enough doctors to serve the citizens of Oklahoma. Except in rare instances, these funds were not forthcoming from a penurious Oklahoma legislature, whose priorities lay in areas such as highway construction, social programs, and local pork barrel projects.

Dean Everett provided a glimpse into the funding woes besetting the Medical Center when he discussed the new Medical Research Building dedicated on March 11, 1961:

> The University of Oklahoma Medical Center was unique . . . in that it combined a private, a state, and a federal institution on its campus, all dependent upon the federal government for matching monies and for many of their research grants (principally from the National Institutes of Health). True, $400,000 of the total construction cost [$800,000] of the new medical research building had been provided by a federal grant, but, since nothing had been appropriated by the state for conducting research there, all work carried on in the building had to be grant-supported; and the unfinished fifth floor had to be completed and equipped with grants-in-aid monies. This was an extraordinary bargain for the taxpayers of Oklahoma but a tall order for the administration and the faculty, since some medical schools were in a better position to lobby for federal assistance than others.[3]

The result of Dean Everett's 1961 trip to Washington was a meeting that would position Oklahoma among the small core of elite medical centers that were "in a better position" to garner federal funding. At the very least, it helped to establish a more positive relationship with the federal granting agencies on which the Medical Center was increasingly dependent. Without that meeting, the Medical Center might never have realized decades of generous matching funds and Hill-Burton medical construction grants.

Prior to the 1961 Washington trip, Dean Everett had often been forced to rely on the kindness of strangers for the Center's operating funds. The strangers in this case were any public or private sources from whom the dean and his cohorts could wheedle financial assistance. Through the good offices of his friend and confidante Lloyd Rader, director of the Oklahoma Department of Public Welfare, the dean had scheduled a meeting with Wilbur J. Cohen, undersecretary of Health, Education and Welfare in the Kennedy administration, concerning the "possibility of congressional action on behalf of medical education . . . and financial operating assistance in particular for schools of medicine in need of such help."[4] Lloyd Rader realized before most Oklahoma politicians the value of "tapping the federal teat"[5] for grants and operating funds not provided by the state legislature. Rader was in the process of elevating a cash-strapped welfare department into Oklahoma's first billion-dollar enterprise by using the same "tap-the-feds" philosophy. He also notified Senators Robert Kerr and Mike Monroney of the dean's visit, and these powerful men vowed to "secure the passage of a bill . . . that will . . . benefit the University of Oklahoma Medical School."[6]

Dean Everett's meeting with Cohen did not occur without a hitch. The busy undersecretary, who was later to serve as the primary architect of Lyndon Johnson's Great Society in his position as secretary of Health, Education and Welfare, was notoriously late for meetings, and the 3:00 P.M. appointment was put off until four, then five, then six. Finally, at a quarter to seven, long after his staff had departed for home, Cohen accompanied patient, always-jovial Dean Everett to the basement snack bar, where the two men shared a dinner of cold sandwiches and warm root beer purchased from vending machines. By the end of the meeting, Cohen had a thorough grasp of the financial straits of Oklahoma medical education, and he vowed to do his utmost to help remedy the situation. The two men departed on a first-name basis, and from that point forward, funding requests from the University of Oklahoma Medical Center were granted at a far higher rate and in larger amounts. As Lloyd Rader put it, "the dean could charm the warts off an Arkansas hog, and I knew if he and Wilbur got together, good things would happen."[7] Rader would later say, "If old Dean Everett hadn't greased the [financial] skids with Wilbur Cohen back in the Kennedy administration, those boys over there [in the Medical Center] wouldn't have a pot to pee in."[8]

Observers of the Oklahoma political scene may challenge the validity of Lloyd Rader's observation, but nobody with even a rudimentary knowledge of the state's medical history will dispute the fact that the University of Oklahoma Medical Center has, throughout much of its remarkable history, had to struggle to receive a viable portion of state funding. In researching this book, we discovered a common theme reverberating throughout the history of the Medical Center: fiscal crisis, funding shortages, budget cuts. Whoever was the governor, no matter who was the dean, and regardless of the health of Oklahoma's economy, the Medical Center rarely received adequate funding to operate a first-class institution for medical education and patient treatment. Yet, in spite of such parsimonious support, Oklahoma politicians, educators, and taxpayers expected a "Harvard on the Plains" medical establishment. This expectation compelled deans such as Mark Everett and James Dennis, as well as department heads such as Stewart Wolf, John Shilling, and Jolly West, to forage for greenbacks in federal and private pastures, leading to a volatile situation in which survival depended upon periodic grants that sometimes constituted as much as 60 percent of the Center's operating budget.

Dr. John Shilling, the first full-time chair of the Department of Surgery at the Medical Center, described how it was in the early days: "Our budget in 1956 for the whole Department, including salaries for me and six others, was $35,000. We had to earn every damn cent above that. Essentially, the university provided only facilities and opportunity. I often wondered why people joined the department under those circumstances, except Mark Everett and all of us had great academic dreams."[9]

Mark R. Everett's tenure as dean and, later, director of the University of Oklahoma Medical Center encompassed seventeen exhilarating years of change, growth, yo-yo funding, shifting medical and educational priorities, and machinations by powerful individuals determined to bend the Center to their will. The fact that several influential legislators, the top bureaucrat among the state's higher education regents, and a coterie of self-aggrandizing physicians in private practice were unable to steer the Center in precisely the direction they desired was a testament not only to the dean's vision and determination but to the brilliant, resourceful department chairs he recruited to Oklahoma from medical centers throughout the country.

However, Dean Everett and the Medical Center paid a price for their vision. The legislature, often under the sway of small-town lawmakers who expected little more from the University of Oklahoma than a competitive football team, funded the Center at a rate that consistently placed it at or near the bottom of the Big 6 (later the Big 8) conference of schools, resulting in a shoddy facility—especially University Hospital—that brought shame to the state. And a number of influential state physicians in private practice, believing that the energetic new clinical chairs at the Medical Center intended to build large practices that would deprive them of patients and income, schemed to defeat key initiatives launched by the Center. In spite of all the powerful opposition arrayed against it, however, the College of Medicine managed to provide a level of patient care and medical education—albeit in rundown buildings and with inadequate equipment—that consistently earned high marks from evaluation committees, licensing boards, and other medical centers that wondered how Oklahoma accomplished so much with so little.

With the retirement of Mark R. Everett in 1964, "the end of an era in Oklahoma medical education was marked with a smile and a tear"[10] as he ended forty years of active association with the Medical Center. The smile, doubtless, was shared by opponents who admired Dr. Everett but were happy to see an indomitable foe depart. The tear was shared by those who had struggled with him to bring the Medical Center to the position it currently occupied—an institution on the threshold of greatness.

Two issues dominated the final years and even months of Dean Everett's service to the University of Oklahoma. First was his struggle with the chancellor of higher education, E. T. Dunlap. Second was his effort to pass State Question 411, the statewide bond issue that would provide $7 million for a new University Hospital to replace the dilapidated horror known—not always affectionately—as Old Main.

THE DEAN AND THE CHANCELLOR

Mark R. Everett became dean of the University of Oklahoma School of Medicine in 1947 and assumed the added title of director of the Medical Center in 1956. E. T. Dunlap was appointed chancellor of the Oklahoma State Regents for Higher Education in 1961. The overlapping years between 1961 and 1964 witnessed a struggle for financial independence by Dean Everett that was countered by an equally urgent struggle for financial control by the chancellor—a conflict that seethed below the surface of Oklahoma politics and education—and was possibly detrimental to both men and their institutions. Although Dunlap was eventually to prevail in his efforts to exert state regent control over the educational expenditures of the Medical Center, his victory came only after Dean Everett had retired and been succeeded by deans who were more susceptible to Dunlap's—and the state legislature's—blandishments.

Pennsylvanian Mark R. Everett came to the University of Oklahoma as a distinguished medical biochemist from Bucknell College (B.S. in Engineering) and Harvard University (Ph.D. in Medicine). He was recruited to Oklahoma as the first chair of Biochemistry and Pharmacology, and his textbook *Medical Biochemistry* served for many years as the standard work for medical schools and colleges throughout the country. Among numerous accomplishments during his tenure at the Medical Center, Dean Everett was most proud of his role in transforming the Medical School faculty from part-time volunteers to full-time staff and recruiting numerous world-class physicians and teachers to the school's faculty.

Native Oklahoman E. T. Dunlap, who served as chancellor of Oklahoma's higher education system for twenty-one years, earned an Ed.D. degree from Oklahoma State University and was a member of the Oklahoma legislature and president of Eastern Oklahoma State University in Wilburton. At Dunlap's funeral service in 1997 U.S. Senator David Boren commended him by stating that the former chancellor "will occupy an important and lasting place in the history of our state. He passionately believed in making higher education accessible and affordable for all Oklahomans" *[DO, 2–1–97]*. Dunlap served during a period in which college enrollments soared in Oklahoma due to the oil boom and increased educational funding by the legislature, much of which he was responsible for generating. He also "oversaw the growth of junior colleges across the state" *[DO, 2–1–97]*.

Not everybody agreed with Senator Boren's assessment of Chancellor Dunlap, however. University of Oklahoma president Paul Sharp, with his oft-quoted accusation that Dunlap was "seeking a common mediocrity" for Oklahoma higher education, was one of many state figures who disagreed with the chancellor's monetary and educational policies. Others felt that Dunlap siphoned funds from the large, research-oriented universities in Norman and Stillwater and directed them to community colleges and rural institutions—to the detriment of Oklahoma's overall educational progress. Dunlap, politician that he was, used such criticism to galvanize support from small-town politicians and powerful school superintendents throughout the state.

The struggle between Everett and Dunlap was based on the simple issue of funding control. Dean Everett insisted on autonomy of money management for his department chairs, while Chancellor Dunlap demanded oversight of all monies coming into the higher education system. Dean Everett felt that, because of persistent underfunding by the Oklahoma legislature, he could achieve his dream of luring brilliant doctors to Oklahoma only by allowing them to apply for grants from the federal government (e.g., research and construction grants) and then, when funding arrived, to allow them to spend it any way they deemed appropriate for building great departments. Chancellor Dunlap, who clearly trusted systems more than individuals, worried that public monies might be spent for private purposes (a belief laden with irony in light of the financial woes that his handpicked successor suffered years later). Raymond Crews, the Medical Center's business manager, put the issue succinctly in a statement to medical historian Robert Hardy: "The basic conflict was over research grants from the National Institutes of Health and other sources. The [Medical Center] administrative attitude was that those research and training grants were made to the individual grantee to carry on his research and his program. The State Regents wanted that [money] included in the general budget of the institution so they could allocate it just as they allocated state appropriated funds, but the university never agreed to that approach."[11]

Chancellor Dunlap was never able, during Everett's tenure, to corral the Medical Center to his satisfaction, and Dean Everett chafed under incessant "interference" by the higher education regents. The irony of the struggle is that, in a manner of speaking, both men were correct in their convictions. Dean Everett could not have successfully recruited his department chairs—and thus built a distinguished Medical Center—without the lures he used; and Chancellor Dunlap could not have satisfied the public's right to know how public monies were spent without a centralized accounting system. The dean operated his Medical Center under the moral precept of an earlier age: A gentleman's word is his bond. The chancellor, perhaps representing the new age, saw a thief under every rock. Dr. John Schilling, chair of Surgery and one of Dean Everett's key recruits, described the dean's funding system: "We didn't have much money, but what we did have went into our academic enterprises. We didn't use it wrongly. I think sometimes we were able to accomplish more that way than with larger budgeted funds over which bureaucratic checks and balances keep you from doing anything with it. Mark [Everett] was quite honest in this regard. Everything was done on faith and what you generated was yours. It was assumed you would use it honestly, the best you could."[12]

The legacy Dean Everett left for his successors was that of a Medical Center with a cadre of departmental chairs who were strong, vigorous leaders, working with a university president—George Cross—who had also served for many years on a university faculty. In particular, the Medical College for the first time could boast of an outstanding group of full-time clinical department chairs in Medicine, Surgery, Pediatrics, Psychiatry, and also had impressive chairs in a significant proportion of the smaller clinical departments. Stewart Wolf, longtime head of Medicine, summarized his relationship with Dean Everett when he was asked why he left the University for the Oklahoma Medical Research Foundation in 1967: "There were just too many committee meetings [under Dr. Everett's successor, James Dennis]. During Mark's tenure, it was almost like heaven. We didn't have any committee meetings. If you wanted to go talk with him, or make a suggestion, he was available. Not only that, he was interested. I loved him. Mark would expedite anything that seemed sensitive to him . . . not just approve it. When I returned from sabbatical in Paris, Mark had resigned. I was so disappointed. I never did understand why he decided to do that."[13]

Dr. Harris D. "Pete" Riley, chair of Pediatrics, expressed the feelings of many of the talented men who served under Dean Everett when he said: "I would be remiss if I didn't say how much Dean Everett helped me. I was young; as a matter of fact, I was the youngest medical school department head in the country when I started. And Dr. Everett helped me in so many ways. He would walk around that desk, put his arm on my shoulder, calm me down, and always come up with something that was helpful. I just really thought the world of him."[14]

STATE QUESTION 411

Dean Everett's last major effort on behalf of the Medical Center was a six-month fight to persuade Oklahoma citizens to pass State Question 411, which provided $7 million in bonds to be issued by the legislature for the purpose of financing construction of a new University Hospital, other capital improvements, and for equipping, remodeling, modernizing, and repairing any and all existing buildings at the Medical Center. Physicians opposed to development of the Medical Center attempted, in an anonymous petition to the Senate, to have the bond issue "reconsidered." Under the leadership of Senators Bryce Baggett and Cleeta John Rogers, this effort was derailed.

Dean Everett appointed Dr. Merlin K. "Monty" DuVal, assistant director of the Medical Center, and Raymond Crews, Medical Center administrator, to assist in the effort to pass State Question 411. According to a memorandum from Dr. DuVal to Dr. Rainey Williams, written in September 1994, DuVal had been asked by Dean Everett

to serve as Assistant Administrator of the Medical Center to one end—getting "us" a new University Hospital. Our first approach was to do this through the bonding authority of the Board of Higher Regents, but their Chancellor, E. T. Dunlap, felt that the size of the issue would make the state-wide bond issue on behalf of all of the state's institutions top-heavy, and so the Regents wouldn't go along. Mark knew that I enjoyed superb relations with the state legislature and encouraged me to "end run" the Regents and seek authorizing legislation for a bond issue on our own. It took two sessions to get it passed, but we got it. (It was later almost derailed by those who resented our success.)[15]

The placing of this bond issue on the 1963 ballot resulted in a three-pronged "study" by the Center's political opponents as well as its suppoorters of the bill and its potential effects. The first study was conducted by a fact-finding committee appointed by Governor Henry Bellmon to assess the present and future needs of the Center and to fully inform the electorate about these needs prior to the election. The committee consisted of Chairman Richard Hough (a pioneering Oklahoma City ear surgeon with great influence among area physicians, especially those at competing hospitals such as Baptist, Presbyterian, and St. Anthony's) and members W. T. "Bill" Paine (president of Big Chief Drilling Company and longtime supporter of the Center) and Senator Louis Ritzhaupt (a Guthrie physician who opposed prosperity or growth at the Center, other than an increase in its indigent patient load).

A second shot was fired at the 1963 bond issue when there was agitation in the legislature to conduct a "comprehensive study" of the Medical Center, a move instigated by "medical experts" within that body. Prominent among those pushing for the study were Senator Ritzhaupt and Senator Richard Stansberry, long-term opponents of the Medical Center and practicing physicians whose motivating force was to assure that the University Hospitals would not compete with private hospitals for paying patients but would confine their role to providing care to indigent patients from throughout the state. This study was given added life when Senator Ritzhaupt realized that he might be outnumbered and outgunned by Medical Center supporters on the governor's fact-finding committee.

A third "study," which had been ordered by the legislature in 1961 but was still incomplete two years later, was being conducted by the Oklahoma State Regents for Higher Education to determine present and future needs for all institutions and agencies of higher learning. Chancellor E. T. Dunlap announced that the study of the Medical Center "had not even commenced and would not be complete until some time in 1964." Dunlap, himself a former member of the legislature and new to the chancellor's office, hoped to delay or postpone the bond issue until this study had been completed. The University of Oklahoma Medical Center Alumni Association felt that Dr. Dunlap, "as chancellor of the State Regents, presents the opportunity to solidify the relationships and understanding between the [University of Oklahoma] Regents and the Legislature to the benefit of the entire State System of Higher Education."[16] However, this concept would never come to fruition because the chancellor, even at this early juncture in his career, devoted his interests and energies primarily to institutions other than the two major state universities. He consistently opposed expenditure of higher education funds earmarked for the Medical Center, and he frequently resorted to requirements for crossing t's and dotting i's seemingly in order to delay consideration and/or approval of requests coming from the University of Oklahoma Board of Regents recommending funds for the Medical Center. He clearly interpreted the thrust for a bond issue for the Medical Center as a means of bypassing the State Regents and their authority.

The governor's study committee endorsed the bond issue, with only Senator Ritzhaupt opposing this position. The comment of Oklahoma City oilman W. T. "Bill" Paine was typical of the committee's attitude after examining University Hospital: "I have been in many hospitals, and hospitals make me sick; only this one made me sicker! The University Hospital needs more beds and more modern beds." The motion for an "investigation" proposed in the state senate was defeated by a thirty to eight vote. The State Regents Study Committee, as noted above, took no stand on the bond issue election. The State Medical Society gave qualified support to it. Opponents of the bond issue included an unnatural alliance of fearful general practitioners affiliated with Oklahoma City hospitals other than University, together with medical specialists who were opposed to full-time faculty at the Medical Center. The specialists contacting the governor, the legislature, and the media were primarily those who previously had declared themselves opponents of Stewart Wolf, chair of Medicine; John Schilling, chair of Surgery; and James Merrill, chair of Gynecology and Obstetrics.

State Question 411 was strongly supported by the Oklahoma Medical Alumni Association, led by Drs. Wayne Starky and Wendell Smith. John Rogers, a Tulsa attorney and member of the Oklahoma Medical Research Foundation, added an important positive voice in the eastern part of the state and garnered support from citizens in that area. The *Daily Oklahoman*, through its positive editorials and feature articles by medical reporters Ray Parr and Claire Conley, was an essential element in the bond issue's ultimate success.

In the view of proponents of the bond issue, reason and progress triumphed over greed and parochialism when, on December 3, 1963, the people of Oklahoma approved State Question 411 by a margin of three to one. Seven million dollars in construction money was assured for a new University Hospital, and history would show that this was the key step in jump-starting a building boom on the Medical Center campus that would continue for decades. Politically, passage of the bond issue was but another in a long line of losses for Senators Ritzhaupt and Stansberry, but it was one of the few major defeats for Chancellor Dunlap in his long career in Oklahoma education.

PICKING A SUCCESSOR

The story of Mark Everett's service at the University of Oklahoma Medical Center is told in volume two of his work, *Medical Education in Oklahoma*. The book, coauthored by his wife Alice, is an articulate, highly detailed account of the College of Medicine from 1932 to 1964, years in which the College grew from little more than a minor branch of the University to an institution of such quality and significance that political commentator Frosty Troy would label it "Oklahoma's best-kept secret."

At the time of Dean Everett's retirement announcement in 1964, there was great pressure on Governor Bellmon and President Cross—by many of the same individuals who had vigorously opposed State Question 411—to assure generous representation of practicing physicians unaffiliated with the University of Oklahoma on the search committee for the new dean. This alliance of physicians, fearing that the charismatic chair of Medicine, Stewart Wolf, might be propelled into the office of the dean, agreed to push for an alternative candidate from the faculty, Dr. S. N. Stone.

S. N. "Newt" Stone was a respected and well-liked practicing surgeon in the community who had trained at the Mayo Clinic and was prominent on the staff of St. Anthony Hospital. At the time of the reorganization of the Medical School curriculum, Dean Everett had appointed Dr. Stone as associate dean for clinical instruction, to supervise the clinical clerkship of medical students during the third and fourth years. Because of the affection and great respect in which Stone was held by the volunteer faculty, those who were opposed to, and feared appointment of, a full-time faculty member as dean—specifically, Stewart Wolf—rallied around Stone as their candidate for permanent dean. In February 1964, the Oklahoma Academy of General Practice unanimously endorsed Dr. Stone as their candidate for dean. They verbalized their hope that the endorsement would counteract the rising support for Dr. Wolf.

That same month, the state Association of General Practitioners "passed a resolution voicing their annual complaint concerning too many specialists being graduated from the medical school."[17] They did not seem to realize that the University granted only the basic M.D. degree and had no control over whatever professional path their graduates chose to follow later in life. On February 11, 186 members of the Oklahoma County Medical Society signed a petition to President Cross supporting Dr. Stone for the deanship. Dr. Cross announced that "a petition is not a good plan with which to select administrators" and stated that he had appointed a representative committee of well qualified individuals whose job it was to recommend a successor to Dean

Everett.[18] The following day, Dr. Rex Kenyon, president of the Oklahoma County Medical Society, announced withdrawal of the petition. Shortly thereafter, the Search Committee reported that they had forwarded four names to the president, none of whom were currently residents of Oklahoma. Included in the list was Dr. James L. Dennis of Arkansas.

In his farewell address to the Medical School faculty, Dr. Everett said: "The present achievements must be maintained and extended by you, in order to further the growth and development of the Medical Center which, at this juncture, rests on the threshold of a great future. To translate the ten-year development plan of the University of Oklahoma Medical Center into reality will be a lengthy task, and will command strong and vigorous leadership."[19]

Fortunately for the Medical Center, the "strong and vigorous leadership" Dean Everett called for would be found not only in the brilliant, energetic faculty he recruited, but in his successor, Dr. James L. Dennis of the University of Arkansas.

1964: THE FINAL MONTHS

Mark Everett's final months as dean and director of the University of Oklahoma Medical Center were spent much like his first: attempting to find funds to operate a quality institution. Fortunately, he and his cohorts were able to scrounge enough money to keep the buildings open while they practiced superior medicine at a grossly inferior University Hospital and taught students the skills they needed to excel in the healing arts. The dean's last few months were eased by the knowledge that grants and gifts to faculty at the Medical Center in 1964 were almost one million dollars more than in the preceding year. Like many other years during Dr. Everett's tenure, the new total for outside funds ($5,386,562) exceeded state appropriations for operation and maintenance of the entire Medical Center. Approximately 80 percent of these funds came from federal sources.[20]

In February 1964, the Oklahoma Academy of General Practice criticized the School of Medicine because there was a "shortage of family doctors" throughout the state. Several members of the Board of Regents, including Dr. Mark Johnson, rejected the criticism, informing the Academy that medical schools cannot tell their graduates what to practice or where to practice. Said Regent James G. Davidson of Tulsa, "It seems to be more of a problem for the medical profession than for the university."[21] Such carping by Oklahoma physicians who did not approve of a "specialist-dominated" Medical Center was common in the 1960s, especially in state medical publications.

Dean Mark R. Everett asked to be relieved as chair of the Department of Biochemistry on March 18, 1964, as soon as additional monies could be found for teaching and research activity in biochemistry. Dr. Everett had served in the dual role of dean of the School of Medicine and chair of Biochemistry for many years. His salary for the combined positions, which as Medical Center director he was responsible for setting, was $18,000 per year—far less than the annual income of most of the chairmen he hired. By comparison, the average salary paid to deans and directors of medical centers in the United States in 1964 was $40,000.[22] Dr. Everett was succeeded as chair of Biochemistry by Dr. Marvin R. Shetlar, chief of the research laboratories in the Oklahoma City Veterans Administration Hospital, at a yearly salary of $21,000.

Dr. Ben I. Heller, professor of Medicine and director of the School of Medical Technology, was appointed head of a new Department of Laboratory Medicine in April 1964. Also appointed at this time were Dr. Sidney P. Traub as professor and head of the Department of Radiology and director of the X-ray department in University Hospital; Dr. James B. Snow Jr. as first chair of the new Department of Otorhinolaryngology; and Dr. Mark Allen Everett, the dean's son, as chair of the Department of Dermatology.

On July 1, 1964, Mark R. Everett retired from the University of Oklahoma Medical Center. During his tenure, which began in 1947, 1,341 students graduated from the School of Medicine. At his retirement, the Medical Center encompassed twenty-three acres of land in northeast Oklahoma City, with a budget of $10,344,699. There were 159 approved internships and residency positions at the Center, while Children's, University, and the Veterans Administration hospitals provided 947 teaching beds. Ninety graduates of the School of Medicine received the M.D. degree in 1964, while 31 were awarded the Bachelor of Science degree in Nursing.[23]

At a retirement banquet in the Skirvin Hotel in Oklahoma City, hundreds of doctors, alumni, and friends witnessed the unveiling by University of Oklahoma President George Cross of a portrait of the dean that would hang in the Medical Center Library. President Cross then appointed a search committee to select a successor to Dr. Everett. Chair of this committee was Dr. Leonard Eliel, president of the Oklahoma Medical Research Foundation. President Cross appointed Dr. Joseph White as interim dean of the School of Medicine and director of the Medical Center until Dean Everett's successor, James L. Dennis, assumed the dual post on September 1.

The legacy Mark R. Everett left to his successor was four-fold: (1) the strong, personal bonds forged between the dean of the College of Medicine and the majority of the practicing community, which prior to 1950 provided nearly all of the clinical teaching faculty; (2) the transformation of the clinical faculty from volunteer to full-time, stimulating amazingly little friction with, and defection of, the volunteer faculty; (3) the good fortune and wisdom to select outstanding clinical departmental chairs who, prior to 1972, were elected by their departmental faculty biannually and thereafter given indefinite appointments by the dean; and (4) the setting of the stage for the vast physical expansion of the campus, which would begin in earnest under his successors, through successful passage of the 1963 bond issue for a new University Hospital.

Chapter II.
Expansion and Struggle:
The Dennis Years,
1965–1969

 James L. Dennis, a native of Oklahoma City and graduate of the University of Oklahoma College of Medicine, had served at the University of Arkansas as associate dean for clinical affairs and director of the Medical Center as well as professor of Pediatrics prior to returning in 1964 as dean and director of the University of Oklahoma Medical Center. Like his predecessor, Mark Everett, he was a pipe-smoking, philosophical physician with strong administrative ability. James Dennis's dream for the Center, however, was different from that of Dr. Everett, who labored to build a College of Medicine in which the best minds taught and practiced the best medicine. Dean Dennis envisioned a comprehensive health sciences center with numerous hospitals, colleges, and institutes on a single campus in Oklahoma City.

Upon arriving at the University of Oklahoma Medical Center, James Dennis inherited the funds from the recently passed bond issue, State Question 411, the seed from which his greatly expanded Center would grow. In addition, he was blessed with a nucleus of strong, full-time clinical department chairs: Stewart Wolf, Medicine; John Schilling, Surgery; Harris D. "Pete" Riley, Pediatrics; Jolly West, Psychiatry; James Merrill, Obstetrics-Gynecology; Mark Allen Everett, Dermatology; and James B. Snow Jr., Otorhinolaryngology. Each of these men, and later Robert M. Bird, professor of Medicine, would play a significant role in his, and subsequent, administrations.

James Dennis spent much of 1965—his first full year as Dean—learning how to operate a large medical complex with inadequate funds doled out by a penurious and frequently hostile legislature. He also learned that not all members of his faculty, the University of Oklahoma Board of Regents, and administrators on the Norman campus shared his goal of a large, multifaceted health sciences center in Oklahoma City.

Much of the autumn following Dean Dennis's arrival was occupied by an acrimonious debate among University regents, the governor, various legislators, and the press over a contract to Benham and Blair Engineering Associates of Oklahoma City in the amount of $225,000 for preparing preliminary plans for construction of the new University Hospital. This contract, awarded prior to the Dean's arrival, had been declared illegal by Attorney General Charles Nesbitt shortly after it was struck. The gist of the argument was that $200,000 of the total amount had been paid from the 1960 Higher Education Bond Issue, whose funds were for a hospital addition at the Medical School, but funds for planning were deemed inappropriate. Settling this debate occupied the Dean's first few months at Oklahoma, leading him to feel that he had stepped into a situation about which he had not been briefed by those who hired him.

1965

The University of Oklahoma Board of Regents opened 1965 on a bright note by resolving the year-long impasse over the Benham contract by the simple act of rescinding it. The regents retrieved the previously paid $225,000 from the Benham Group, then paid a similar amount from the University revolving fund to purchase the preliminary plans. Although this act appeared like mere card shuffling to many, the 5–2 vote of the Board smoothed the ruffled feathers of individuals who insisted on following the letter of the law. Then, by a 6–0 vote, a consulting contract with the California hospital planning firm of Lester Gorsline Associates was authorized to assist a committee chaired by Robert Bird, professor of Medicine, in the planning for a new hospital.

Robert Montgomery Bird, a 1939 graduate of the University of Virginia Medical School, had worked at Cornell University with Dr. Stewart Wolf. He served the University of Oklahoma as professor and vice chair of Medicine (1952–1974); associate dean for planning and development (1965–70); and dean of the College of Medicine (1970–1974). He became director of the Lester Hill Institute at the National Library of Medicine in Washington, D.C., in 1973 and served in that capacity until his death. He was a sixth-generation Virginian whose ancestor and namesake had written the first American novel. A silver-haired and silver-tongued gentleman, he was a life-long bachelor who quickly became fast friends with, and virtually part of the family of, Anatomy professor Ernst Lachmann and his wife Anya. Soft spoken but resolutely firm, Dr. Bird suffered from frequent migraine headaches that were a constant impediment to his work and life. Some faculty members credit Dr. Bird with originating the "health sciences center" concept that would be championed so vigorously and successfully by James Dennis.

Dean Dennis made his first significant change in Medical Center personnel when he hired Robert Terrill to replace Raymond Crews as University Hospital administrator. Crews, who had served simultaneously as the business administrator of both the Medical Center and University Hospital since 1959, was a quiet man whose honesty was legendary. Crews was resolutely loyal to the Center, but when questioned by friends or the press about the comings and goings at University Hospital, he could be counted on for a good quote. Queried years later by the authors about the increasing control Oklahoma welfare director Lloyd Rader was exercising over the Center's hospitals in the 1970s, Crews responded: "Yes, he was taking over. So what? He had the power, and he had the wherewithal. You sure as hell didn't see us turning any of his money back."

In March 1965 a committee chaired by William Morgan Cain, president of Cain's Coffee Company and a long-term Medical Center supporter, recommended that Presbyterian Hospital relocate from central Oklahoma City to the Medical Center campus. Presbyterian's decision to move to the Center came only after the fears of its board and key physicians could be quelled about "medical school control" and "moving over to the east [i.e., 'Black'] side" of town *[DO, 5–8–65]*. Drs. William Rucks, Ben Nicholson, and Charles Bielstein, all members of the Oklahoma City Clinic staff, were instrumental in moving the decision forward. It was among the last efforts of Dr. Bielstein, who died suddenly on May 6.

The Medical School commencement for 1965 was held in May on the Norman campus at Holmberg Hall. Dr. William S. Middleton, former dean of the University of Wisconsin Medical School and national director of the Veterans Administration, gave the address. Dr. Middleton had spent the 1963–1964 academic year at the Medical Center as visiting professor of Medicine during the sabbatical of Dr. Stewart Wolf.

Dean Dennis learned that his honeymoon at the University of Oklahoma would be short-lived when, at the June regents meeting, there was a heated exchange regarding the consultant contract with Lester Gorsline Associates. This contract, sanctioned "in principle" at the January meeting, had not yet been officially approved, largely due to opposition by Regents Davidson and Calvert. Davidson had also led the opposition to solving the Benham Group planning controversy the previous December. An annoyed Dr. Dennis said, "You people didn't tell me about your architectural contract troubles when I signed my contract. I didn't know about it. There are 12 new medical centers going up in this country right now. We are investigated right and left and audited right and left and criticized right and left. I want your help and I need to know now if you can't give it to me" *[DO, 6–1–65]*.

The dean pointed out that the 1963 bond issue for $7 million still had not been activated by the state legislature because the senate had failed to approve the action taken sometime previously by the house as HB 1010. Senators habitually opposed to the Medical Center were successfully delaying action in an attempt to be certain that any new facilities would not be used for "private" patients of the full-time faculty. President Cross agreed with his new dean: "You said just what needed to be said" *[RM, 8198]*. The regents, at the urging of their president, Julian Rothbaum, quickly passed the Gorsline contract by a 4–0 vote, with Regent Davidson abstaining.

Regents President Julian Rothbaum was a prominent Tulsa businessman whose success had occurred principally in the oil business. He had grown up and attended high school in Hartshorne, in eastern Oklahoma, with Carl Albert, who was then speaker of the U.S. House of Representatives. Rothbaum, a plain-spoken man with a strong sense of justice and intense loyalty to the University, was the first appointment to the University of Oklahoma Board of Regents by Governor J. Howard Edmondson, whose family was also from eastern Oklahoma. One of the rare regents to be appointed to two terms, he served again when appointed by Governor David Hall in 1979.

The day following the acrimonious June regents meeting, House Speaker J. D. McCarty said, "I have high praise for Dr. Dennis and I believe he has exhibited ability and courage toward problems affecting the Medical Center. I will personally enter into negotiations between the House and Senate to resolve the difficulty at the earliest possible time" *[DO, 6–12–65]*. Representative John McCune of Tulsa said, "An element of Oklahoma City doctors is trying to embarrass the school's Dean." He further indicated that "certain financial interests" had prevailed upon the senate committee to amend the bill to provide that bonds must be sold to private investors, costing an additional $2.5 to $5 million in interest, as well as inserting the clause requiring that construction must be for a hospital "primarily used for charity and indigent patients" *[DO, 6–12–65]*. On June 16 however, the Senate-House Conference Committee agreed to the house version, and on June 17 this report was adopted and the bill sent to the governor for his signature. The $7 million voted by the public some eighteen months earlier in State Question 411 suddenly became available for the new dean.

Passage of this bill was another blow to the habitual senate malcontents who immediately proposed yet another "investigation" of the Medical Center.

Senator Bryce Baggett, a long-time supporter of the Center, made a bitter attack on the proposed investigation, which had been initiated by Senator Richard Stansberry, saying, "I am ashamed of some of the things that have gone on to get votes for this resolution. A small group of physicians have notions about how the Medical Center should be run. I would be embarrassed for the Senate to bring these deals out here on the floor" *[DO, 7–7–65]*. There was unusual agreement among the senators, various medical organizations, and the educational community that the intent of the so-called senate "study" was actually an attempt at harassment. The house passed a resolution condemning the senate resolution. Senator Stansberry, in his zeal to derail the proposal, self-importantly stated "My integrity in this matter is being questioned. Repealing the resolution would be one of the worst things this senate could do. I consider this action a personal insult to me" *[DO, 7–20–65]*. On July 8, the senate passed a resolution by Senator Hal Muldrow of Norman effectively killing any legislative study for the present. At the same time, the State Regents for Higher Education finally published its "Self Study" on education in Oklahoma which proved generally supportive of programs at the Medical Center.

In August, a committee headed by Dr. Richard A. Clay proposed the organization of an Oklahoma Eye Foundation to cooperate with and support the School of Medicine. The development of such an institute, combined with the impending arrival of privately owned Presbyterian Hospital on the Medical Center campus, would constitute the first steps in Dean Dennis's full-service health sciences center. In looking back at the dean's plans for expanding the Center, Dr. Stewart Wolf commented, "Dean Everett was primarily interested in the quality of medical teaching and health care; Jim Dennis was interested in expansion. Under Jim, we had to have a dental school, a pharmacy school, anything that was expansion."[1]

Stewart Wolf was a graduate of Johns Hopkins University School of Medicine who had trained at New York Hospital in Medicine, and became an associate professor at Cornell. According to Mrs. Mark R. Everett, he arrived as chair of the Department of Medicine in 1952 "like a wind storm on the prairie!" Full of ideas, he served the College of Medicine until 1967, when he moved across the street to the Oklahoma Medical Research Foundation (OMRF), retaining his base salary and professorship in the department. This move was at the urging of Dr. Dennis, who had reservations about criticism regarding expenditure of funds in the Department of Medicine, especially in regard to operation of the Tott's Gap farm in Pennsylvania, where Wolf had a summer research operation. Stuart Wolf's entire life was dedicated to excellence, and he was disappointed when this desire was absent in others.

Surgeon G. Rainey Williams was a great admirer of Dr. Wolf: "I give Stewart Wolf credit for establishing a clinical esprit de corps [at the Center] which was beyond measure. He got good people to work in dismal surroundings [University Hospital]. The first years were a struggle, but they were made pleasant by the feeling that we were going to do something good, something adventurous. Stewart Wolf led that. He motivated people—led them to believe that they could do things that they previously thought they couldn't possibly do! And, of course, he would not have come here without the support of Dean Everett."[2]

Early in September 1965 Governor Henry Bellmon appointed a committee, chaired by Oklahoma City oilman Dean A. McGee, to draft an organizational plan for an "Oklahoma Health Sciences Foundation," whose initial purpose would be to galvanize support for an additional bond issue that would provide money to complete the campus master plan. At the first meeting of the directors in March 1966 Governor Bellmon praised the Foundation and its forty-eight trustees as business, professional, and educational leaders who would preside over the development of a great medical-science complex. Later, the Foundation became the vehicle for the acquisition of additional land for the Center as well as an organization for exchange of information and coordination of plans by the numerous entities on the campus. Another part of its vision was that the Oklahoma Health Center might assist various institutions on the campus and sponsor campus-wide services such as an expanded medical library.

Dr. William Thurman, Medical Center provost in the 1970s, recalled that the initiative to form an Oklahoma Health Sciences Foundation "provided a legal means for raising money all over the state. It also was a legal way to buy land that would be needed in the future by the Center."[3] As a result, the Foundation began buying lots throughout the Medical Center area. Dr. Don O'Donoghue was titular head of the Foundation and Robert Hardy the executive director. Hardy hoped that his position might eventually evolve into a "presidency" of the entire campus, but that was not to be. The University of Oklahoma was the dominant player in the Medical Center, and the executive vice president and director (later the provost), would inevitably be its leader. When Dr. Stewart Wolf became aware of these expansionist plans, he stated: "I liked it to be the 'University of Oklahoma Medical Center.' The 'Health Sciences Center' was not the purpose of the thing. The whole purpose was to get more doctors for Oklahoma. When Dean Everett and President Cross were working together, the idea was to develop a stronger school, a stronger campus, and start those full-time clinical chairs . . . with lots of pep. We needed more buildings; but we didn't need a Health Sciences Center."[4]

According to Dr. William Thurman, it became clear that the heads of the various organizations on the campus needed a forum for exchange, and "either Dean [McGee] or Stanton [Young] said, 'Why don't we just incorporate that function here [in the Health Sciences Foundation]? That's the way to get the work done.' There were some people, not from the Medical Center, who had no real function. It was a super suggestion, whoever made it, so we moved the Foundation physically out here and held all the meetings out here. . . . It's a liaison with the community. Half of the board is made up of the community, and the other half from the Medical Center."[5]

Dean A. McGee was a prominent Oklahoma oilman, partner of Senator Robert S. Kerr in the Kerr-McGee Oil Company, and constant booster of Oklahoma business. He had an enduring interest in the Medical Center and was instrumental in developing the 1965 comprehensive plan for the campus, gaining support of the Oklahoma City Chamber of Commerce, dealing with politicians locally and nationally, and supporting the development of Presbyterian Hospital, the Eye Institute (named in his honor), the Health Sciences Foundation, and the actions of the Oklahoma City Urban Renewal Authority on the campus. He would also give future critical support to a series of provosts, deans, and vice presidents.

In November 1995 Dean Dennis suggested publicly that there might be a need for an additional bond issue to finance the subsequent construction needed to implement the recommendations of the Gorsline "Medical Center Master Plan." His statements automatically unleashed vocal opposition from the senate's resident "experts" on health care, Senators Stansberry and Ritzhaupt. Their negative comments were countered by Dr. Robert Ellis, chair of the Legislative Committee of the Oklahoma Medical Alumni Association, who summarized for the public the critical needs of the Center. The Ellis statement, while not silencing the critics at the state capitol, had the effect of increasing public perception of the major shortcomings at Oklahoma's only resource for health care practitioners. Some years later, the key element in the Gorsline master plan—a new adult and children's hospital linked together on a service podium containing laboratories, X-ray facilities, etc.—would be superceded and rendered obsolete when Lloyd Rader, director of the Department of Human Services, would say, "The federal government takes too long. I have $19 million and I'm going to start the investment in Children's Hospital tomorrow!" Dr. Ronald Elkins, senior thoracic surgeon and long-time faculty member, believed that if somebody had persuaded Mr. Rader to use that money to build a new tower adjacent to the new University Hospital at that time, the Center would never have had the long-standing problem of duplication of facilities and services it experienced. In the opinion of Dr. Elkins and others an entirely new Children's Hospital, rather than the Nicholson and Bielstein Towers in a reworked hospital, would have been much more efficient.[6]

1966

Dean Dennis quietly worked on his goal of expanding the Medical Center throughout 1965 and into 1966, pushing for more physical space, new buildings, and housing on campus for additional organizations. The year proved less politically boisterous and far less stressful than his first year, and he spent much of it behind the scenes laying the groundwork for achieving his vision of a great medical complex.

On the Norman campus, January 1966 witnessed the addition of the millionth volume at the Bizzell Library, marking a milestone in University of Oklahoma intellectual development. Like the library, the Department of Psychiatry, Neurology and Behavioral Medicine in Oklahoma City also experienced academic expansion. A Ph.D. program in Biological Psychology was approved; Eugene Pumpian-Mindlin, a nationally prominent analytical psychiatrist, was named as associate chair of the department; and Oscar Parsons, Ph.D., was made director of the new doctoral program. Parsons was later responsible for the department devoting significant resources to research rather than exclusively to clinical care.

In February, the newly incorporated Health Sciences Foundation requested from the Oklahoma City Urban Renewal Authority approval to expand the land dedicated for use by the Medical Center from the original 50 acres to 240 acres. This proposal, to include all the land bounded by 8th Street, 13th Street, Lottie, and the Crosstown Expressway, was approved by the Authority and would become what would be known as the Oklahoma Health Center. Governor Henry Bellmon, who spoke at the first meeting of the Directors of the Health Sciences Foundation on March 2 said, "We could develop a medical sciences complex which will likely become one of the greatest in the nation" *[DO, 3–3–66]*.

Early in May 1966 the University of Oklahoma Board of Regents approved a policy document which recognized both "private" and "service" patients as essential to the educational mission of the University Hospital. Up to this time, patients had traditionally consisted of an indigent or "welfare" core. This decision would quickly rouse the opposition and enmity of many physicians in private practice, as well as their legislative supporters.

At the same May meeting, regents approved construction of a swimming pool by the Medical Center Faculty Club on land labeled the "Houghton Property." The Houghton house had been purchased by the regents in 1961 "in order for the extension division to have facilities for continuing education in the medical sciences" *[RM, 9083]*. Although many a lazy summer afternoon would be whiled away by faculty members and their families at the pool, there was very little evidence that actual educational activities ever took place there. The Houghton house had been immediately mortgaged to the University regents (May, 1961), a transaction that was not completed until 1967, when it was "paid in full and the Faculty House Association . . . executed a deed to the property and delivered it to the President's office" *[RM, 9084]*. During construction of the Faculty House swimming pool, the secretary of the Capital Improvement and Zoning Board, Mr. Irvin Hurst, ordered a temporary stop to construction, saying that the facility was being built "without proper authority." Mr. Hurst and his board frequently exercised "legal oversight" in the area by opposing Medical Center construction projects.

The Houghton house purchase was notable for reasons other than construction of a swimming pool. Several years previously, the Kellogg Foundation had made a grant to the University for construction of a postgraduate education facility on the Medical Center campus. Although the details are somewhat hazy, many faculty members thought that the funds from this grant were actually used to construct the University of Oklahoma Press building on the Norman campus, and the Houghton house was purchased as a much less expensive "substitute" for a continuing education center on the Oklahoma City campus. (The Kellogg Center on the Norman campus was built several years later.) Since the house was totally unsuitable for instructional activities, it was never seriously utilized for postgraduate activities.

In June, regents approved the razing of the old School of Nursing building, constructed in 1946. This was done in order to make way for the proposed new University Hospital which, in the Gorsline plan, occupied that particular plot of land. The Nursing School building was a symbol of the "health sciences center" concept that viewed nursing as an endeavor that could be taught and practiced independently of the hospitals and independently of a School of Medicine. Proponents of nursing independence—who were some of the earliest harbingers of the still-dormant women's movement locally and nationwide—hoped to see a College of Nursing that would be considered on par with the College of Medicine and vocally opposed the destruction of the building.

Another educational expansion for the Medical Center occurred in July when regents approved the development of a School of Health. At the same meeting, an affiliation agreement with Presbyterian Hospital to build on the Medical Center campus was approved.

Leaders of the Mercy Hospital medical staff announced to the *Daily Oklahoman* in November that their hospital also planned a move to the Medical Center campus. This proposal never achieved reality because the Mercy Hospital staff, unlike that of Presbyterian Hospital, consisted predominantly of non-specialist physicians, many of whom feared the strong specialist makeup of the University medical staff, and to a lesser extent, that of Presbyterian. When the proposal was brought before the full Mercy Hospital staff, it was defeated, setting the stage for the later move of this hospital to far northwest Oklahoma City.

1967

The year 1967 began with tragedy and fear striking the Medical Center campus following the January 13 murder of medical student Jeanette Morrone in her apartment two blocks from University Hospital. As a result of this brutal crime, medical students visited the city council and police officials asking for greater protection and better lighting in the area. The tragic incident once again brought to the fore the long-neglected issue of safe, affordable campus housing for students. On January 16 a man named Howard Gaddis was charged with the murder of Ms. Morrone (as well as another woman the previous December). Gaddis was sentenced to death, but his sentence was later commuted to life in prison.

Among several buildings the Medical Center desperately needed was a facility that it could devote to teaching the basic sciences, and 1967 witnessed the torturous gyrations necessary to have such a structure funded and built. At their December 1966 meeting, the Board of Regents had approved plans for construction of a "Student Education Building" on the Oklahoma City campus with funds remaining from the 1963 bond issue. Subsequently, on January 19, 1967, the federal government announced an award of more than $2 million for construction of the Basic Sciences Education Building, and in May, regents approved plans and specifications for the "Basic Sciences Teaching Building" (later known as the Basic Science Education Building) at an estimated cost of $3.7 million. Finally, on September 14, regents accepted the bid of contractor Blount-Barfell-Dennehy Inc. to construct a building designed by the architectural firm of Frankfurt-Short-Emery-McKinley. In August, the federal government announced a $4.9 million grant for construction of the new University

Hospital. These structures would be the first of an array of federally subsidized buildings which would transform the campus during the next decade.

In March the Oklahoma Health Sciences Foundation approved a "final revised model" for their proposed $185 million medical complex, including $90 million in state facilities, of which $40 million would be federal matching money. Included in this model were: a library and computer facility, the new University Hospital, a building housing the State Department of Health, graduate colleges of Dentistry, Pharmacy, Nursing, and Public Health, a student center, student housing, and Presbyterian Hospital. Ultimately all but the College of Health Building would be built.

In addition to the beginning of the Medical Center's building boom, 1967 witnessed increased agitation for a more important role for "family medicine," not only because of the personal interest on the part of Dean Dennis but as a focus of concern by the Oklahoma legislature, which was keenly interested in bringing more general practitioners to rural areas of the state. The Center's commitment to this program was evidenced by approval of plans for a $300,000 Family Medicine Clinic to be built adjacent to the campus, and the signing of an agreement with the University of Oklahoma Foundation Authority to construct and equip the facility at 815 N. E. 15th Street. The previous February had seen the long-awaited opening of the Family Medicine Clinic in a temporary building adjacent to the building site designated for the new building specified in the Campus Master Plan. A contract with the University of Oklahoma Foundation Authority was signed in April, and construction of this new facility began on August 3, 1967.

A Medical Center audit in June showed a larger unencumbered balance than anticipated in the Center's revolving fund due to increased reimbursement for hospital services, especially by the Department of Public Welfare. Use of these funds to address the critical need to raise employee salaries to the national minimum wage of $1.25 per hour was voted by the regents, subject to approval by the State Regents. This action was in stark contrast to the state's continued squeeze on appropriated funds as evidenced by the governor's "no out of state travel" decree that same month.

Throughout the spring and summer of 1967, there was great campus-wide concern regarding a potential significant loss of federal funds for student loans due to the absence of matching money in the Medical Center budget. In September the Sarkey's Foundation agreed to provide the necessary funds for this match in student loans.

October saw the return of Dr. Louis J. West, professor and head of Psychiatry, Neurolgy and Behavioral Sciences, from a year's leave of absence. Dr. West, a popular teacher as well as flamboyant campus character, had been missed by the local press as much as by the Center's students. At the same time, longtime University of Oklahoma President George Cross began to hint at retirement, forcing regents to seek a replacement and providing deans of important colleges an opportunity to solidify positions and build empires.

George Lynn Cross, a distinguished botanist from South Dakota who served as University of Oklahoma president longer than any other individual, was a warm, caring individual who preached that students were the sole purpose for the university's existence and that its only function was to meet their educational needs. He was a man of wit, charm, and reason, and he used these qualities to move the University forward through the turbulence of a postwar student boom, chronic underfunding by the state legislature, racial integration on campus, and increasing student activism. It remains one of life's little ironies that the man many consider the University's greatest president is remembered best by the general public for his sarcastic quip to a legislator that he needed funds to build a university the football team could be proud of.

Senator Bryce Baggett, always a strong supporter of the Medical Center, introduced Senate Joint Resolution 26 on March 1, proposing a $47.3 million bond issue for construction at the Medical Center to be funded with an additional one cent tax on cigarettes (Senate Joint Resolution 25). One month later, Governor Dewey Bartlett asked that the bill authored by Senator Baggett be shelved and that a study of the needs for all of the state's higher education institutions be undertaken. Senator Baggett announced that he would not push his legislation if the governor objected. Many citizens believed that because the governor and his family had been educated in private schools and institutions, he frequently provided only luke-warm support for increases in public higher education funding.

On March 17, the University of Oklahoma Board of Regents honored Dr. Ernst Lachman as a regents professor in recognition of his service as chairman of the Department of Anatomy for more than twenty years. Ernst Lachmann was a refugee from Hitler's Germany who joined the medical faculty in 1934. He had served as chair of Anatomy since February 1945. The Regents' proclamation stated, "His students and former students hold him in the greatest affection, and his colleagues equally love and respect him. His leadership has brought to our Department of Anatomy the respect of the world of medical education; his scholarship has been widely published and has brought him international repute. A University is fortunate indeed whose faculty is graced by such a scholar and gentleman" *[RM, 8829]*.

A graduate of the University of Breslau in East Germany, Ernst Lachmann had spent the ensuing years in Berlin, principally in radiology with some of the international pioneers in the use of X-ray. An anatomist and radiologist who rapidly adopted Oklahoma as his home and who served the University for decades, he and his wife Anya were lovers of cats and of classical music. Anya was a native Russian whose fractured English was a constant delight to all who knew her, and even she sometimes chuckled at her own mispronunciations. Once during a summer faculty picnic at the Oklahoma City Zoo, she was heard to mutter, "Eet ees hot like hell" as she chewed on a hot dog and drank forbidden wine (Oklahoma was a "dry" state until well after World War II). Anya was also noted for her low opinion of the Oklahoma City cultural scene. More than once following a standing ovation for an indifferent performance at a symphony concert, she was heard to mutter loudly, "Hicks! Hicks!" as she sat hunched in her chair, practically invisible among the standing, cheering throngs surrounding her.

On May 11, 1967, the title of James Dennis was changed from Dean and Director of the Medical Center to that of Dean and Vice President for Medical Center Affairs and Director of the Medical Center *[RM, 8914]*. This action, with its many implications for the future, passed unanimously without comment by the regents, and was taken in anticipation of the imminent retirement of President Cross and installation of a new University president. At the same meeting, the plans for the Biomedical Science Building for Medical Education were presented with the intent that a construction bid would be issued in July.

A final May action by the University's Board of Regents established the School of Health Related Professions, as recommended by the State Regents' earlier "Self Study." This school would consolidate what were formerly hospital certificate programs and Norman campus pre-clinical programs on the Medical Center campus (e.g., medical technology, radiology, various chemistry courses, and physical therapy).

At a special meeting of the Board of Regents on May 22, 1967, the new president-designate of the University, John Herbert Hollomon, U.S. undersecretary of commerce, was introduced. The regents voted unanimously to appoint Dr. Hollomon at a salary of $35,000, with additional perks of a house, automobile, $7,500 annual maintenance allowance, and fringe benefits. The appointment was to be effective on July 1, 1968.

June witnessed, for the first time, a suggestion by Medical Center staff to conduct a separate commencement exercise in Oklahoma City for medical students only *[RM, 8951]*. This idea would be broached several times before regents would agree to it. Many regents, and the Norman campus in general, opposed the idea on the basis that a majority of medical students had never attended, nor even visited, the main campus. Because of this, it was felt that they should have at least this minimal connection to the parent University.

In July the Oklahoma State Regents for Higher Education sought approval from a special study committee appointed by governor Bartlet for support of a $100 million bond issue to construct new facilities on many state campuses, including some $30 million for the Medical Center. These actions culminated in the "HERO" bond issue of 1968 (discussed later in this chapter).

On August 1 federal agencies notified the Medical Center that nearly $5 million in federal matching money would be available for construction of the new University Hospital. This grant, together with the balance from the 1963 Medical Center bond issue for University Hospital, would fund construction of what would become "Everett Tower."

In faculty personnel actions during the summer of 1966, regents promoted Dr. Edward N. Brandt to full professor and gave him the additional title of assistant to the vice president for medical affairs. Dr. Bertha Levy was promoted to the rank of clinical professor of Pediatrics, while Dr. A. L. "Larry" Dee, chair of Pathology, Dr. B. Connor Johnson, chair of Biochemistry, and Dr. A. Kurt Weiss, professor of Physiology, were granted academic tenure.

Autumn was a busy time at the Medical Center, as Dr. Walter Whitcomb moved from the School of Medicine to full-time service as the Veterans Administration Hospital chief of staff, and nearly all of the faculty in Preventive Medicine and Public Health were given parallel appointments in the new School of Health. The regents approved an additional contract with Lester Gorsline Associates to develop plans for a School of Dentistry on the campus. A request by Dr. William Schottstaedt, acting dean of the School of Health, that the faculty be permitted to fund an additional study by Gorsline Associates was submitted and recommended to the regents by Dean Dennis. Underlying "turf" tensions were exposed when new University President Hollomon suggested that such consultants should participate "as appropriate" within an overall University study, which his own office was undertaking. This suggestion was the first public sign of developing friction between Hollomon and Dennis.

Late in 1967 regents voted to extend Norman campus retirement benefit programs to Medical Center personnel, an action sought by the faculty and Dean Dennis, and later implemented by University of Oklahoma President Paul Sharp. Dr. Sharp would later consider this one of his most significant accomplishments for the Medical Center.

November saw Dr. James F. Hammarsten appointed to replace Dr. Stewart Wolf as chair of the Department of Medicine. The latter was named regents professor. In the same month, Dr. Faye Sheppard, the first female faculty member of the School of Medicine, was promoted from instructor to assistant professor of Biochemistry after service as an assistant in Biochemistry and Pharmacology since 1926—nearly forty-one years! The only other woman on the full-time medical faculty at this time was Dr. Jeanne Green in Pathology.

The number of administrative employees at the Center remained relatively small at this time, with Robert C. Terrill serving as administrator of the University Hospitals, Raymond Crews as the business administrator, and Ralph Stump as the controller. In a related personnel matter, the year closed on a negative note when the governor's office ordered yet another "freeze" on hiring and travel because of a shortage of state funds. All travel out of state was to require prior approval by Vice President Pete McCarter.

Faculty salaries, which had stayed in relative check under the administration of Dean Everett, began to rise rapidly in 1967. As late as 1965 salaries of full professors in clinical departments had ranged from $1,200 to $1,800 per month. Not until 1967 was the $20,000 per-year barrier breached, with the recruitment of renowned pathologist Dr. Paul Kimmelstiel at an annual salary of $24,000. His remuneration constituted a new record, but one that was to be broken three months later when Dr. Nelson Ordway, a pediatrician and neonatologist, was hired at an annual salary of $29,000.

1968

Dean James Dennis continued to build his administrative staff and solidify his position as undisputed leader of the Medical Center during the early months of 1968. The new University president, Herbert Hollomon, took issue with the dean in a number of areas, revealing a fissure that would eventually develop into a great chasm between both men before the end of the decade.

In January 1968 Dr. William W. Schottstaedt, the acting dean of the School of Health, was appointed as that institution's permanent dean. In July he became administrator of the School of Health Related Professions.

The University of Oklahoma Board of Regents approved preliminary plans for construction of three hundred housing units for students on the Medical Center campus in February. In June, construction of two twenty-story apartment towers would also be approved. Like proposals for student housing that preceded—and followed—this one, the plans would not come to fruition.

February also saw the regents approve Dr. Boyd Gunning's recommendation that a branch office of the University of Oklahoma Foundation be located on the Health Sciences Center campus. Unlike the Foundation on the Norman campus, regents approved the transfer to this office of "all the research and training contracts and grants except where there is a legal or other compelling reason to the contrary" *[RM, 9228]*. This action was taken following a request from Dean Dennis. It was notable that the action took place just prior to Dr. Hollomon becoming president of the University.

On the political front in the spring, Senator Richard Stansberry attempted to amend the recently voter-approved Higher Education Building Bond Issue to mandate funds for a Tulsa School of Medicine. The Medical Center's Student Council (whose president was a Tulsa resident) wrote to the legislature opposing this action. The *Daily Oklahoman* editorialized against establishing a medical school in Tulsa on both fiscal and educational grounds, a conclusion reached also by Dr. Charles Edwards, a consultant from Booz, Allen and Hamilton *[DO, 3–24–68]*.

In personnel moves during early March, Dr. Joseph White accepted the position of vice president and dean of the University of Texas Medical Branch at Houston, and his appointment at the Center was terminated in May *[RM, 9335]*. Meanwhile, Drs. Eugene Jacobson (Physiology), James Hammarsten (Medicine), and Paul Kimmelstiel (Medicine) were granted tenure. Dr. William Felts was named chair of Anatomy, while Dr. Donald Halverstadt was appointed as assistant professor of Urology (Pediatrics section) in early April. In May, Drs. R. Timothy Coussons and Patrick McKee were named instructors in Medicine. Both of these high-quality individuals would remain at the Center for many years and become significant players in its political and educational futures. Dr. Ernest Lachmann and assistant professor of Biochemistry Faye Sheppard retired on the first day of July, and Drs. C. G. Gunn and Thomas N. Lynn were promoted to the rank of full professor. Dr. Jeanne Green, the College of Medicine's second full-time female faculty member, was promoted from assistant to associate professor of Pathology.

By the end of June, Dean Dennis had solidified his administration with the appointment of Dr. Edward N. Brandt as assistant to the vice president and director of the Computer Center, and Dr. Robert M. Bird (professor of Medicine) as associate dean of the College of Medicine. In addition, he recruited Dr. Tom Bruce to the Department of Medicine. These men would play key roles in his administration. The dean also drew the attention of President Hollomon and the local press when the University of Oklahoma Development Authority purchased for his use an elaborate $178,000 home of 6,000 square feet, located at a prominent Nichols Hills address. In response to questions and outright public criticism, Boyd Gunning, a spokesman for the University of Oklahoma Foundation, said, "For some time, the Medical Center has been anxious to secure a suitable home for the dean of the Center."[7] John Houchin, chair of the regents, said, "Anything that's done for Jim [Dennis] that helps ensure that he stays with us is commendable" *[DO, 6–3–68]*. The purchase of this home coincided with the regents' purchase of a $100,000 home in Norman for President Hollomon.

Dr. Herbert Hollomon assumed the presidency of the University of Oklahoma on July 1. On the same date, Dr. Mark Allen Everett was elected chair of the Department of Dermatology and Robert H. Bayley was named a research professor of Medicine. At the recommendation of the Faculty Board, Neurology was separated from the Department of Psychiatry, Neurology and Behavioral Science and given full departmental status. The word "neurology" was simultaneously dropped from the title of the previous department.

Dr. Walter Joel, the colorful and popular professor of Pathology, retired from the faculty on August 1, and a week later Dr. John D. Chase, professor of Medicine and chief of staff of the Veterans Administration Hospital, resigned and moved to the central Veterans Administration office in Washington, D.C.

Nineteen sixty-eight proved fiscally rewarding for the Medical Center staff when more than $800,000 in new state funds were appropriated in June, the entire sum earmarked for faculty salaries. This represented an 80 percent increase over the previous year in new state funds for salaries.

On September 25 longtime and much-loved professor of Pediatrics Dr. Ben Nicholson died suddenly. One of the sections of the new Children's Hospital was named in his honor by Lloyd Rader, director of the Department of Human Services. A month later, William W. Schottstaedt, M.D., dean of the School of Health, was formally named head of the School of Health Related Professions.

Perhaps the most significant event of 1968 was approval by Oklahoma taxpayers of the $99 million "HERO" bond issue ("Higher Education for a Richer Oklahoma"), from which the Medical Center garnered $27 million for new buildings and programs. Governor Dewey Bartlett's Advisory Council on Capital Expenditures had recommended the bond issue (State Question 463) for construction projects at state institutions, of which more than one-fourth was reserved for the Medical Center. In spite of an effort by Senator Richard Stansberry of Oklahoma City to amend the issue to provide for a Tulsa Medical School, Governor Bartlett and legislative leaders rallied to the aid of the Medical Center and defeated his proposals *[DO, 3–22– 68, 3–24–68]*. The Medical Alumni Association and physicians throughout the state joined with educators and enthusiastic media, especially a very supportive *Daily Oklahoman*, to assist both vocally and financially in the successful pursuit of the November vote. Citizens easily approved State Question 463 and the dream of a greatly expanded Medical Center became an assured reality. Dean Dennis would recall several decades later, "From the start, our philosophy was to 'think big' and compromise later—if we must—but to plan for the excellence of faculty, students and patients" *[DO, 2–1–99]*. Not long after passage of the bond issue, the Medical Alumni Association gave a "Thanks for the $27 Million for Health" dinner for the political leadership of the state, the press, television, and statewide health-related associations. (The positive leadership role of the Medical Alumni Association, under the vigorous direction of its secretary, Lawrence W. Rember, would play a vital role in developing support for the Center and its programs throughout the 1960s and 1970s.)

1969

Nineteen sixty-nine arrived cold and windy on the plains of Oklahoma, and with it many new problems and trials for the University and its Medical Center. When he was not knocking heads with the press, the legislature, or even his own Board of Regents, Hollomon was locking horns with Dr. James Dennis in a power struggle that, while initially remaining below the surface, consumed the energies of both men and interfered with the orderly flow of business at the institutions they represented.

The year began with the hospitalization of Margaret Hollomon, wife of President Hollomon, for "general studies," a term which led to much campus speculation and rumor. This gossip was fed by the increasing notoriety of Dr. Hollomon himself, a figure of growing controversy in Oklahoma educational and medical circles.

Herbert H. Hollomon, a Massachusetts Institute of Technology and Harvard University graduate in Engineering, had served as manager of the General Electric Research Laboratory (1961–1962) and assistant secretary for science and technology in the Department of Commerce from 1962 to 1967. According to Regent Julian Rothbaum, Hollomon had a superior education and was a highly intelligent man whose background had not prepared him for Oklahoma's culture or mores. Rothbaum recalled that: "one autumn Saturday, Herb was serving bloody Marys in the morning . . . outside . . . in full view of football game attendees. I said, 'Mr. President, this is a kinda church-going state, and folks that drink like to do a *lot* of drinking, but they pull the shades down—kind of drink in the bedroom.' 'No, sir,' he said, 'I'm not going to hide it. I'm going to serve these folks drinks out here in the open.' I said, 'Well then, alright, you do that.' I was just trying to give him some good Oklahoma advice. He sure was ahead of himself."[8]

Dr. Hollomon's penchant for shooting himself in the foot socially was demonstrated by his reaction to John Kirkpatrick, a prominent Oklahoma City philanthropist, Annapolis and West Point graduate, and oilman, who recalled that someone introduced him to Dr. Hollomon as "Admiral Kirkpatrick." "After I extended my hand to him," Kirkpatrick said, "he turned his back on me—snubbed me—muttering something about 'lock-step education.'"[9] This was not a very effective way to gain the interest and esteem of a man who, in the ensuing years, donated hundreds of millions of dollars to various charities and educational institutions throughout the state. It was possibly as a consequence of this encounter that very little of the Kirkpatrick fortune ever found its way to the University of Oklahoma. Hollomon, who served as University chief during a period in which the U. S. government was maligned for its involvement in Vietnam, frequently was unable to conceal his distaste for the military "as evidenced by his handling of the anti-war demonstration at the annual ROTC review, an event much criticized by Governor Bartlett and many Oklahoma politicians and citizens" *[DO, 6-11-70].*

Life continued at the Medical Center, however, and on March 1 associate professor Gordon Deckert was made vice-chair of the Department of Psychiatry and Behavioral Science following the resignation of prominent Psychoanalyst Eugene Pumpian-Mindlin. Deckert was awarded tenure the following month when Dr. Jolly West, chair of Psychiatry, resigned to become head of the same department at the University of California at Los Angeles. Also in March, William Brown, a graduate of the University of Michigan Dental School, was named dean of the new University of Oklahoma School of Dentistry. Later in the month, the Department of Physical Medicine was dissolved after functioning without a chairperson for several years.

The month of May saw professor Eugene Nordby of the School of Engineering named University of Oklahoma vice-president for administration and finance, an action deemed uncongenial to the Medical Center by many physicians and Center administrators, especially when the fiscal crisis on the Oklahoma City Campus became apparent in the fall. Later, Nordby was to play a leading role in the drive of the central University administration to gain control over all Health Sciences Center finances. Also in May, civic leader Stanton Young, president of the Oklahoma City Chamber of Commerce, visited Washington, D.C., to lobby for enlargement of the Oklahoma City Urban

Renewal Area and future building space for the Medical Center. At about the same time, Dr. Edward Brandt was named associate dean of the Medical Center.

Edward N. Brandt Jr., was an Oklahoma City native and University of Oklahoma graduate who had established the Biostatistical Laboratories on the Medical Center campus, and who rapidly advanced up the ladder of medical administration. In July 1970 he left Oklahoma to become dean of the University of Texas School of Medicine at Galveston and, then, vice president for medical affairs for the Texas State Higher Education System in Austin. He later served as assistant secretary of health, education and welfare in the Reagan administration. Ultimately, Dr. Brandt would return to Oklahoma as dean of the College of Medicine.

On June 12 Dean Dennis informed the University regents that in the coming year there would be a financial crisis on the Oklahoma City campus requiring layoffs of personnel, reductions in services, and restrictions on departmental budgets. This fiscal crisis was due to the continued low level of state funding and national and local inflationary trends, including an increase in the minimum wage paid to Center employees, as well as a significant reduction in funding for the Regional Medical Program (Heart-Cancer-Stroke block grant).

The Oklahoma Regional Medical Program

The Oklahoma Regional Medical Program had originated as a grant from the U.S. Department of Health, Education and Welfare, which bundled together a large number of small but dissimilar health-related programs for which the University provided assistance and consultation, including agreements with the Oklahoma American Cancer Society, Valley View Hospital in Ada, the Oklahoma Health Planning Commission, Newman Memorial Hospital in Shattuck, the Oklahoma City Area Hospital Council, and the Oklahoma State University Tech campus in Oklahoma City *[RM, 13201]*. The federal government approved an additional year of funding for this program, and also funded renewed contracts for various shared services (such as Radiology, Cardiology, laboratory, etc) with hospitals in Ardmore, Ada (Valley View), and Lawton (Southwestern). Included in this program were projects at Northwestern University at Enid, Jane Phillips at Bartlesville, Oklahoma State University Technical Institute (Nurse Teleconference Project), Oklahoma Trauma Research Society in Tulsa (Emergency Medical Services), Oklahoma Council for Health Careers, Northern Oklahoma Development Association, Southwestern Oklahoma Development Association, Oklahoma Health Planning Commission, and the Rheumatology Section at the University of Oklahoma Health Sciences Center *[RM, 13471]*. A virtual grab bag of federal goodies was included in these programs. Throughout the 1970s, the Department of Health, Education and Welfare's generosity to institutional program proposals led to inflated budgets of the sponsoring universities; and at the University of Oklahoma Health Sciences Center, as elsewhere, termination of funding for these federally sponsored programs led to fiscal crises. Provost William G. Thurman remembered that the unpredictability of such funds, as well as uncertainty regarding the flow of money from the Department of Human Services, led to many of the problems which the Health Sciences Center campus has experienced to the present day.[10] The crisis was addressed at the July 24 regents meeting when it was noted that, without a considerable increase in either revenues or state appropriations, there would have to be a serious curtailment in hospital services. Although the Center had already canceled all outstanding faculty vacancies in the Medical School and granted few salary increases, the fact that many tenure-track faculty positions had previously been funded from the Regional Medical Program severely strained the College budget. Additionally, the regents were concerned that significant College reserves had been expended on what they viewed as elaborate administrative offices in the Rogers Building. Dean Lynn would later prohibit the use of "soft" funding for base salaries of tenured faculty.

Plans for construction of student housing on the Oklahoma City campus were once again discussed by the regents at their June meeting. In a related matter, regents voted that the Medical Center Power Plant, to be built for providing chilled water and steam to the entire campus, was to utilize natural gas rather than electricity.

Just Grow, Baby!

If the motto of the University of Oklahoma's football coach in the 1970s and 80s was "Just win, baby!" the motto of Medical Center Dean James Dennis could just as easily have been "Just grow, baby!" While the dean continued to tighten his administrative and financial control of the Medical Center in 1969, he was a persistent advocate of campus growth, and if medical departments were able to fund new structures that were not mandated by the central administration or the Board of Regents, or funded by the legislature, so be it. The Department of Dermatology provided a good example of a small department taking matters into its own hands when the physical resources provided by the Medical Center proved frustratingly inadequate. Early in 1969 the Dermatology faculty had expanded to such an extent that the space allotted to it was insufficient for maintaining offices, laboratories, and clinics for full-time faculty, never mind physicians on part-time status. No clinic facilities were dedicated entirely to Dermatology, which conducted out-patient activities in the north portion of the University Hospital Emergency Room (located in the relatively new North Pavilion building, which housed Radiology and other clinics) in the mornings when emergency traffic was low. The only teaching and office space assigned to Dermatology was a single room in the old School of Nursing dormitory on Phillips Avenue.

Dr. Mark Allen Everett, Dermatology chair, resolved to build a facility to provide sufficient clinic, teaching, and office space for his expanding faculty, as well as for third- and fourth-year medical student use. Moving the Dermatology Clinic out of the hospital required formal approval of the University Hospital Board. The board initially postponed a decision due to the reservations of several of its members about letting a clinic leave the hospital. It ultimately acquiesced in the proposal following personal visits to each member by Dr. Everett.

The new building's 4,500-square-foot, two-story structure was constructed on land purchased by Dr. Everett and subsequently donated to the University. Funds were derived from bonds issued by the University of Oklahoma Development Authority, a division of the University of Oklahoma Foundation, and purchased by C. A. Vose, president of the First National Bank of Oklahoma City. The initial offer for the bonds, to be repaid by revenue from Dr. Everett's private practice, was for 7.5 percent tax-exempt bonds. Believing that the offered rate was too high to be financed by his practice, Dr. Everett visited Mr. Vose. Vose agreed to buy the bonds personally because of the long-standing friendship between Dr. Everett and Mr. Vose's daughter and son-in-law, Dr. and Mrs. G. Rainey Williams.

The new Dermatology building was an innovative, contemporary structure of poured cement, designed and engineered by Seminoff, Bowman and Bodie from sketches provided by Dr. Mark Everett. Everett had been inspired by the construction of the new addition to the library at Trinity University in Dublin, Ireland. On June 18, 1970, the newly completed building was dedicated at 619 N.E. 13th Street. Speakers on the occasion included H. O. Harden, chair of the University of Oklahoma Foundation, Ruben Sparks, chair of the Board of Regents, and Dean Dennis. Dr. Everett would transfer his highly successful downtown practice of Dermatology to the new campus structure in July 1970 when his faculty status was changed from part- to full-time. This departmental move to a free-standing building was in the vanguard of the transfer of other practices and private entities to the campus, including the Presbyterian Hospital (1974), the Dean McGee Eye Institute (1975), the Oklahoma City Clinic (1978) and the Oklahoma Allergy and Asthma Clinic (1980).

The successful operation of the Dermatology Clinic over the next year with a growth in, rather than a loss of, private patients was a positive sign for these other institutions. It strengthened their resolve to make the move to the Health Sciences Center campus. The Oklahoma City Clinic staff had always constituted the core of the Presbyterian Hospital staff, and had initiated the hospital's move to the campus. The Oklahoma Allergy and Asthma Clinic was a partnership of internists and pediatricians, all of whom were dedicated volunteer faculty. Founded in 1926 by Dr. Ray Balyeat as the Oklahoma Allergy Clinic, in 1979 the president was his step-son, Dr. Robert Ellis, who with Drs. Charles Haunshchild, George Winn, Jim Wells, John Bozalis, and Lyle Burroughs, underwrote the note for construction of the building at Lindsay and Thirteenth Streets. Ellis had for many years been a close friend of Drs. Rainey Williams and Mark Allen Everett, while Dr. John Bozalis, like Dr. Ellis, had served as president of the medical alumni organization. Together with his father, Dr. George Bozalis, John originated the Evening of Excellence annual dinners in support of medical research in the College of Medicine.

Additions to the Dermatology building, dedicated on November 20, 1981 by President Banowsky, and on May 13, 1993 by President Van Horn, resulted in first doubling and then tripling the size of the original building. Each of these additions was constructed exclusively from funds earned in private practice by Dermatology faculty, and with generous gifts from alumni and departmental friends, especially Mr. Richard Fleischaker, a philanthropist, oilman, and champion of the Medical Center. No state appropriations or federal grant funds were employed in building this structure. When the initial bond issue was paid off, it would be deeded to the University with the proviso that it must always be used exclusively for Dermatology, or title would revert to the Stovall Museum of Natural History in Norman.

In August, the Norman campus was abuzz as President Hollomon filed for divorce from his wife Margaret. At the same time, the fiscal crisis on the Oklahoma City campus deepened. Costs of equipment and supplies had escalated, and the recent federal mandate of a minimum wage of $1.50 per hour added almost $100,000 in costs to the reduced Medical Center budget. Personnel were laid off and services drastically cut to operate under a budget of $14.3 million.

The Medical Center suffered additional blows in August when Drs. Stewart Wolf and Ed Brandt announced their departure for new positions at the

University of Texas in Galveston. At the same time, intrigue continued at the regents' meetings as the board voted to separate the positions of dean and vice-president for medical affairs into separate entities following protests from other University colleges that their deans, under the current arrangement, were technically subject to the Medical College dean.

In November "Monty's Ditch"—a huge culvert to divert water from an underground stream beneath University Hospital and the source of frequent floods in the basement of the north wing—was completed. The project had earned this moniker when the culvert was conceived and championed by former Associate Dean Monte Du Val years earlier because of flooding in his and other departments.

At the end of November, Dr. Len Eliel resigned as vice-president and director of the Oklahoma Medical Research Foundation, a position he had held since 1965. In his resignation statement, Eliel declared that "new blood" was needed to keep the Foundation in the forefront of medical research. Eliel's resignation was forced by members of the Board of Directors, who believed he was steering the organization too much in the direction of support for the College of Medicine and its faculty. The leading candidates to replace Eliel were Stewart Wolf and Robert H. Furman, director of the In-patient Clinical Unit. The latter was supported by Paul Condit, who had been recruited by Eliel to head the cancer section at the OMRF some years previously. Additionally, Furman was the personal physician for two of the most vocal members of the board of directors. Accordingly, Harvey Everest, chair of the board, asked Wolf if he would, in effect, share authority with Furman, who was opposed to closer cooperation with the College of Medicine. Wolf refused this offer and Furman then ran the institution until a new president was appointed. His influence with board members continued for many years. Colin MacLeod, the new president appointed in 1971, was a distinguished research scientist who suddenly died of a coronary occlusion while in England some nine months later. This was attributed by some to circumstances surrounding the sudden resignation of the executive vice-president for fiscal affairs, Reece McGee.

1970

Severe budgetary problems continued unabated into 1970, while the political infighting between the University president and the Medical Center dean flared on almost a weekly basis—exacerbated in considerable part by a lack of state funds needed for institutional growth and educational programs. The struggle finally erupted into the full glare of media scrutiny during the year, culminating in public name calling, state officials taking sides, accusations and counter accusations, and, before the year was out, the more or less forced resignation of both men.

January 1970 witnessed the appointment of David Mock as associate dean for student affairs. An accessible and highly principled man, Dr. Mock dealt with curriculum problems and managed student affairs for many years at the Medical Center, earning the gratitude of hundreds of physicians who sought his insights and guidance during their student years.

In February Dr. Jack Metcoff was appointed professor of Pediatrics, while Dr. John Colmore was named acting associate dean of the College of Medicine. In a few months, Colmore's appointment would play a role in the power struggle between President Hollomon and Dean Dennis.

Dr. Tom Bruce and Dr. Donald Halverstadt were granted tenure in March— Bruce as professor of Medicine and Halverstadt as assistant professor of Urology. At the same time, Mary Schottstaedt, wife of the dean of the School of Health Related Professions, was removed from the list of faculty tenure candidates because of the fear of nepotism relating to her husband's position. Lester Gorsline Associates was once again hired as a building consultant, this time to plan the new College of Dentistry building. Also in March, the Computer Management Corporation (CMC) was hired over International Business Machines (IBM) to provide a billing system for University Hospital. This was the first in a long line of what many Medical Center personnel felt was unwise contract awarding. CMC at this time had little experience in the areas of consultation and development of medical computing technology, whereas IBM was an acknowledged leader in the field.

At the end of March controversy erupted between the State Regents for Higher Education and the State Nursing Board over control of nursing education curricula in the state of Oklahoma. Under existing law, the regents had absolute control over all nursing courses and course content in state-supported institutions. However, the Nursing Board maintained that criteria for licensure meant de facto control over criteria for the nursing degree.

Late in May the legislature initiated another study of medical staffing needs for the state of Oklahoma. The impetus for the latest study came from rural communities convinced that their medical needs were not being met because physicians graduating from the Medical Center were opting for specialization and avoiding small-town general practice. The complainants chose to blame the Center rather than the real "culprit" in at least 50 percent of these cases: spouses of graduating physicians elected to avoid small-town life in rural Oklahoma.

Dennis vs. Hollomon

The political struggle between Dean James Dennis and President Herbert Hollomon continued at midyear with rumors that Dr. Dennis might take a position at the University of Arkansas in Little Rock because, as the *Daily Oklahoman* reported, "In the two years that Dr. Hollomon has been OU President, the two have differed over the operations, responsibility and philosophy of the medical center and medical school. 'I will make up my own mind in three or four weeks,' Dennis said" *[DO, 3–27–70]*. In a related matter, the *Oklahoman* reported that Governor Dewey Bartlett's appointment of Dr. V. M. Lockard of Bartlesville to the Board of Regents "apparently will hold the key to Dr. J. Herbert Hollomon's future as president of the University" *[DO, 6–11–70]*. It was public knowledge that Governor Bartlett despised President Hollomon and hoped to fire him, using a Board of Regents that supported his desires. On June 16 the *Oklahoman* reported that Dean Dennis was considering another job, although "Bartlett hinted . . . that OU regents might oust Hollomon" and that the governor had "called Dennis several times to urge him to keep the director's job" in spite of the fact that the Dean had "been at odds with Dr. Hollomon" for several months. The *Daily Oklahoman*, in reviewing the squabble years later, would state that "in fact, the two were incompatible in both personality and management style. Hollomon resented the medical campus' independence" *[DO, 2–1–99]*.

The flap between Dennis and Hollomon reached the editorial page when, on June 20, the *Daily Oklahoman* stated that: "Governor Bartlett is charged with exerting improper influence on the regents when he discussed the problems between the dean and the president with a potential new regent. Differences between Dr. Hollomon and Dr. Dennis . . . have been over basic policies that the regents will have to consider. . . . It would seem incumbent on the governor at least to advise a new regent that he also may face hard decisions on other issues, too, such as campus disorder."

Governor Bartlett and several state legislators had been particularly critical of Hollomon's handling of student political disturbances in the spring. On the other hand, there were those who felt that Hollomon had handled student unrest during this troubled era with great skill. There were no Berkley riots or Kent State shooting scenes in Norman. Former Regents Chair James G.

Davidson of Tulsa, who was one of Hollomon's staunchest defenders, said, "The problem with people who want to get rid of Hollomon is they don't know what's really going on at the university. . . . They are uninformed about the total university and what Herb has done to upgrade it and make it a national symbol" *[DO, 6–25–70]*. Dennis contended that repercussions from student unrest were spilling over from Norman to Oklahoma City, particularly when it came to the issues of budgets and administration. In actuality, student unrest on the Medical Center campus was not related to the national Vietnam protest movement, but to the threat that the current state of fiscal austerity might result in closure of educational programs in the Colleges of Health and Health Related Professions, as well as a rise in tuition throughout the campus.

On June 24 President Hollomon announced that he had "reached an agreement on the responsibilities and authorities of Dr. James Dennis." John Houchin, a former regents' chair, predicted that "if Hollomon did not resign, he would be fired. Unfortunately, Hollomon has a faculty for generating controversy" *[DO, 6–24–70]*. Regent Julian Rothbaum summarized the situation in his own inimitable way: "Hollomon seemed to have great trouble in Oklahoma. You have to be like Bill Clinton when he tried to change the health [Medicare] laws. Instead of doing it in one big swoop, like he secretly wanted to, you have to kinda nibble at it and go kinda slow sometimes. You need to present an idea and let people digest it for a while. Hollomon always wanted to do things yesterday."[11]

At their June 25 meeting, the Board of Regents established, for the first time in history, a permanent Medical Center Committee consisting of Horace Calvert as chair, with Nancy J. Davies and Huston Huffman as members. Upon recommendation of President Hollomon, the regents also changed the title of Dean Dennis to executive vice president of the University for medical affairs, and effectively separated the Health Center budget from the Norman campus budget. This action was undoubtedly an end result of the power playing by regents, the governor, President Hollomon, and Dean Dennis. According to the *Minutes* of the June 25 meeting, Dr. Dennis stated that he "would like to express [his] gratification for this action" and that he: "was appalled at the implication in the press that I was personally trying to get the president fired. I never at any time made such a request and to describe [sic] the crisis that exists here today to a personality clash between me and the President is evading the issue, and the issue as far as I am concerned is the integrity and the future of the Medical Center. I have challenged only the policies of the President that I feel are not in the best interests of the Medical Center."

Following the Dennis declaration, Regents Chairman Calvert, stated, "I believe that for the best interests of the University, the Board of Regents should not retain Dr. Hollomon." Although the *Daily Oklahoman* on June 25 had predicted a 7–0 vote against retaining the president, the regents reaffirmed confidence in President Hollomon by a 4–1–1 vote and supported his continued employment. Calvert was the lone dissenting vote, while Regent Lockhart abstained. President Hollomon then made a passionate, if rambling, statement:

Obviously, I appreciate deeply the honesty and consideration, care and concern which this board has taken with respect to the matter before them. . . . There are deep divisions in our country . . . differences which have often led to hatred and violence. In many ways I feel that the Nation itself is threatened. The State is threatened. The University is threatened. I've told this Board privately, which I should now say publicly, the only thing I have to give is to try and protect the deepest values of our place, which is openness, due process, justice under the law, equal opportunity for those independent of race, creed, or color, and the freedom and openness of this institution; I will give my life, and that's all I have to say.

Hollomon also "immediately pledged himself to try to bring the many divergent forces on campus into harmony" *[DO, 6–26–70]*.

On July 7 Dean Dennis tendered his resignation, accusing President J. Herbert Hollomon of violating trusts and agreements concerning the operation of the Medical Center. His resignation came in spite of the fact that at the June 25 meeting of the regents he had been given most of the powers and authority that roughly parallel the position of chancellor at other large, multicampus state university systems. "Dennis acknowledged that he told Hollomon on June 25, prior to the regents meeting, 'I don't trust you.' Dennis was to become vice president for Health Sciences at the University of Arkansas" *[DO, 7–8–70]*. Decades later, James Dennis would admit that his abrupt departure was probably too hasty *[DO, 2–1–99]*.

Before the dust had settled from the James Dennis resignation, another bombshell dropped. In spite of the vote of confidence President Hollomon had received less than a month earlier from the regents, he startled the board with his resignation on July 23. The president said, "Assaults by the Governor on the President and values of the University make it abundantly clear that any member of the faculty, any student, or any employee may be persecuted or threatened for his way of life or his beliefs. These threats to the integrity of this University and its members starkly represent the spirit of repression now running rampant without reason among us" *[DO, 7–24–70]*.

The *Daily Oklahoman* editorialized that "The turmoil that has plagued the university in recent months has proved costly to the school, the state and to many individuals. The bitterness that marked Dr. Hollomon's prepared statement to the regents reflected the deepening divisions over university administration and policy" *[DO, 7–24–70]*. Regent Reuben Sparks had absented himself from the July 23 meeting, proclaiming that he stayed away because he might have said something he should not say. He suffered a fatal heart attack shortly after, and Governor Bartlett named Robert Lollard as a replacement for Sparks. President Hollomon indicated that this appointment was an indication to him that "Assaults on the university and on me personally were to continue." Dr. Dennis, in his resignation, "also expressed personal bitterness. And Dennis's statements did nothing to heal the discontent over university affairs" *[DO, 7–24–70]*. The regents named Dr. Pete Kyle McCarter, Norman campus provost, as acting president of the university.

Dr. John P. Colmore was selected to replace James Dennis at the Medical Center and was named interim executive vice president for medical affairs at the July 23 regents' meeting. Dr. Colmore had served as a University of Oklahoma medical faculty member since 1952. The 48-year-old professor of Medicine and Pharmacology had been acting associate dean since February, an appointment which was now made permanent. A Tennessee native and Princeton and Columbia graduate, he was named interim executive vice president in order that he might have as long a period as possible of orientation with Dr. Dennis prior to his departure. James Dennis's appointment, however, would be terminated on September 15, 1970.

On July 27 President Hollomon "lashed out against his critics, including Governor Bartlett and Dr. James Dennis, OU vice president for medical center affairs," saying that the governor had "blessed out" the regents after their vote of confidence in him and said that Dr. Dennis had never contacted him personally regarding his dissatisfaction with the administration. "I couldn't understand what was bothering Dennis because he never said anything to me. The strategy in this state seems to be that if you can't get your way, go public" *[DO, 7–28–70]*.

More disturbing news came on August 13 when it was learned that the former wife of President Hollomon had died in Boston at age 50 after an apparent heart attack. A decree of divorce had been issued on May 18. The situation worsened in November when it was announced that Dr. John Colmore was gravely ill and had been hospitalized since November 18 at

University Hospital. Dr. Leonard Eliel was authorized to act on Dr. Colmore's behalf during the illness. However, Dr. Colmore died of chronic relapsing hepatitis the day following this announcement. He was 49. His replacement was Dr. Eliel, who was appointed interim executive vice president effective December 1.

Leonard Paul Eliel, a California native and Harvard University graduate who trained in Internal Medicine at Massachusetts General Hospital, was a scholarly, soft-spoken medical investigator. He had come to the Oklahoma Medical Research Foundation in 1951 to head the cancer research division. He became acting director of research in 1954, director in 1955, and vice president and director of research after having served as executive director from 1962 to 1965. His tenure was complicated by a division of authority between himself and a lay administrator—initially Hugh Payne and later Reece McGee. Lay directors were unhappy with his belief that closer relations should be developed with the School of Medicine. Business leader and OMRF Chair Harvey Everest said, "I think it's time for you to go." Eliel then resumed his position as a vice-president and director of research while at the same time becoming a member of the Department of Medicine faculty. In 1971 he was named interim executive director of the Medical Center, and later as director, vice-president for health science affairs, and provost. Several University administrators believed that Leonard Eliel was a "duck out of water" in the position as the leader of a comprehensive Medical Center— and "probably unsuited to the appointment." However, Dr. Eliel filled a controversial post at a difficult time and tried to maintain equanimity in a period of great crisis. Perhaps his greatest weakness was a tendency to avoid issues rather than face them head on, a quality that sometimes increased turmoil rather than quelled it.

In November 1970 bonds for the Steam and Chilled Water Plant were issued after the Center's clinical chairs were coerced into pledging private practice revenue in the Oklahoma Medical Center Trust to underwrite repayment of the bonds until such time as the plant was "up and running" and earning revenue. This method of financing was employed because the facility would supply power for non-state entities (i.e., private institutions on the campus), and University income from state sources could not legally be used for this purpose. Construction on the plant began the following February.

Also in November, the College of Pharmacy was ordered by the State Regents to move from the small southwestern town of Weatherford, Oklahoma, to the Medical Center campus. Many people believed that one school of pharmacy was more than sufficient to provide for the needs of the state.

However, rural legislators had prevented earlier attempts to consolidate the Norman and Weatherford pharmacy schools. They would succeed once more in sustaining duplicate facilities for the sake of political expediency.

About this time, an incident occurred that did not reflect well on the Medical Center or the University and was precursor to several similar events in subsequent years. Dean Emeritus Mark Everett, following his retirement in 1965, had been provided a spacious office on the first floor of the old Medical School building to write a second volume of his history of the Medical Center. Several years later, without prior warning, he was directed to vacate these quarters and move to an office not much larger than a closet, without windows, near the auditorium. Then, in 1970, he was informed by Medical School administrators that he would have to relinquish even this small space, that was now needed "for other purposes." Phil Jackson, a long-term employee who served as construction superintendent of the new University Hospital, had chatted with "the old dean" and provided him with a hard hat so that he could visit safely the various construction sites on the campus. One day Jackson observed Dean Everett and his secretary packing boxes to leave their cramped quarters. Upon inquiry he learned that the departure was forced. Feeling that this was a heartless way to treat someone who had served the University for forty years, Jackson approached Dr. Mark Allen Everett and asked, "Don't you have room in your new Dermatology building for the old dean?" Dean Everett was immediately provided with offices for himself and his secretary, with a fine view over 13th Street to the new Presbyterian Hospital grounds. The old dean remained in this office for ten years, writing the second volume of *Medical Education in Oklahoma* with the help of his wife Alice Allen Everett.

As a tumultuous 1970 came to an end, former President Herbert Hollomon married Ms. Nancy Gade in a ceremony in Guilderland, New York. Ms. Gade had been an assistant professor of drama at the University of Oklahoma during Hollomon's tenure as president. The two had met following a faculty appreciation banquet at which Ms. Gade was honored. The President was escorting Ms. Gade home, when he was notified that a potentially dangerous political protest by students was underway in front of his house in Norman, forcing him to spend the night in what he deemed safer quarters.

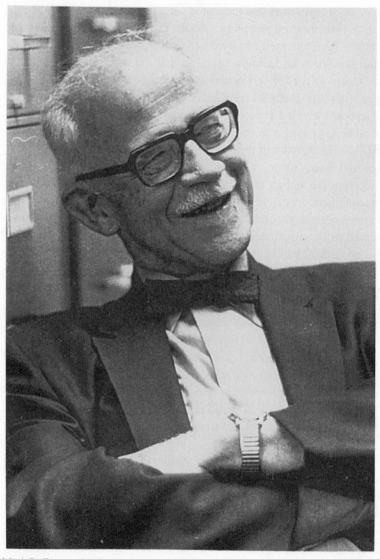

Mark R. Everett, Ph.D., Dean of the University of Oklahoma College of Medicine and Director of the Medical Center. (AAE)

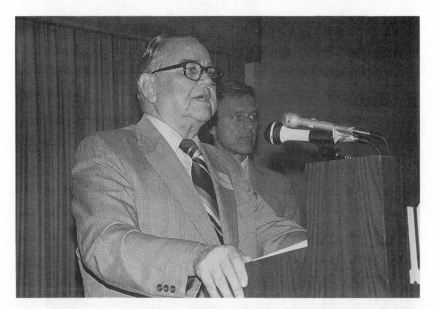

E. T. Dunlap, Ed.d., Chancellor of the Oklahoma State Regents for Higher Education, with William Banowsky. (OUPA)

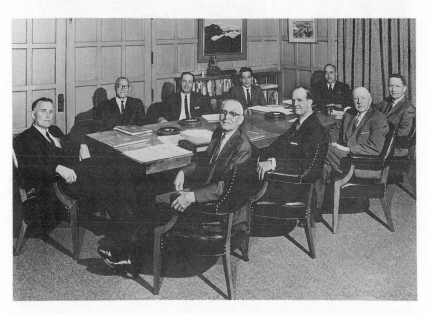

The University of Oklahoma Board of Regents with President George Lynn Cross (far left). Courtesy Western History Collections, University of Oklahoma Libraries. (OUPA)

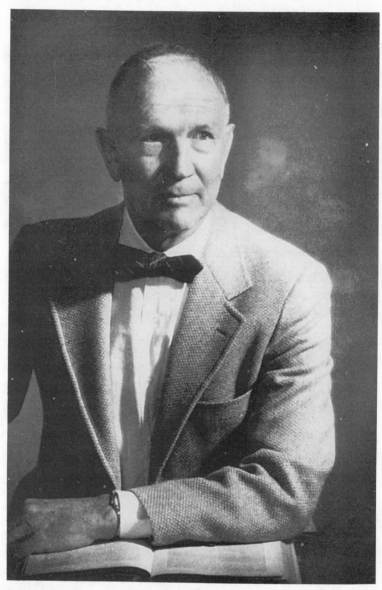

John Schilling, M.D., first full-time Chair of the Department of Surgery and second Chair of the Faculty Board. (AAE)

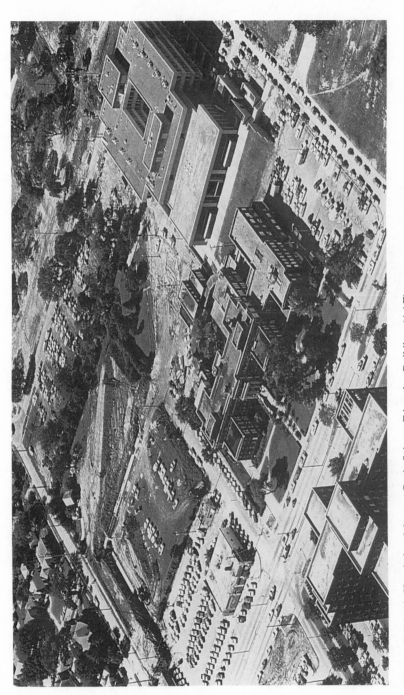

The old Children's Hospital and the new Basic Science Education Building. (AAE)

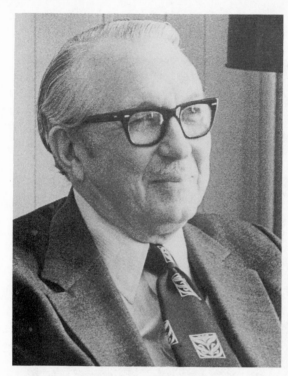

James Dennis, M.D.,
Dean of the College of
Medicine, Director of the
Medical Center, and
Executive Vice-president
for Medical Affairs.
(OUHSC)

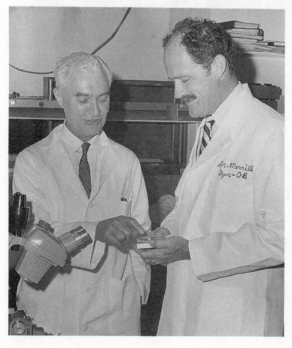

Robert M. Bird, M.D.,
Professor of Medicine
and Dean of the College
of Medicine, and James
M. Merrill, M.D.,
Professor and Chair of
the Department of
Gynecology and
Obstetrics. (AAE)

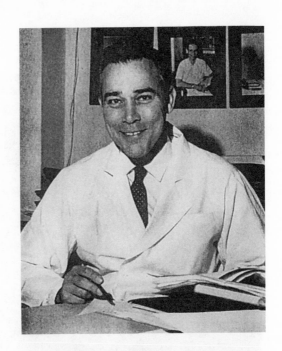

Stewart G. Wolf, M.D.,
Professor and Chair of the
Department of Medicine.
(AAE)

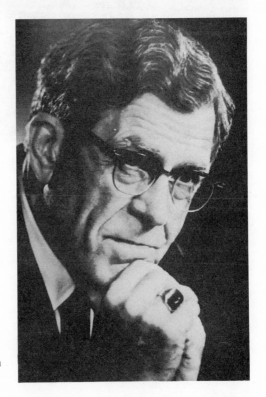

Dean A. McGee, Oklahoma City
oil man, civic leader, and
prominent supporter of the Health
Sciences Center. (OUHSC)

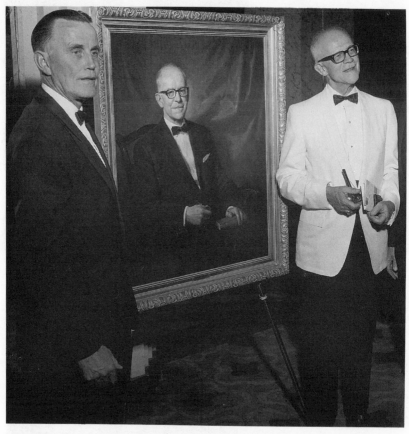

George Lynn Cross, Ph.D., President of the University of Oklahoma, at the presentation of Dr. Mark R. Everett's portrait. (AAE)

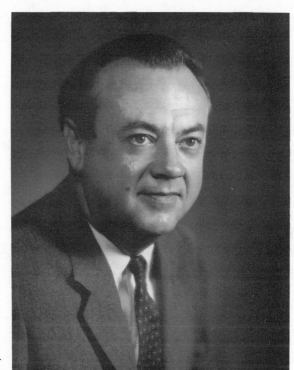

Herbert A. Hollomon,
Ph.D., President of the
University of Oklahoma.
(OUPA)

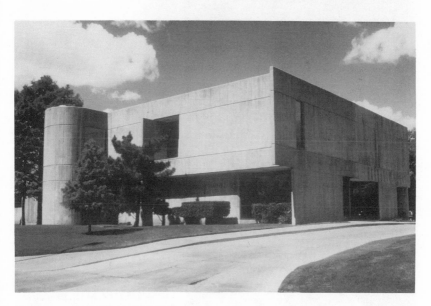

The Dermatology Clinic. (OUHSC)

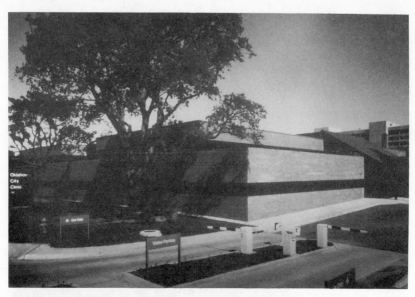

The Oklahoma City Clinic. (OUHSC)

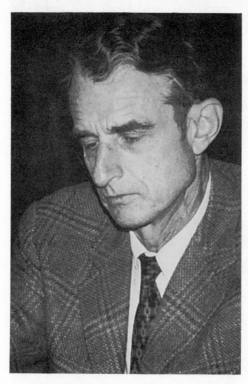

Leonard P. Eliel, M.D., Executive
Vice-president of the Health
Sciences Center. (AAE)

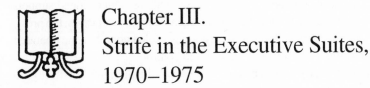

Chapter III.
Strife in the Executive Suites,
1970–1975

 The widely publicized conflict between Medical Center Dean James Dennis and University President Herbert Hollomon resulted in consequences far greater than the simple departure of both men from the University of Oklahoma. It led to a loss of power, if not respect, for their offices and a temporary "bunker" mentality among the executives who succeeded them. This mentality lasted for a relatively brief period on the Norman campus, as new president Paul Sharp was dragged into the public spotlight—albeit a less glaring and personal one than his predecessor had wilted under—by the sheer press of events and insatiable demands on the chief executive of a large university. At the Medical Center, however, the effects of the Dennis-Hollomon struggle were far more profound and led to consequences that took considerably longer to overcome. Some of the consequences are with us to this day.

Physicists like to say that nature abhors a vacuum, and the University of Oklahoma Medical Center illustrated this principle immediately after the departure of James Dennis. The vacuum created by the withdrawal of the dean, combined with the continuing financial crises that focused budget needs on clinical income rather than legislative appropriations, led to the rise of a new force that had lain relatively dormant. Going about its business effectively, creatively, but usually out of the bright glare of publicity, this new force was the faculty itself, led by its brilliant clinical chairs.

The dean of the College of Medicine was, historically, the most powerful individual at the University of Oklahoma Medical Center, exercising near-absolute control over faculty appointments, salaries, clinic space, and most other important matters. There was never a question of "who is in charge," in spite of the fact that Dean Everett had practiced a kind of genteel, laissez-faire management, and his successor, James Dennis, allowed trusted cohorts to operate little empires in specialties such as Medicine, Surgery, Psychiatry, and

Obstetrics/Gynecology. The dean historically had the unquestioned support of the University of Oklahoma Board of Regents and, in most cases, the president of the University. As long as these entities smiled upon him, he operated with unquestioned authority, autonomy, and control.

When the power struggle between Dennis and Hollomon burst into the public consciousness, the special relationship between the Medical Center and the University began to wither. The first sign of danger appeared when the regents changed the title of James Dennis from dean and director of the Medical Center to executive vice-president for Medical Center affairs in June 1970 with the subsequent deletion of his title of dean of the School of Medicine. Suddenly the Medical Center had a vice-president but not a dean. The regents would quickly appoint a replacement—Dr. Robert M. Bird—who would be, in essence, a dean-once-removed. He would answer to the new vice-president rather than to the University president and the Board of Regents. No longer would he be in charge of campus development, budget management, political and social relationships with the outside world, and countless other functions deans had historically performed for the Medical Center.

In the opinion of the authors, this dramatic change in titles was sought by James Dennis because he feared that Herbert Hollomon planned to oust him or, at least, to eviscerate his power as Medical Center dean. In his mind, a promotion to a vice-presidency would ensure that the Center would continue to be represented at the highest levels of the University bureaucracy. Unfortunately, by failing to anticipate the problems he was creating for his successors, James Dennis accomplished the exact opposite of what he intended for the deanship. Not only had this maneuver ousted Dean Dennis personally from his role on the Oklahoma City campus, it forever removed all subsequent deans from the special, direct, unfettered relationship they had enjoyed with the president of the University and its Board of Regents. Never again would the dean's office participate in a Mark Everett-George Cross type of relationship; indeed, it would move farther and farther from this model as provosts, assistant provosts, and other bureaucratic layers were added over the years.

As though the schism between the Medical Center and the University were not damaging enough, two other key events occurred in rapid succession that, when added to the Dennis-Hollomon fiasco and the continuing legislative refusal to fund the Medical Center adequately, opened the door to the emergence of a new force. These events were, first, the ascension of Dr. John Colmore to interim, and then permanent, medical director, followed by his terminal illness (and subsequent death), which prevented him from exercising any effective leadership. Second was the selection of Dr. Leonard P. Eliel as permanent executive vice president for medical affairs. Doctor Eliel was a fine man and an excellent researcher, but he was not a strong administrator and never seemed comfortable in the role of leadership. This combination of events led to a continuing power vacuum in which responsibility for the Medical Center shifted from the offices of the dean and the executive vice president/provost to the circle of strong clinical chairs who constituted the majority of the Center's Faculty Board.

THE FACULTY BOARD

The Faculty Board was created in 1948 by Medical Center Dean Mark Everett to provide, at the request of the dean, advice on a wide variety of issues regarding the School of Medicine. It consisted of the departmental chairs plus several elected members of the volunteer and full-time faculty. From 1960 to1970, the role of the board became increasingly formal. In addition to its role as advisor to the dean, it assumed responsibility for all the faculty committees, including the committees for curriculum, promotion, and tenure. With the creation of the Faculty Board Advisory Council by Dean Dennis, this new body assumed direct responsibility for committees related to curriculum, but submitted its recommendations directly to the Faculty Board rather than to the dean.

First in importance among faculty committees was the Curriculum Committee, initially chaired by Dr. Ben Nicholson (Pediatrics), then by Dr. Jim Merrill (Obstetrics-Gynecology), and later, under various other names, by Dr. Gordon Deckert (Psychiatry), Dr. Patrick McKee (Internal Medicine) and Dr. Dennis Weigand (Dermatology). The Faculty Board's first chair, subject to election biannually, was Dr. Don H. O'Donoghue, chair of the Department of Orthopedics. He served through June 1973 and was succeeded by Dr. John Schilling, who served for exactly one year. His elected successor was Dr. Mark Allen Everett, head of Dermatology, who chaired the board for the next seventeen years. Later, the faculty by-laws would be altered by Dean Donald G. Kassebaum to preclude the re-election of Dr. Everett, who, though lacking the power of formal administrative office, wielded great influence on behalf of the faculty and the College of Medicine.

Mark Allen Everett, a 1951 graduate of the University of Oklahoma College of Medicine, studied pediatrics and dermatology at the University of Michigan, public health at Tulane, and served for two years in the United States Air Force in Germany as chief of preventive medicine for the Twelfth Air Force. Returning to the University of Oklahoma in 1957, he established the research and residency training programs for the Department of Dermatology, was elected its chair in 1965, served as interim chair of the Department of Pathology, and was later appointed Chief of Staff of University Hospital from 1980–1985. He served as chair of the Faculty Board during a period in which that board exercised its greatest influence at the Health Sciences Center.

During Dr. Everett's tenure as chair, the Faculty Board undertook a wide range of studies of administrative structure, codes for student behavior, changes in the curriculum, minority issues, relationships with the hospitals, criteria for admission to the College, standards for promotion and graduation, makeup of the Medical School admissions board, names and status of individual departments, and revisions of the faculty bylaws. The board also strongly defended the well defined prerogatives and duties of the faculty regarding definition of standards of admission, courses of instruction, requirements for graduation, content of the educational programs of the College, and recommendations of students for the degree of Doctor of Medicine. In addition, the board had the obligation to recommend to the faculty any matters requiring its attention, as well as to consider interdepartmental matters requiring action, advice, and/or arbitration. The board also acted as an executive advisory board to the dean, resulting in constant interaction between the dean, his associates, and the chair of the Faculty Board.

Dr. Rainey Williams, professor of Surgery, succeeded Dr. Everett as chair of the Faculty Board in 1990, and was followed by Dr. Fred Silva, chair of Pathology. Under Deans Everett and Dennis, the Faculty Board functioned primarily in an advisory capacity; during the regimes of Provosts Eliel, Thurman, and Rich, the board usually served as the primary interface between the faculty and the university administration, with the dean becoming gradually more of a representative of administration than of the faculty, and the board being less decisive in decision making.

THE NATIONAL BOARD EXAMINATIONS

At the end of 1970 the Faculty Board, at the recommendation of the Academic Council, voted to adopt a proposal that "successful completion of the National Board Examinations, Part I and Part II, be prerequisites for advancement and graduation respectively. The department or departments involved may, at their discretion, determine the passing level" *[FBM, 12–9–70]*. This resolution was originally proposed at a Faculty Board retreat at Fountainhead Lodge in the eastern lake region of Oklahoma. Dr. James Merrill (OB–GYN) recalls an amusing incident at the retreat: "As the meeting broke up on the third morning, there were four or five of us waiting for the elevator, including Joe Kopta, chairman of Orthopedics. When the elevator arrived, out stepped a second year orthopedic resident with an attractive 'non-wife.' This guy was spending the weekend at the resort with this tootsie, not knowing that his school's Faculty Board was having a retreat in the same building—including the chairman of his department! I remember he punched the 'up' button several times rapidly, trying to get out of there."[1]

The National Board exam proposal was strongly supported by Drs. Merrill, Snow, Schilling and Everett, with Dr. Merrill its chief architect. Months later, on June 16, 1971, in a memorandum to Dr. David Mock, Dean Robert M. Bird ordered that the National Board Exams be implemented in the academic year 1972–73. This requirement was to become a frequent bone of contention among students who failed the test, among the faculty, and to administrators who were bombarded with complaints from students requesting reversal of their failures.

Doctor James Merril was a graduate of the University of California at Berkeley (1945) and the University of California at San Francisco (M.D. 1948). During the 1950s, he studied at Harvard and served in the United States Air Force. He returned to the San Francisco faculty in 1958, where he served as an assistant and associate professor until his selection as chair at Oklahoma in 1961. Merrill occupied the position of secretary-treasurer of the American Board of Gynecology and Obstetrics from 1976 to 1984. A Markle scholar, he had great influence on the medical curriculum in his role as chair of the Curriculum Committee. He seemed always to come round to an institutional rather than a parochial view. Originally opposed to Family Practice residents in the clinics, he later facilitated their training in obstetrics (while denying them privileges to do "C" sections). He was a strong supporter of a centralized Professional Practice Plan. Like Dr. John Schilling, he had a stern, demanding personality, insisting upon high standards for himself and others. Always a champion of excellence on campus, he resigned his position as chair at Oklahoma in 1983, saying that no chair should serve for more than twenty years. He moved to Seattle, Washington in 1984, where he served as Executive Director of the American Board of Gynecology and Obstetrics.

In January 1971 it was announced that the National Institutes of Health had awarded matching grants for construction of the Biomedical Sciences building and the Medical Center Library, in the full amount of $18 million requested by the regents. An additional $10 million would be derived from the HERO Bond Issue. At the request of Acting University President Pete McCarter, regents approved a resolution to condemn whatever nearby land was needed for all future building plans. A suit filed by the landowner regarding condemnation was to result in a court judgment of $145,000 against the University only a few months later. Also in January, regents took up the long-standing issue of housing for students on the Oklahoma City campus and approved plans for 147 apartments at a cost of $4.1 million. An application to the U.S. Department of Housing and Urban Development for financial support for this project was suggested and voted. Later, in February 1972, the housing plan would be revised to include 300 two-story town houses. Still later, the entire housing project would fail due to problems in financing state bonds and a lessened interest by students, most of whom now had families and preferred to commute from suburban areas such as Edmond and Norman.

The curriculum for the new College of Dentistry was approved at the request of the Medical Center provost in January, although concern over decreasing federal grants cast a shadow over plans for the opening of this College in the autumn of 1972. The regents also reluctantly granted permission to hold the Medical Center graduation ceremonies in Oklahoma City rather than in Norman, fearing that the already tenuous relationship of the Center's students to the parent University would be further lessened, and some students might leave without ever having seen the Norman campus. The vote specified that the permission was for one year only. Little did the regents dream that this seemingly one-time permission would become the rule and tradition on the Oklahoma City campus.

The month of January also witnessed a special meeting of the Board of Regents that resulted in the selection of Dr. Paul Sharp as ninth president of the University of Oklahoma. Sharp was a conciliatory, even-tempered leader whose presidency was characterized by the presence of over-ambitious vice presidents and often hostile regents and legislators. He would serve with bravery throughout the difficult financial and political vagaries of the 1970s, showing himself to be a strong advocate of science and scholarship on the Oklahoma City campus while defending the Center against political attacks and attempts to reduce the medical complex to little more than a trade school. A former dean praised Sharp for always trying to do the right thing, saying that "it is better to have a president who tries to do the right thing than one who always *knows* he is doing it."[2] He and his wife Rose participated fully in the life of the University and were regarded with affection by faculty and students.

(In 1998, the beautiful Performance Hall in the new Cattlet Music Center on the Norman campus was named for him.)

In March, the regents contracted with the Central Oklahoma Transportation and Parking Authority (COTPA) to develop and manage parking structures on the campus. Many on the faculty thought this an unwise decision from a fiscal point of view because the Authority would pay only token rent to the University. In addition, COTPA would be able to levy large parking fees on faculty, staff, and visitors. As part of the agreement, the University was expected to make a commitment to the effect that it would pay the cost of operating and amortizing these structures. Eventually, a separate authority called Medical Technology and Research Authority (MTRA) would assume control of all campus parking.

In April 1971 tenure was granted to Dr. Leonard Eliel (Medicine), Dr. Mark Allen Everett (Dermatology), and Dr. Everett Rhoades (Family Practice and a specialist in American Indian health programs). Dr. Eugene Jacobson, professor of Physiology, resigned his position, effective at the end of August. Former Dean and Director Mark R. Everett was made an Emeritus Regents Professor of Medical Science.

An agreement of affiliation was signed between the College of Medicine and St. Anthony's Hospital in June 1971 recognizing the role of this community hospital in the education of medical students. Since World War II, students had rotated on Internal Medicine and Surgery services, and as a result of this agreement, Family Medicine became an additional rotation service.

In July, Dr. Ben Heller, chair of the Department of Laboratory Medicine, resigned his position and moved out of state. Dr. Heller had long been a political activist, playing an important role in the national presidential campaign of U.S. Senator Eugene McCarthy. Heller was the last chair of the short-lived Department of Laboratory Medicine, which soon would be abolished and its functions returned to the Department of Pathology.

Also in July, the state legislature passed a resolution asking the University of Oklahoma Board of Regents to "extend services of the OU Medical School to provide leadership in the development and coordination of medical education services in Tulsa." In urging this action, state Senator Finis Smith told the regents that "the future is very bright for establishing a health training center in Tulsa" *[DO, 7–21–71]*.

An external review of the Department of Biochemistry was received by the Faculty Board in late July. Recommendations included rigorous review of faculty research at regular intervals, examination of the Medical Center's relationship with the Oklahoma Medical Research Foundation, regular review of space requirements associated with research, and more scrutiny of tenured faculty. This report presaged a persistent discomfort within Medical Center departments that contained a large percentage of faculty who possessed full-time faculty appointments but were housed in, and paid directly by, the Oklahoma Medical Research Foundation. This was a situation which would lead to continual friction in the future.

In August, President Sharp named Leonard P. Eliel as executive vice president for Medical Center affairs, and in September the title was changed from "interim" to "permanent executive vice president for Medical Center affairs." Later, in November, the State Regents for Higher Education approved a change in name of the Medical Center to the University of Oklahoma Health Sciences Center *[RM, 11183]*. At the same time, the various "schools" at the Center were changed to "colleges": Dentistry, Health, Allied Health Professions, Medicine, and Nursing. These changes presaged a later radical reorganization of the Health Center's administration. *[Note: As a result of these formal actions by the Oklahoma State Regents for Higher Education, henceforth in this history the University of Oklahoma "Medical Center" will be called the "Health Sciences Center," and the "Medical School" and "School of Medicine" will be called the "College of Medicine."]*

On August 23 former Dean James Dennis returned to Oklahoma City for a meeting of the Oklahoma Health Sciences Foundation Board, saying that all health service officials at universities "feel extremely frustrated" at the tightening of state and federal funds which put all university medical centers in a financial bind. He stated that the Oklahoma City campus "is a model that is being emulated in many areas" *[DO, 8–24–71]*. Dr. Dennis, with then-Governor Bellmon and oilman Dean McGee, had been the principal champions of the "health campus" concept.

Also in August, regents heard a pessimistic forecast regarding the financial outlook for health care institutions as federal grants began to dry up. The University's grandiose plans for a new School of Health seemed to disappear overnight with the decision that the school, now a college, would remain in the old College of Medicine building because the prospect for federal funding in support of a new building was now practically nil.

The names of the various departments and divisions in the College of Dentistry were approved by the regents at their October meeting. In November, they approved the first revisions of the Faculty of Medicine bylaws since 1953. Both the original and revised versions of the bylaws were prepared by a committee composed of Drs. Mark Everett and Rainey Williams, and had already been approved by the Faculty Board. In a final November action, the regents announced an increase of $2.3 million in the cost of the Ambulatory Medical Clinic addition to University Hospital.

During 1971, the salaries of the deans of Medicine and Dentistry were raised to $2,875 per month, while that of the dean of Health Related Professions was elevated to $2,375—incomes identical to that of Gordon Deckert, chair of Psychiatry. Other salaries in 1971 were: chair of Medicine, $2,385 per month; chair of Biochemistry and Molecular Biology $2,169; and chair of Pediatrics $2,489. The administrator of the University Hospitals was paid $2,083 per month. (Readers surprised at these relatively penurious salaries may be equally amazed at the mind-boggling figures that have been carved out for the same positions late in this century. Although inflation rose approximately 110 percent from 1979 to 1996, Health Sciences Center executive salaries advanced more than 1,000 percent!)

Regents completed 1971 with an announcement from the National Institutes of Health of a grant of $1.19 million for construction of a third floor on the Biomedical Sciences building, a site intended for dental instruction. The regents also announced, for a second time, that the Health Sciences Center's commencement would be held at the Oklahoma City Civic Center Music Hall. In a final December action, following more than a year of preparation, regents presented the "Report of the Task Force for Long Range Planning" for the Health Sciences Center. The chief conclusions of the report, presented but not discussed by the Board until the following February, were: (1) service (direct patient care) and education of students are the first priority of the Center; (2) emphasis on medical care must be on excellence, not indigent care—a conclusion that would require a change in image as well as in state legislation mandating payments to the Center's hospitals by counties or the state for indigents; (3) the Center's departmental policies should be in harmony with University policy, although the vice president and his staff should primarily develop rules that are Center-wide and not merely College or departmental activities; and (4) more effective liaison with the public, alumni, and the legislature must be developed.

1972

Nineteen seventy-two opened with growing agitation by civic groups as well as by state and federal government entities for larger College of Medicine classes and increased minority representation in medical specialties. Recently passed federal health manpower legislation (HB 8629) introduced *capitation grants*, which provided support funds to medical schools based upon the increased number of students admitted to entering classes. These grants would be given to medical schools for the purpose of encouraging expansion of class sizes, since national studies had convinced the deep thinkers in Washington that there was a serious pending doctor shortage in the country.

On January 5 the Health Sciences Center Faculty Board, acting for the faculty, voted that the number of students in the entering class be increased to qualify for the capitation grants. With national discussions centering around shortening the medical curriculum to three years as well as expanding class sizes, the Faculty Board in February, as part of a broad review of College of Medicine admission policies, increased the English prerequisite to nine hours while agreeing to consider students for admission after three years of college. At this same meeting, the use of faculty-student interview teams for prospective students was implemented, and it was suggested that workshops be held for premedical advisors at various colleges throughout the state.

Additionally, the need to recruit minority students without subjecting them to dual academic standards was emphasized. The Robert Wood Johnson foundation granted $119,000 in scholarship aid for minority students in September 1972. Time would demonstrate that such grants were essential to the recruitment of high-quality minority students to the University of Oklahoma Health Sciences Center. A special project grant from the federal government (directed by Dr. Harris D. Riley, with the help of Dr. Joseph Feretti) was obtained to help in the recruitment of American Indian students. These changes were stimulated by an in-depth report from a committee headed by Dr. Mary Frances Schottstaedt, following an investigation of minority recruitment in the College of Medicine.

At the January regents' meeting, it was determined that temporary quarters must be found to meet the needs of the Dental and Nursing Colleges since their facilities would not be completed in time for scheduled classes, primarily because of a delay in receipt of federal matching funds. To ease the need for space, construction of what was to be known as the Interim Building was begun, a structure just east of the Children's Hospital. Consequently, the Allied Health Professions building, planned but awarded no matching funds, would be reduced in priority in the University's Master Plan and its place taken by the Interim Building. The $800,000 of HERO Bond money earmarked for the Allied Health building would almost exactly fund the total construction of the Interim Building. Although it was planned that upon completion of the Dental and Nursing Buildings, the Interim Building would be used as the first phase of the Allied Health Facility, this was never accomplished. First used by the Department of Psychiatry as an in-patient building, the Interim Building was then used jointly with the Department of Human Services for information management services, and, later, exclusively for the department's computers. In an interview years later, Provost Thurman recalled that Lloyd Rader needed the Interim Building for his computer facility to back up Medicare and Medicaid paperwork:

> They needed a building to house all those big computers and we needed a service center. That was when the University—not DHS—was running everything from the viewpoint of buildings and grounds. We acquired the first floor of Moon Elementary School from the School Board, but had no money to fix it up. . . . There is no doubt that the Moon-Interim Building exchange was one of the better things I did for the campus.[3]

Vice-chancellor Gary Smith later recalled that "We traded the Interim Building to the Department of Human Services in exchange for Lloyd Rader completely gutting and rebuilding the interior of the Moon Building. It seems we also got something in addition—maybe some cash."

On January 18 another problem related to the opening of the College of Dentistry was addressed by the Faculty Board: the provision of basic science education by the basic science faculty. The board recommended that the basic science departments of the College of Medicine be made joint departments in both colleges. On February 10, 1972, the regents approved naming the following departments as "conjoint" departments between Medicine and Dentistry: Anatomical Sciences, Anesthesiology, Biochemistry and Molecular Biology, Community Health (later Family Practice and Community Medicine and Dentistry), Microbiology and Immunology; Pathology, Pharmacology, Physiology and Biophysics, and Psychiatry and Behavioral Sciences.

Family Medicine

In Oklahoma, there was long-standing, strong sentiment for educating all medical students in what later came to be known as "family medicine." Until after World War II, almost all University of Oklahoma graduates usually entered Family Practice either just after their internship or after an additional year of study in Pediatrics, Medicine, or Surgery. In 1947 Dean Everett and the faculty initiated the policy that all medical students would take a *preceptorship* of at least one month's duration, during which there would be assignment to a general practitioner in one of the smaller cities or towns of Oklahoma. Hobart, Pauls Valley, and Durant were prominent and long-standing examples of Oklahoma towns in which preceptorships were taken. The program was assigned to and directed by a Health Sciences Center assistant dean. In the 1970s, many requests were made to substitute other rotations for this service in non-rural or non-family practice. All such requests were rejected by the faculty. The Faculty Board, through the Academic Council, recommended in 1973 that this program be emphasized and strengthened, and when Family Medicine became a full department, the preceptorship program was transferred to it for administrative purposes. A division of Family Medicine was established in 1965 and was placed within the Department of Preventive Medicine and Public Health when none of the existing clinical departments in the College of Medicine was willing to include the program. Dean Dennis, believing that physicians with long experience in the private practice of medicine were essential to the educational program, recruited his old medical school roommate, Dr. Thomas Points, to co-ordinate establishment of family medicine clinics for teaching medical students and to develop outreach programs in family medicine continuing education throughout the state (e.g., the Wakita clinic). Dr. Points also attempted to arrange the education of physicians interested in family practice within clinics of the various specialty departments in the hospital. Without participation in the selection process by Dr. Points, the dean recruited Dr. Roger Lienke in 1966 to head a Family Medicine residency program within the division. Points suffered a coronary occlusion in 1968 and subsequently was no longer actively directing the programs. Dr. Thomas Lynn, appointed to head the Department (a joint operation of both the Colleges of Medicine and Health) in 1968, recalled that "to gain more credibility and support from the legislature, something had to be done with Family Medicine." At his recommendation, and with enthusiastic support of President Sharp and Dr. Lienke, the name of the department was changed to the Department of Family Medicine and Community Health in 1969. In 1972 Dr. Leonard Eliel suggested that "divisional status at the present time isolates and limits Family Medicine," and with the approval of Dr. Lynn, the divisional status was terminated and a separate department created *[RM, 11292]*. Administration of the preceptorship program was transferred to it in 1973. By that time, the Family Medicine residency program, which had begun as a clinic in the hospital in 1969 with three residents, had grown to a ten-resident program, with a probable seventeen new residents to arrive in July 1972 *[DO, 1–23–72]*.

In February, regents accepted the newly completed Mark R. Everett Tower (University Hospital) and approved construction of the Biomedical Sciences building with HERO bond funds and federal grants. The month concluded with enormous shock among the Oklahoma City medical community when it was announced that Dr. Colin M. MacLeod, the new president and scientific director of the Oklahoma Medical Research Foundation, died during a visit to London.

The Budget Crisis

By the spring of 1972, the Health Sciences Center had accumulated a $2.3 million deficit. It was estimated that the move into the new Everett Tower would cost an additional $1 million plus $500,000 per year in additional operating expenses. Furthermore, the federal government had discontinued nearly $1 million per year in training grants and the legislature had mandated numerous new (and unfunded) programs. A programmatic study of the "mission, goals, and objectives of the Health Sciences Center, relating to the health resources of the State of Oklahoma," directed by the regents in March 1971, was received and accepted at the April meeting. Apparently the urgency for the study, seen initially by Interim University President McCarter, was no longer present, since no action was taken by the regents or by President Sharp. Simultaneously, two additional Health Sciences Center evaluations were being undertaken, one by the State Regents, the other at the direction of the governor. Both were initiated in response to the continuing budget crisis exemplified by the $2.3 million deficit in Center operating funds—a crisis resulting from expanding programs and static revenue, especially from the state, and the regents' strong reaction to the crisis *[DO, 4–11–72]*. The findings of the study groups were scheduled for presentation at the end of July 1972. Their recommendations were anxiously awaited because of a regents' resolution, initiated by the regents' Health Sciences Center Committee, presented by Ms. Nancy Davies, and passed on April 13, which stated in part:

As we initiate new programs and enlarge enrollments in the College of Medicine and other colleges, in response to actions and plans of the State Legislature and State Regents, we must rely on increased resources. Although we have presented our needs realistically, these resources have not been forthcoming. Therefore, we propose the following action: (1) Consolidate Children's Memorial Hospital by moving patient care activities to the main University Hospital, and close seventy-eight (78) beds in the hospitals beginning September 15, 1972. (2) Close the University Hospital Emergency Room beginning October 1, 1972. (3) Close other non-paying services in the hospitals on a selective and sequential basis *[RM, 11419]*.

These bold moves by the regents were largely spearheaded by Ms. Davies and Mr. Huston Huffman, who also initiated strong and ongoing contacts with legislative leaders. Additionally, Ms. Davies expressed regret at the loss of nationally known faculty members, who seemed to be leaving the Center in droves. President Sharp said, "The University on both campuses is now losing, and will continue to lose, the finest of its professors whose teaching and research have attracted regional and national attention. This is the price we pay and the erosion of quality that is the consequence of underfinancing" *[RM, 11419]*. Needless to say, these recommendations, especially the proposal to close the Children's Hospital, brought considerable attention to the Center from throughout the state. Dr. Jephtha Dalston, University Hospital administrator, later said, "This proposal met with sharp and immediate adverse reaction by the population of the state and its political leadership, and also precipitated a series of politically based investigations which extended over the ensuing eight months."[4] Governor Hall, opposing closure of the University Hospital Emergency Room, blamed the legislature, which had pared his tax increase program by $42 million. He pointed out that the legislature appropriated only $2.3 million in new funds for twenty institutions. The governor, because of the turmoil on the Oklahoma City campus, announced the appointment of Robert Richardson as an "inspector general" to investigate the Health Sciences Center. Richardson, a professor in the College of Law, spearheaded an investigation into departmental policies and finances which stemmed from a suspicion on the part of some legislators that Health Sciences Center physicians were "pocketing money" from patient care which properly belonged to the University. The investigation led to more than a little anger and hostility in the medical community.

Reacting to Governor Hall's statement as well as to widespread criticism of inadequate legislative funding of the Health Sciences Center, state senator James Hamilton, as usual, responded, "It is a complete subterfuge to tell the public that this facility is not being adequately funded by the legislature" *[DO, 4–19–72]*. He described the crisis as a "so-called financial plight." Said Hamilton, "The crisis simply would not exist if the administration would take steps to properly administer funds that are on hand." In an editorial, the *Daily*

Oklahoman noted that "the Medical Center receives less than half its total operating budget from state-appropriated funds" and "the Center has been given responsibility by the legislature itself for starting several new schools and programs" *[DO,4–20–72]*. The response of both the State Regents, under Chancellor E. T. Dunlap, and the legislature, dominated by Senator Hamilton, was to institute yet more studies of the Health Sciences Center. Compounding the problem was the fact that the legislature, under the leadership of Senator Hamilton, mandated yet another costly program at the Health Sciences Center: the establishment of a College of Medicine branch in Tulsa! Governor Hall blamed legislators for the cutbacks in higher education in general and the Health Sciences Center in particular: "Their names are in the records of the House of Representatives and Senate and should be published on the front pages," he said *[DO, 4–18–72]*. With newly added schools, burgeoning educational programs, and diminished appropriations, the investigations and solutions suggested by the triumvirate of Hall, Hamilton, and Dunlap was all higher education needed!

Lloyd Rader, "The Director"

There was another individual who was to play a more important and far more highly constructive role in Oklahoma medical education than the three men mentioned above. He was Lloyd E. Rader, director of the Department of Human Services, appointed by Governor Johnston Murray on November 12, 1952. Rader was born in Bridgeport, in western Oklahoma, attended what became Southwestern State University in Weatherford, and had operated a small business in Binger, Oklahoma, before going to work as an accountant at the Oklahoma Tax Commission. He was a longtime friend and colleague of former Medical Center Dean Mark Everett. Together, they had served on the Crippled Children's Commission and, after numerous battles, engineered the incorporation of that commission into the Department of Public Welfare, where a continuous and more predictable flow of funds was assured for Children's Hospital (through Senate Bill 20, signed by Governor Howard Edmondson on June 24, 1959). Mr. Rader was to be the principal advocate for Children's Hospital, and later the adult hospital, bringing the immense resources of the Department of Public Welfare to the development of the Health Sciences Center. Bruce Perry, administrator of the University Hospital in the mid 1970s, was amazed that there seemed to be no vocal constituency for the Children's Hospital at this time. Fortunately, Lloyd Rader would provide a constituency that perhaps no other Oklahoman could have matched. In Perry's words, "Lloyd Rader worked for it, he fought for it, and he spent money on it—a lot of money."[5] Rader's work was his life, and he strove incessantly for what he believed to be the good of the people and the state of Oklahoma. He derived his power from the resources of the state welfare department—especially the earmarked two percent state sales tax—and from the love and good will of the people he helped through the years. Fortunately for the Health Sciences Center, Lloyd Rader was totally dedicated to caring for children and for the sick.

Dr. Harris D. "Pete" Riley, chair of Pediatrics at the time, recalled that when the proposed closure of the Children's Hospital was announced, he told Provost Len Eliel: "I think that it is the worst thing that could be done, because every child's care is completely paid for. What happened in those days, money would come into the Children's Hospital program and it would get spread over the entire Center, particularly to the adult [University] hospital. So I went to see Dr. George Garrison, who was, since Dr. Nicholson's death, chairman of the advisory committee to the Department of Human Services. He did not become incensed very often, but he sure was over that proposal. He said, 'I think we should do everything possible to prevent it.'"[6]

Dr. Riley then called Lloyd Rader and arranged to have breakfast early the following morning.

When I told him all about it [the proposed closure], he couldn't believe it. He went back to his office and got on the phone and had Vera [his secretary] call everybody he could get hold of, including his chief lawyer, Harry Johnson. Before the day was over, a letter was sent to Dr. Eliel. Basically, it said, 'You can't do this. It isn't going to happen.' Lloyd warned that cutbacks ordered by the Board of Regents could cost the Medical Center millions of dollars in state and federal funds and suggested that federal law might prohibit the proposed closings. Nothing happened, except increased funding for the Children's Hospital by the Department of Human Services.[7]

The state of Oklahoma seemed, in these years, always on the verge of bankruptcy. The 1972–1973 budget crisis was complicated by: (1) continued controversy over the proportion of "new" funds available to the State Regents which were reallocated to the University of Oklahoma campuses; (2) mandated increases in federal Social Security and income tax withholding on payrolls; (3) and the unacceptability of the current extremely low wage scale for entry-level workers. There was also a fear that the new appropriations might not be distributed to higher educational institutions on a percentile basis similar to the past—i.e., the high end of the 16.5–22 percent of total higher education appropriations traditionally devolving to the Health Sciences Center. There was fear that the appropriation to the State Regents for Higher Education might adopt a different formula, a more politically popular one which would favor the small, non-research colleges and junior colleges. Finally, the completion of construction of the many new buildings at the Center would inevitably lead to even higher operating costs and a greater financial crisis.

In May, the State Regents, in a document called "Resolution 800," launched a "thorough study of the financial needs of the OU Medical Center and an inventory of the functions and educational programs operated therein, with the view of establishing a level of financial support which must be provided if the institution is to operate its programs at a quality level expected by the people" *[RM, 11471]*. July 1, 1972, was selected as the due date for completion of this study. A similar study had also been mandated by the legislature several months earlier.

On a happier mid-year note, the University Hospital Board, the Health Sciences Center administration, and the president of the University recommended that: "the new University Hospital building be named the 'Mark R. Everett Tower,' to honor Mark R. Everett, Dean Emeritus of the College of Medicine and the first Director of the Medical Center. The concept and plans for the new University Hospital took shape while Dr. Everett was Dean, and the first state bond issue in support of the hospital was also passed prior to his retirement from office. Dr. Everett has made a lasting contribution to our campus and is most deserving of this tribute" *[RM, 11430; DO, 4–16–72]*.

At this same time in May, the pending construction of the $1.3 million Dean A. McGee Eye Institute was announced at a luncheon of two hundred civic and business leaders in Oklahoma City. An address was given by former professor of surgery and Associate Dean Merlin K. DuVal, now the United States assistant secretary of HEW for health and scientific affairs *[DO, 4–22–72]*. May also witnessed a group of resident physicians alleging that conditions at University Hospital had deteriorated to the point that they were forced "to follow unacceptable medical practices." They feared that "political moves to keep the hospital from closing Children's Memorial Hospital and emergency room services will cause further funding shortages, which could make it impossible to care properly for patients or maintain accreditation in some areas." Dermatologist Raymond Cornelison stated that, "Lighting is so poor in some areas that I am unable to see the patient's skin." He continued, "We [the College of Medicine] came from a second-rate school in the 1950s and became a first-rate school. What we're afraid of is we are losing everything that was gained" *[DO, 5–21–72]*. Dr. Cornelison would later become president of the Oklahoma County Medical Association and then Secretary of the Oklahoma State Medical Association.

A grass roots movement in Seminole, Oklahoma, in June raised $42,000 to assist the Health Sciences Center and "show the state legislature that citizens across the state are in support of finding better methods of financing health care" *[DO, 6–8–72]*. In an editorial several weeks later, the *Daily Oklahoman* stated that the legislature not only short-changed the Center some $5 million, but also "diverted an appropriation of $100,000 to a non-existent college of medicine in Tulsa," urging Governor Hall to "make good" on his promise to "beef up facilities at OU and OSU, and up-grade graduate facilities" *[DO, 6–25–72]*. At the end of June, the regents approved a "shortfall, standstill" education and general budget for the Center, over the opposition of regent Bob G. Mitchell. The services that would have to be cut at the Center were to be decided after the State Regents' and the legislative studies became available.

Faculty Practice Income and the "Practice Plan"

In July 1972 Provost Leonard Eliel announced that the administrative reorganization of the Health Sciences Center was complete, saying: "It was apparent last year . . . that the Health Sciences Center was in need of administrative reorganization because its management techniques were outdated and no longer appropriate to an institution which was enlarging and growing so rapidly, and which had become so complex. We recognized that there was no central fiscal control. After a search, Mr. Gerald Gillman was named Director of Administrative Affairs, and Mr. Tom Tucker was hired as the Health Sciences Center's first full-time University counsel" *[RM, 11590]*.

Later, Dr. Eliel would say, "We can document these needs to the University regents, the State Regents, and the state legislature. . . . Within one office we will be able to have complete accountability, responsibility and visibility pertaining to all of our funds" *[RM, 11590–91]*. The key phrase consisted of the last four words, which suggested that any income earned by the faculty would now be recorded for public scrutiny. Concluded Dr. Eliel: "The Medical Center Physicians' Trust, which, because of its complexity, has been difficult to understand and a source of a great deal of misunderstanding, you might say, will be reorganized into a practice plan which will provide centralized accountability and complete visibility of its resources. We expect to have this reorganization complete by October 1" *[RM, 11590–91]*.

Throughout the current financial crisis, the increasing dependence of the Health Sciences Center budget on the flow of faculty practice funds was almost never publicly recognized. There was muttering and rampant rumor-mongering about the private income of faculty physicians, including sugges-tions that the majority of these funds were not flowing through the University system but were being put to private use by the physicians. Dr. William Thurman recalls, "When I was interviewed for the position [of provost], I was told that over half of the faculty were pocketing the patient money."[8] There was no acknowledgment of the large percentage of this pool of money being spent by the faculty on University facilities and activities. For example, the faculty provided funds for underwriting such new construction projects as the Dermatology building (built in 1969–1970 with $250,000 of faculty money); the Radiological Sciences Addition (built in 1969 with $290,000 of faculty income); and the entire Steam and Chilled Water Plant. Dr. Gordon Deckert, chair of Psychiatry, who was the last faculty-elected chief of staff of Univer-sity Hospital under University of Oklahoma management (1970–72), later commented on the phenomenon of faculty members providing personal income to construct buildings for the benefit and permanent use of the Health Sciences Center: "I can't imagine that happening now; it was such a phenom-enal thing. I remember [Leonard] Eliel calling us all together, saying, 'The only way we can get that water and power plant is for us to put it together, underwrite it with faculty practice income.' And we agreed to do that. Can you imagine the current [1997] group of chairmen agreeing to that, or even thinking about doing that?"[9]

Gordon Deckert was born in a Mennonite community in South Dakota in 1930. A 1955 graduate of Northwestern University Medical School, he had completed his training in psychiatry at Oklahoma in 1962. He served as chair of the Psychiatry Department from 1969 to 1987, succeeding nationally prominent L. J. "Jolly" West, who had been the first full-time head of the department from 1954 to1969. Deckert was chief of staff of University Hos-pital from 1970–1972. Throughout the 1970s and 1980s he played a vocal, constructive, and prominent role in the academic, political, and fiscal affairs of the hospitals and the College. He was a "process" man, as opposed to his predecessor, Dr. West, whom he considered an "innovator." Together with Drs. Schilling, Merrill, Everett and, later, Williams and McKee, he was one of the chief Health Sciences Center leaders for over two decades.

The Professional Practice Plan

Two factors led to the developing pressure on the Center to implement, under the auspices of the University of Oklahoma, a Professional Practice Plan that would control and account for all private faculty income. First, there was an increasing need for supplemental funds, as state appropriations did not keep up with operational costs for new programs and facilities, especially as federal subsidies were declining; and secondly, the faculty practice funds were not visible to the money men at the State Regents and in the legislature. As early as April 1963, state Senator Louis Ritzhaupt of Guthrie, a habitual critic of the College of Medicine, had asked the State Examiner and Inspector to make a complete audit of the school because "the department of welfare paid $1 million to the school for medical care . . . and about $500,000 of this was deposited in a special fund which," he understood, "was to be spent at the discretion of doctors." He said that he wanted an audit to determine how the money was spent *[DO, 4–5–63]*. At this point in history, practice funds were typically deposited into the Physicians' Trust Account at the Oklahoma Medical Research Foundation, and from there dispensed for departmental operations, supplementation of faculty income, and general improvements at the Center. The focus on outside control of faculty income was a source of great irritation to the faculty, which, by and large, had felt that income from their practice was primarily benefitting the Center rather than themselves.

Throughout the summer and autumn of 1972, the Faculty Board struggled to develop a Practice Plan acceptable to State Regents, the legislature, the University of Oklahoma Regents, and the Health Sciences Center faculty. A first draft of a plan was made by a committee consisting of Dr. Schilling and Dr. Merrill, in conjunction with F. C. Love, formerly an attorney for the Kerr McGee Corporation. A proposal was presented to the Faculty Board in early September. Criticism of the proposal was exemplified by the memorandum of Dr. Ronald Elkins, professor of Surgery, written to his chair, Dr. Schilling. He emphasized that the control proposed would actually discourage, not support, clinical practice by faculty; and that the plan in no way indicated how an environment conducive to high quality clinical practice was to be developed. He objected to the use of faculty income to "enrich" the ability of the dean of the College of Medicine to assist developing programs, believing that assuring an adequate income for faculty members and fostering the development of needed programs was a duty of the dean and the administration and not the responsibility of the clinical faculty. He further predicted, correctly as it turned out, that the proposed 10 percent tax for billing and collecting would inevitably grow, and with it the accompanying additional large bureaucracy, without in any way improving the collection rate or enhancing the interface with patients. The concept that clinical departments should earn, through clinical income, the funds to pay all departmental overhead he considered to be likewise an abdication of responsibility on the part of the administration. The suggestion that clinical faculty should earn all or even part of their base University salary was also opposed. He concluded, "Dr. Schilling, I am deeply opposed to this present plan. I am opposed to the philosophy of the plan, which primarily consists of how to divide up the income earned by faculty members (in private practice). There is no approach suggesting that serious thought has been given to efforts to improve our clinical setting and our ability to practice medicine. As long as the major intent of the plan is how to divide the funds earned by the faculty so that various individuals who in no way contribute to the earning of this fund get their share, I am unalterably opposed" *[FBM, 9–14–72]*.

On November 17, Provost Eliel met with the Health Sciences Center Trust Fund administrators (chairs of the clinical departments and divisions who collectively supervised all private patient income that was deposited in an Oklahoma Medical Research Foundation account) to explain why he had placed a moratorium on the expenditure of departmental trust funds, and to address rumors that departmental trust funds were in imminent danger of being seized by the administration to offset the deficits which increasingly threatened the Health Sciences Center. Dr. Eliel said he had been informed that the departments were not entitled to the trust fund money and that neither he nor anyone else in the room had legal access to it, except for the (dean's) enrichment funds. The provost also discussed the critical situation regarding the proposed opening of Everett Tower, the fact that the Center was operating without a budget, the various investigations in progress, and his plans to meet on a daily "crisis" basis with Dr. Deckert (chief of staff at University Hospital), the three deans, and the Center's consultant, John Dumas.[10]

"Site of Practice" Policy

A second source of irritation to the Health Sciences Center faculty was increasing emphasis on a "Site of Practice" policy, which obligated faculty physicians to place their private patients in campus hospitals—i.e. University, Children's, the Veteran's Administration Hospital, and the small hospital which was then operated in the Oklahoma Medical Research Foundation. This policy was implicit in the Medical College by-laws of 1971 which required that full-time faculty "center all patient care in the University of Oklahoma Health Sciences Center, including, if appropriate, those affiliated hospitals and clinics where part of the academic program of the University is conducted. Faculty members may not render patient care on a continuing basis elsewhere."[11] Many of the faculty believed that this restriction limited their ability to render quality care. This belief was supported, tangentially, by a consultant report from Baldwin G. Lamson, M.D., Director of Hospitals and Clinics at the University of California at Los Angeles. Initiated by Dr. Eliel, Lamson's study of the Oklahoma Medical Center had one major recommendation: "I advise you to do everything in your power to avoid curtailment at this juncture, and to take the first steps toward building the Center's capacity to provide medical services to the private sector. Although locally there is an image associated with indigent patient care, hopefully, with the opening of the new facility [Everett Tower], this image will be quickly altered, although time will be required to develop the full reputation of the Center at a local level comparable to that already enjoyed on a national basis."[12]

From April 1972 until November 1973, the Faculty Board struggled over a written Site of Practice policy which would be acceptable to faculty critics as well as to the regents, and yet one that would have sufficient flexibility to permit patients to be treated in other institutions when it was to their medical advantage. Wording that specifically outlined the procedure for exceptions to the general policy was initially developed by a committee of Drs. Schilling, Everett, and Deckert, approved by the regents in March, restudied, and again approved and forwarded to the regents by the Faculty Board on October 17, 1973. The issue was revisited in September 1974 as the move of Presbyterian Hospital to the Health Sciences Center campus became imminent. Programmatic exceptions to the policy were recognized, and the Faculty Board strongly recommended relaxing the requirement that all patients in the 15–21 year age group be hospitalized at Children's Hospital. This was especially indicated in the case of gynecology and obstetrics patients *[FBM, 9–18–74]*.

In August, surgical nurses at the Health Sciences Center threatened to resign unless certain expectations were met, including salary increases. Regents expressed regret at their inability to increase salaries, saying that increases were justified and deserved, but deferred any action pending reports from the State Regents and the Governor's Study Committees. The nurses stated that they would defer any action until September. The recommendations made the preceding April regarding closure and/or consolidations of the Center's hospitals were likewise deferred until September.

Several other less pressing matters also received regents' attention in August. For the coming academic year space was rented at a variety of Oklahoma City locations for Nursing, Dentistry, and the executive vice president's staff from the Oklahoma Health Science Facility, Inc. Approval was granted for the sale of $2,100,000 of Health Sciences Center parking facility bonds by the Central Oklahoma Transportation and Parking Authority. And construction of the new Presbyterian Hospital at Northeast 13th and Lincoln Boulevard was begun late in August.

In September, Dr. James B. Snow Jr., chair of Otorhinolaryngology and nationally known faculty member at the Health Sciences Center, resigned to take a similar position at the prestigious Pennsylvania University Hospital in Philadelphia. Many faculty resignations during this period were due to Center under funding, the public suspicion surrounding faculty practice funds and their use, and the imposition of the new faculty Practice Plan.

Also in September, the College of Medicine enrolled its largest class in history with one hundred forty-eight students. Of this total, twenty-six were women, a record number to this point. At the same time, the College of Dentistry announced the formation of its inaugural class with the enrollment of twenty-four dental students.

The increasing dependence of the Health Sciences Center budget upon the generosity of the Department of Institutions, Social and Rehabilitative Services (DISRS), and its director Lloyd Rader, was attested to by the fact that at the September regents' meeting, "Mr. Lloyd Rader has arranged to fund previously unreimbursed services in the University Hospitals. . . ." *[RM, 11650]*. Simultaneously, Senator Henry Bellmon's office announced the award of $15 million in federal construction funds for clinical sciences and biomedical science buildings for the Colleges of Medicine and Dentistry.

Later in September, Provost Eliel stated, "I am recommending to the Regents today that the previous request to consolidate and curtail services [at the Center's hospitals] be withdrawn" *[RM, 11650]*. In a not-unrelated matter, Eliel announced that a study of Children's and University Hospitals was underway, the purpose of which was to develop a "specific proposal within the next two months for reorganization of the hospitals." Dr. Eliel continued: "We would like to emphasize that reorganization . . . is to be accomplished within the framework of the University and under its Regents. There is not a quality medical school in the country that does not have its own teaching hospital. To remove the hospitals from the University, as some have suggested . . . would lead to their demise as first class patient care and teaching institutions; the academic units which depend on the hospitals as training laboratories would soon follow in the inevitable decline" *[RM, 11651]*.

The State Regents' report on the "Financial Needs of the Health Sciences Center" was presented to the University of Oklahoma Board of Regents in July, but no discussion of it was recorded in either the July or September minutes! The minutes did, however, reflect that yet another prominent faculty member had tendered a resignation, this time Dr. Eleanor Knudson, dean of the Nursing School.

In September, Dr. Thomas Acers was named professor and head of the Department of Ophthalmology. In addition, the Central Oklahoma Parking and Transportation Authority bond issue for a parking structure was canceled because "it would not be feasible for the University to participate in this project" *[RM, 11679]*. A scaled-down surface parking lot for 750 cars was approved "subject to the availability of funds from reserve accounts on the Norman Campus," a project that presumably would be financed again from faculty practice income [RM, 11680].

At the request of President Sharp, the regents in September "assigned to one office the responsibility and authority for all activities involving our relationships with the public generally and particularly the groups which have a special interest in the University's well being and continued progress" *[RM, 11684]*. This action was thought to mean that Health Sciences Center faculty were to keep hands off donors who might give to the overall University and let vice-president John Dean do it! (John Dean was a University vice-president and former banker, among whose duties was major fund raising.) The concept that certain affluent donors—whether individual or institutional—should be within the purview of senior administrators only, and should never be approached by mere faculty, was a cardinal principal of fund raising at the University at this time. Thus, organizations such as the Kerr Foundation or the Noble Foundation could not be solicited by individual faculty members or departments.

The regents' Health Center Committee, under chair of Huston Huffman, held their first monthly meeting in the new Everett Tower in November. At this meeting, Ron Martin, president of the Student Council, "expressed the general feeling of frustration because nothing had been done in four or five years [about student housing], although there had been much conversation" *[RM, 11791]*. Mr. Huffman explained that the regents needed legislative action in order to handle the financing for student housing. As recently as April, regents had approved an item on their agenda that specified an October 9 construction date for student housing on the Health Center campus—a project that would not see the light of day.

A graduate program awarding a Master of Science degree in Nursing was approved in November. In addition, the first sharing agreement with the Veterans Administration Hospital was sanctioned. By this agreement services available at one hospital were shared with other hospitals on a contractual basis. Sharing allowed joint utilization of services by institutions, with reimbursement of the providing institution by the receiving one. Many laboratory and radiologic services would eventually be provided more extensively and at less cost as a result of this agreement.

Also in November, a Bachelor of Science program in Occupational Therapy was approved for the School of Health Related Professions, upon receipt of a five-year HEW special grant for this purpose. The month also witnessed the continuing saga of faculty and staff departures. Valued hospital administrators Ed Schwartz and Robert Terrill left the University for other prestigious schools, as did dermatologist Julian Swann.

The long anticipated "Proposed Practice Plan for Geographic Full-Time Faculty of the College of Medicine" was presented in December. The essential elements of the plan were: (1) all full-time faculty were required to participate in the Practice Plan; (2) all professional income must be deposited to University accounts and be "contractually controlled" by the University, which would specify processes for billing, collecting, etc.; (3) each participant in the plan would have a written contract with the regents each year; and (4) "full implementation of the plan must be accomplished in phases to insure cooperation of all participants and preserve the current level of contributions to the H. C. from professional practice earnings" *[RM, 11842–11845]*. Dr. Merrill recalled that Dr. Elkins, in spite of the contrary view of his chair, Dr. Schilling, fought successfully to omit a section limiting the amount of time which could be spent in private practice. Additionally, it was decided that practice income would not be paid as part of the University salary, but as a supplement to the physician, without withholding tax, and as "schedule C" rather than salary income. Merrill thought that "the removal of the time restriction related to the high percent of billing for supervised care, rather than for genuine private practice."[13] It was estimated that, under the supervision of Herman Smith Associates, it would take 90–120 days to set up the billing office specified in the plan and accomplish contracts with each faculty member. Regents Braly and Mitchell urged prompt approval and implementation of the plan.

A busy 1972 concluded with agreements with the State Health Department for joint operation of the Child Study Center and for participation of resident training in Surgery, Internal Medicine, and Radiology at Griffin Memorial Hospital in Norman. The latter agreement initiated what would be a long association of the two agencies in the provision of care and training of residents at Griffin. Also in December, regents endorsed "the right of college and university students to listen to anyone whom they wish to hear, . . . and any person who is presented by a recognized student or faculty organization should be allowed to speak" on the campus. Simultaneously, "all members of the academic community must respect the dignity of others. The expression of dissent . . . may not be carried out in ways which injure individuals or damage institutional facilities or disrupt classes. Speakers on campus must . . . be protected from violence . . . and must be given an opportunity to be heard" *[RM, 11860]*. Finally in December, an Affirmative Action plan and Equal Employment Opportunity program were initiated for the University.

Milestones for 1972 at the Health Sciences Center included: completion of the new Everett Tower of University Hospital, opening of the College of Dentistry, expansion of the College of Nursing with a new graduate program, beginning construction of the Presbyterian Hospital, announcement of the formation of the Dean A. McGee Eye Foundation, an increase in class size for the College of Medicine, and the beginning of the end for a Professional Practice Plan controlled by individual members of the medical college faculty—although the reason for initiation of the plan in the first place (inadequate state funding) was not yet publically addressed. Finally, perhaps the single item of greatest future impact on the Health Sciences Center resulted from the creation, by legislative action, of two new medical institutions in Tulsa.

1973

The Tulsa Connection

In March 1972 the legislature passed two bills permanently changing the medical education landscape of the state by mandating the establishment of the Oklahoma College of Osteopathic Medicine and Surgery (Senate Bill 461) in Tulsa and establishing a Tulsa branch of the University of Oklahoma College of Medicine for the final two years of clinical work (Senate Bill 453). Employing their typical fiscal wizardry, the legislature expected all of this to be accomplished without appropriate state funding for either the Oklahoma City campus or the newly mandated Tulsa institutions. This resulted in a severe financial crisis on the Health Sciences Center campus. For more than twelve months, the chaos and fiscal shortcomings on the Oklahoma City campus were complicated by continuing debate on how the University could find funds for two "nonexistent Tulsa schools," as the *Daily Oklahoman* put it, while at the same time dealing with the mounting debt in Oklahoma City.

Senate Bill 453 established the Tulsa College of Medicine and mandated the position of "resident dean" as the chief executive officer of the operation. This action, in spite of the lack of support by the University of Oklahoma, its College of Medicine, and the University of Oklahoma Board of Regents, resulted from agitation for the establishment of a College of Medicine in Tulsa by the Tulsa Medical Education Foundation. The groundswell of pressure on the legislature was led by Dr. Wendell Smith, the administrators of the three Tulsa hospitals, as well as by physicians practicing in Tulsa, many of whom feared the probable influence of the newly instituted College of Osteopathic Medicine in their city. The State Regents for Higher Education, although aware of the movement in the legislature, did not oppose the bill.

Tulsa Regent Julian Rothbaum felt that the real power behind the establishment of a Tulsa branch was state Senator Finis Smith, a parochial eastern Oklahoma legislator who later became President Pro Tempore: "He [Smith] simply had enough power to get it located over here. That's all there was to it. He did it for Tulsa economic reasons. Finis had enough political clout to get it here, in spite of all the medical education experts saying all these things needed to be in one spot. After it got over here, and started creating jobs and taking care of indigent people—making a contribution to the people—then it got support of the Chamber of Commerce and all the power structure in Tulsa."[14]

Dr. William Thurman would later recall:

There was a running argument about whether to put in a Tulsa College of Medicine. A lot of people were opposed to it. It was never clear why the regents were so polarized. At one point they withdrew the application [for construction funds]. Tom Brett, a regent from Tulsa, said: 'Wait a minute, this is not an issue; we have a state law that says we're going to do it.' On the other side, the regents said we can control the speed of development of the Tulsa Medical College as it relates to funding, and control the relationship to this campus. It was pointed out during that discussion that the chairs here would also be the chairs there, with the associate chairs appointed over there. However, some Tulsa people wanted just the opposite: the head of surgery over there wanted to be chairman of Surgery [for the entire College of Medicine]. Rainey [Williams, chairman of Surgery] did his best to be accommodating—to let the Tulsa chairman feel independent, etc. But the guy asked Rainey to stop coming over to do grand rounds! This was the kind of problem that surfaced over the regents' decision.[15]

In spite of the regents' perception of how the Tulsa branch would develop, it was quite clear that until the summer of 1974, following a critical site visit by the Liaison Committee on Graduate Medical Education, the faculty and administration at Tulsa, as well as many senators and representatives in the legislature, believed that they had established an independent institution—a free-standing College of Medicine offering years three and four of a curriculum leading to the degree of Doctor of Medicine. Once again, the Oklahoma legislature ignored fiscal reality and showed that the path for accreditation of schools of medicine was just as political as legislating new institutions of higher education in Oklahoma.

The debate over the Tulsa medical facilities proceeded full speed into 1973. By March, legislative leaders felt that there would be enough money available to solve the Health Sciences Center crisis and, at the same time, launch the Tulsa College of Medicine and Osteopathic School. While reluctant to fund the new institutions entirely out of the state's general fund, the legislature hoped that federal grants (Representative Willis' theory) or bond issue money (Senator Hamilton's theory) would become available *[DO, 3–9–73]*.

A preview of the Herman Smith Study of the Health Sciences Center hospitals was provided to key members of the University administration, the governor's office, and the legislature in February. Senator Phil Smalley of Norman said the review indicated that the legislature should take "a hard new look at priorities" in view of comments from Jack Dumas, leader of the Herman Smith team. Smalley said that the Tulsa Osteopathic School training project and the Tulsa College of Medicine should be included in the reevaluation, but Senator James Hamilton of Poteau (the senate president pro tempore), Representative William P. Willis of Talequah (speaker of the house), and Senator Finis Smith of Tulsa (former senate president pro tempore) favored going ahead with the Tulsa medical plans independently of any problems or needs on the Oklahoma City campus. This example of Oklahoma "politics as usual" was largely attributable to the fact that legislators from eastern Oklahoma felt that money appropriated for indigent care at the University hospitals primarily benefitted Oklahoma County, and that there was no state subsidy, directly or through educational funds, for indigent care in Tulsa *[DO, 2–15–73]*.

In spite of the fiscal crisis and lack of financial support, higher regents Chancellor E. T. Dunlap on February 26 requested the "we proceed with the implementation of the plans for the College of Medicine in Tulsa in accordance with Senate Bill 453 of the 1972 legislature" *[RM, 12002]*. President Sharp said, "This new College must be subject to the receipt of sufficient funds to establish and operate the program," adding that he "does not recommend commencement of this branch of its future operation will be at the expense of vital programs at the existing Health Sciences Center" *[RM, 12003]*. The *Daily Oklahoman*, in an editorial on March 14 stated that "Establishment of medical and osteopathic training facilities in Tulsa seems a long way from reality, given the present uncertain availability of financing" and the estimated $2.8 million and $1 million annual operating costs at the Tulsa Medical and Osteopathic Schools, respectively *[DO, 3–14–73]*. This judgment clearly did not take into account the legislative habit of instituting programs without providing operating funds for them. A Policy Statement proposed by the Chancellor envisioned the granting of a degree in Human Medicine by the College of Clinical Medicine in Tulsa *[RM, 12004]*. Applicants to the College of Medicine were to declare their intention to matriculate to the Tulsa branch at the time of application, in effect mandating a dual pathway for admissions.

Much of the "Tulsa problem" was due to factors other than the important point that two schools were not needed to satisfy the medical staffing needs for Oklahoma; nor was there enough money being appropriated to run even one school effectively. The lack of consensus among the University regents, as well as constant opinion changes by one or two regents, magnified the problem. This acrimony lasted much longer than necessary. According to Dr. Thurman, "a lot of feelings were hurt and a lot of damage was created for the Medical College among the Tulsa community's perception of what was going on. It took a long time to overcome."[15] State Senator George Miller summed up the Tulsa issue when he said, "Although the legislature cannot justify a Tulsa medical facility from a fiscal point of view, with the political situation being what it is, the train is fired up and going full throttle in this direction" *[RM, 11929]*.

Meanwhile, the Oklahoma City campus was experiencing a pleasant infusion of money from a source that provided, for a number of years, the deepest of deep pockets. The first of many large expenditures on Children's Hospital by Lloyd Rader and the Department of Institutions, Social and Rehabilitative Services (DISRS) was undertaken in January. A memorandum agreement between the regents and DISRS provided that the Department would pay for remodeling and equipment of "surgical suites, intensive care units, recovery rooms and related areas" at a cost of $350,000, to be paid by the Department and to be jointly overseen by the University and the Department

[RM, 11911]. The architectural firm of Hudgins, Tompkins, and Ball was named as supervisory architects.

A senate committee consisting of Senators Hamilton, Miller, and Richard Stansberry was formed to study the feasibility of creating a nonprofit governmental corporation to operate the University hospitals and to make other recommendations. The committee urged President Sharp and Vice President John Dean to present their recommendations promptly in order to permit action in the current legislative session. Sharp indicated that specific recommendations would follow receipt of the Herman Smith Associates' report.

Although Children's Hospital had found a patron saint in Lloyd Rader, funding shortages continued to bedevil the Medical Center on other fronts. The program in Family Practice at the small community of Wakita, Oklahoma, had been an early effort at outreach to rural Oklahoma, but the 1969 agreement with the Wakita Community Health Center, whereby the University's Board of Regents agreed to assume responsibility for three years' duty as the governing body of the facility, proved to be a costly one for the Health Sciences Center and University budget. In November 1972 President Sharp said that the project must be discontinued by July 1, 1973, unless "it can be made fiscally sound" *[RM, 11796–11798]*. At their March meeting, the regents tabled a request for the approval of educational programs at the Wakita Family Practice facility because: (1) it was being illegally operated out of revolving fund income for capital improvements; (2) the consent of the State Regents would imply a retrospective approval of previous illegal acts; and (3) the cost return factor was "too high" *[RM, 11929]*. President Sharp "called attention to the fact that appropriated state funds (E&G funds) have been used to liquidate a capital investment on this facility, and this should not have been done" *[RM, 11937]*. He said the only question to consider for the program was the termination date. The entire program was terminated in February by a vote of 5 to 2, with regents Neustadt and Brett dissenting. This action occurred in spite of an impassioned plea from Wakita representatives, including John Day Williams, president of the local bank. Termination effective June 30 was confirmed by the State Regents on March 29.

The "Richardson Report," the Hospitals, and Physician Income

Beginning in October 1972, a task force directed by Robert E. Lee Richardson, a University of Oklahoma law professor appointed as an "inspector general" by Governor David Hall, had undertaken an investigation of the Health Sciences

Center at the request of the legislature and the governor. Dr. William Thurman recalled that the genesis of this effort was Senator Gene Howard, who felt strongly that something was very wrong on the campus, probably related to physician's billing for patient care, and that "something needed to be done." Said Thurman: "The moment legislators heard that some physicians on the campus were charging patients and putting the money into private bank accounts, they assumed that everybody was doing it and that it must be illegal. In all honesty, when you look back on the budget situation then [1972], it was more that we didn't get the NIH funding we expected than the [low] level of state funding. The latter did not go down then; it just stayed the same. The NIH funding just went POOF! Everybody lost it; not just OU."[16]

Raymond Crews, the Center's operations director, told Dr. Thurman that "over 90 percent of the practice money came back to the University, with a mere 10 percent going to the people who generated it."[17] All private practice income was deposited in the Physicians' Trust Fund account at the Oklahoma Medical Research Foundation, the directors of which were the chairs of the clinical departments. Robert E. Lee Richardson conducted his investigation in a hostile and intrusive manner, alienating most of the faculty, and sought to uncover wrong-doing rather than analyze problems. The source of Richardson's animosity to the Center was never understood, although some conjectured that he was hostile because Medical College faculty members usually earned considerably more money than did he and his fellow professors in Norman.

In November, Provost Eliel charged that "the governor's task force probe of the Medical Center is using gestapo tactics and disrupting the morale of medical center employees" *[DO, 11–16–72]*. Needless to say, this claim focused even more media attention on what was happening at the hospitals. Richardson's report, presented in late January 1973: (1) emphasized the failure of the Health Sciences Center administration (i.e., Dr. Eliel and Dr. Bird) to answer twenty-four questions asked by the task force; (2) indicated that financial problems are "minimal compared to those which will occur in future years"; (3) severely criticized financial and management practices at the Center, including individuals on the payroll who were "not working for the state," including Dr. Wilson D. Steen, who directed Oklahoma Health Sciences Facilities, Inc. while serving as acting head of the Department of Family Practice and Community Medicine and Dentistry, and also Oklahoma Health Center President Robert C. Hardy; (4) commented adversely upon rental of space for the Nursing School from employees of the Governor's office and the State Tax Commission; (5) faulted the "very high accounts receivable" in the

University Hospital budget; and (6) indicated that the Oklahoma City medical community was rapidly approaching a bed surplus. The report did not identify indigent care as a major contributor to deficits, although "most experts have long recognized it as a major source of financial trouble at the center" [*DO, 2–1–73*].

The reaction of Governor David Hall to the Richardson Report was typical of his approach to all problems in higher education—i.e., that "There are some bad facts, some problems of management, of the handling of funds. This legislature and this administration are going to have an accounting of how the tax dollars are spent and see that they are spent in the best way for the health care of the people. I am thankful that this problem didn't start in my administration" [*DO, 1–31–73*]. Governor Hall clearly was concerned more with accounting for Health Science Center funds than he was with accounting for his own income, given his continuing widely publicized fiscal problems with the U. S. Internal Revenue Service.

Even University administrators shied away from the Richardson task force's attack. Vice president Eliel noted that "Governor Hall said Tuesday he had inherited the financial troubles of the Center when he became Governor two years ago." Eliel pointed out that both he and President Paul F. Sharp took over their present jobs after Hall became Governor" [*DO, 2–1–73*]. State Senator Phil Watson said he "was disappointed with the thirty page report" from Richardson, and believed that "it stirred emotions that didn't need to be stirred at this time" [*DO, 2–2–73*]. He said he was looking forward to the Herman Smith Associates report, which he hoped would suggest solutions as well as delineate problems. Watson then asked Dr. Eliel if there "were any conflict between him and Dr. Robert Bird, Dean of the College of Medicine, who is on a one month's leave?" He further said that Governor Hall's televised speech "was made in a negative vein so far as the problem was concerned" [*DO, 2–2–73*]. The supporters of the Richardson findings thought that Dean Bird was the principal villain in the financial accountability controversy and that Dr. Eliel was protecting him. Bird was accused of shielding the faculty who were opposed to full implementation of the practice plan. The Health Sciences Center Student Association presented a resolution urging Dean Bird's return from leave at the earliest possible date.

According to Dr. Ronald Elkins, Bird was basically fired as a result of protecting faculty interests, while ironically, Dean Lynn was later praised for having done the same—i.e., protecting faculty members. Elkins recalled that at the height of the Site of Practice controversy, "Someone reported that I had performed an operation at Presbyterian Hospital. Dr. Bird told me that I could not do that again. I replied that if the occasion arose, I would do it again if it was in the best medical interest of my patient, and accordingly, you should fire me. Dean Bird walked over to the sink and drank an entire bottle of Malox!"[18] Little did Dr. Elkins realize that his statement had precipitated an angina attack!

An analysis by the *Daily Oklahoman* found that the Richardson report listed "30 solid pages of things wrong with the Center but did not make a single recommendation about putting things right" *[DO, 2–1–73]*. Only on March 15 did the *Oklahoman* learn that the task force had recommended razing the old University Hospital and had "pooh-poohed" the role of indigent care in the fiscal crisis *[DO, 3–16–73]*. The turmoil surrounding the Richardson report stemmed from legislative hostility to the Health Sciences Center and, especially, the suspicion that faculty physicians were "pocketing money right and left" *[DO, 3–16–73]*, primarily, it was thought, through the mechanisms of the Oklahoma Health Sciences Facilities Inc. and the Physicians' Trust Fund at the Oklahoma Medical Research Foundation. A consequence of the report was an atmosphere of fear and rejection engendered in medical faculty by the actions and statements of the governor and legislators (especially some vitriolic members of the senate). In addition, there was an aura of fiscal crisis at the Center stemming primarily from the fact that the legislature and the State Regents, following their usual practices, mandated too many medical services while providing too little money with which to provide them. The Center's adult hospital was requiring increased appropriations primarily due to deficits resulting from unsubsidized indigent care, the coming on line of newly constructed buildings for which no operational funds had been provided, and, according to Dr. Thurman, the slowing flow of federal subsidies for medical education.[19] About this time, the provost was notified that although the funds for the College of Health building had been approved in Washington, President Nixon had sequestered all of the money earmarked for health facility construction in the country. This would prove a further blow to campus expansion.

Because of the ensuing squeeze on the Health Sciences Center budget, legislators cast a covetous eye on funds generated via the faculty Practice Plan. Senator George Miller made clear to the State Regents that he believed that: (1) the Hamilton Bill (Senate Bill 113) did not require the deposit of revolving funds with the state; (2) "definitely the legislature was not on a witch hunt with regard to the inquiries that are being made into operations at the Health Sciences Center"; (3) the regents and the administration are candidly and actively cooperating with state officials and the legislature in an effort to solve the problem and find solutions; (4) very serious reservations exist about the use of revenue sharing funds for continuing operations, and this should be studied very carefully before the State Regents recommend such an employment of funds; (5) unequivocally, the Health Center cannot continue to operate the hospitals for indigent care out of educational funds; and (6) "although the legislature cannot possibly justify the Tulsa operation, nonetheless it is a political reality" *[RM, 11929]*.

At this same time in February, three hundred students on the University campus signed a petition to Regent Huffman commending the physicians in the Center for "voluntarily and generously contributing their incomes to the support of the H. C." The petition also stated that "the State Legislature has continually failed to meet their clear public responsibility to assist in providing health care to Oklahoma's growing numbers of medically indigent population" and urged that the other Oklahoma hospitals begin sharing the burden of indigent care, "which they had conspicuously failed to do" *[DO, 2–10–73]*.

Dean Robert Bird asked Dr. Mark Allen Everett, chair of the Faculty Board, and Dr. James Merrill, vice chair, to spearhead preparation of a suitable reaffirmation of the Site of Practice policy acceptable to the regents. The latter board approved the subsequent resolution in September, with the additional statement that "Exceptions to these regulations will be rare and shall be authorized only by the University Administration in consultation with the appropriate hospital governing boards and professional staff" *[FBM, 10–17–73]*. The agitation for this latter statement came primarily from the hospitals recently separated from the University—i.e., the Children's Hospital, which was transferred to DISRS on March 17, 1973 (effective July 1) via Senate Bill 316—and from University Hospital, which was placed under a separate board of trustees in May 1973. The director of each hospital feared that revenue from private patients might be diverted to other hospitals, especially to Presbyterian Hospital when it became operational on the campus. Furthermore, the faculty was concerned that a DISRS directive requiring all patients under twenty-one years be admitted only to Children's Hospital would preclude provision of services that were only available at University Hospital to those under twenty-one. This policy was especially onerous for the Obstetrics/Gynecology faculty, since all obstetrical deliveries took place in the University and none at Children's, while many of the mothers were under twenty-one years of age. The turmoil associated with the Site of Practice policy and the centralization of faculty practice income contributed to the resignation and departure of several faculty members, including Dr. Paul T. Condit, head of the Oklahoma Medical Research Foundation's cancer section since 1964, and

Dr. Donald B. Halverstadt, professor of Pediatric Urology. Halverstadt was to later play an important role as chief of staff of Children's Hospital and of all the DISRS hospitals, and even later as interim provost and a University regent.

The unhealthy tension between the State Regents for Higher Education and the University of Oklahoma Board of Regents was attested to by the fact that when the University purchased two properties on Elm Street in Norman from the University of Oklahoma Foundation, "two State Regents wondered if there was any profiteering going on as a result of the transaction" *[RM, 11928]*.

Sending a Political Message

In March 1973, University President and Mrs. Rose Sharp awakened at 2:00 A.M. to the sound of what they thought was hail on the roof of their house. They quickly discovered, however, that the crackling sounds were actually a fire consuming the doors to their home! Four gasoline firebombs had been set by parties unknown, one at each of the house's outside doors. The Sharps fled to the hotel at the University Conference Center, where they spent the next six weeks as repairs were made to their heavily smoke-damaged home.

The Federal Bureau of Investigation and campus police believed initailly that the attack on the Sharp home was the work of the same group of students who had been setting small paper fires in front of campus buildings over the previous three months, ostensibly to draw attention to the "plight" of Black students on campus. Later, it was learned that the fires were the work of five former students, three men and two women, who had traveled from California to "show the locals how to set fires." The group rented a car in Oklahoma City with stolen credit cards and then drove to Norman where they attacked the Sharp home. Although no action was taken by the FBI or the local police because the students could not be found, months later one of them was discovered in a mental hospital in Ohio. She informed officials that the others had fled to the Gulf and to the West Coast.

As a result of this incident, there was an outpouring of support and sympathy for the president from the faculty, student body, and the Norman community. Prior to the incident, students had been extremely anti-administration. Afterwards there was an obvious sea-change in the attitudes of each of these groups. The hatred of authority that had become manifest during the administration of Herbert Hollomon was finally dissipating. At a subsequent regents' meeting, the president pointed out that the bombing, when added to the Health Sciences Center's financial crisis, had placed an enormous burden on the senior administrative staff and that the sacrifices made to deal with both situations was a "demonstration of the finest qualities of dedication to the University" *[RM, 11986]*.

Some months earlier than this incident, in response to criticism from practicing physicians from around the state, the College of Medicine Admissions Board was reconstituted by direction of the regents so that the majority of the board would be practicing physicians from the seventy-seven counties, with a decrease in the number of full-time Health Sciences Center faculty members. Dr. Eliel pointed out that although they were eager to serve, many of these out-of-town physicians were unable to commit a sufficient amount of time to interviewing candidates, substantially slowing the admissions process. He recommended the addition of three faculty members to the board in order to facilitate interviews. Regent Santee opposed the addition, suggesting a greater number of members be included from Tulsa. As a compromise, the three full-time faculty were added for only sixty days! This action was but yet another example of the hostility, distrust, and fear of some physicians that Health Sciences Center faculty would compete with the non-faculty physicians for private paying patients, and it lay at the heart of much of the antagonism in the legislature, among medical groups, and within governing bodies such as the regents.

Also in March, a Statement of Functions of the Tulsa Clinical Medicine Facility was adopted by the regents, which included the concept of a separate admissions track to the Tulsa branch. Additionally, a Practice Plan Policy Statement, developed by the College of Medicine faculty, under the leadership of Dr. Schilling, Dr. Deckert, and Dr. Everett, was approved. The motion for approval was made by Regent Huston Huffman. The statement, called Policy for Operation and Governance of the Professional Service Auxiliary of the College of Medicine, emphasized the need for: (1) involvement of faculty in direct patient care; (2) an upper limit on the time which faculty could devote to such care; (3) improved referral sources for patients to the center; (4) a uniform procedure for accounting for all faculty patient income; (5) adequate reporting and auditing of receipts and disbursements; (6) providing for income enhancement as well as limits; (7) assuring effective university control of all patient-care income [RM, 12009–12018]. During this same regents' meeting, the accounting firm of Touche-Ross was hired to audit the entire Health Sciences Center.

The Herman Smith Report

At a special meeting of the Board of Regents on March 17, 1973, a report was delivered by Herman Smith Associates on management problems at the University's hospitals. An "existing management vacuum" was found responsible for the fact that "the administrative and fiscal affairs of the hospitals are in serious disarray" *[RM, 12056]*. The firm proposed that in order to serve appropriately as consultants, they should assume management functions of the hospitals for a brief period of time. The report was presented by Jack Dumas of the Smith Associates and had been prepared at the request of the regents to address the findings of the Senate Committee for Investigation and Study of Health Care Facilities in Oklahoma, created by Senate Resolution 9 (the infamous Richardson Report). The Dumas report found that: (1) "the management and fiscal affairs of the University of Oklahoma Hospitals have been effectively stabilized"; (2) "the brief time and attention the University Hospitals can elicit from a board of regents faced with the problems of a vast university community is unacceptable"; and (3) ". . . the larger problem . . . begins with the total governance of the University of Oklahoma" and the significant elements of mismanagement have obscured "the broader and more responsible issue of the overlapping roles, conflicts and competitiveness" of the governor's office, the state legislature, the State Regents, the University of Oklahoma Regents, and the Health Center administration. These agencies, continued the report, will:

> need to reexamine seriously and conscientiously the basis of authority and responsibility for each of the above bodies and the processes for decision making and communication. Most faculty members at the H.C. have been demoralized and dismayed by previous mandates to develop needed programs of instruction for which they were required to provide the leadership necessary to secure financial support. Now they are criticized, if not vilified, as financial support is removed with little or no forewarning, leaving the faculty in the posture of being the mismanagers, when in fact, it was the decision-making process of the legislative and educational leadership that prompted them to develop these programs in the first instance *[RM, 12058]*.

The Herman Smith report also charged that changing the title of the vice president for medical center affairs and director of the Medical Center to executive vice president for Medical Center affairs and director of the Medical Center "placed the president of the University in the position of ceremonial head . . . and further confused the accountability of the OUHSC. By exercising this expediency, the University Of Oklahoma abdicated its responsibility for the schools of the health professions for which it is now paying a severe price" *[RM, 12059]*. Furthermore, continued the Smith Report, creation of the Oklahoma Health Center has "further complicated the planning and decision-making process at the H. C. to a substantial degree" *[RM, 12060]*. Because of "unrealistic planning in relation to resources and a lack of appreciation of the relationships required to achieve a distinguished health sciences center," the Smith Report labeled the Center's plans for expansion as "a two hundred million dollar dream—or delusion?" *[RM, 12061]*.

According to the Smith Report, "A myriad of funding mechanisms and absence of an effective accounting system" had resulted in fiscal insolvency. Solutions recommended included: (1) an interim legislative appropriation of $1.7 million; (2) substantially greater operating funds in subsequent years; (3) a separate board of trustees for University Hospital which will devote sufficient time to solving problems; (4) elimination of archaic and arbitrary rules and regulations which impede operation of a short term acute care teaching hospital; (5) institution of a joint conference committee between medical staff and their governing body; (6) a sufficient budget to open and operate the Everett Tower; (7) sustained preferential utilization of Children's Hospital by DISRS (Senate Bill 20) or transfer of the Children's Hospital to the State Welfare Commission; and (8) operation of Everett Tower as a private referral hospital for surgery, obstetrics, and gynecology, while delegating all other responsibilities to community hospitals throughout the state *[RM, 12066]*.

The Smith report, endorsed by University administration, the provost, and the president, was approved by the regents. In response, the board took a number of actions. They: (1) forwarded to the governor and the legislature a request for a supplemental appropriation of $778,000; (2) requested an additional sum of $955,000 for operating and equipping Everett tower; (3) changed the title of Dr. Eliel from executive vice president for Health Sciences to that of provost (thereby removing him as the chief executive officer and making all campus colleges responsible to the Norman campus with regard to finances); (4) voted to separate the University Hospitals organizationally and functionally from the academic programs at the Center; (5) requested the State Welfare Commission to assume control of the Children's Hospital; and (6) voted to request an increase of $9.3 million in operating funds for the hospital for fiscal 1973–74 *[RM, 12089; DO, 3–14–73]*. The regents took no action on the proposed long-range solutions of independent governance, providing for adult indigent care, the role of the Presbyterian Hospital, and recognizing that an essential role of University Hospital is that of a tertiary specialized referral center. On March 20 Senator Stansberry filed a bill to transfer the Children's Memorial Hospital to DISRS. This bill was passed by the Senate on March 26 and by the House on April 17.

Predictably, legislators from the central and western parts of the state— e.g., Senator Phil Smalley of Norman—believed that any comprehensive solution of Health Sciences Center problems must include a reevaluation of the Tulsa College of Medicine and the Osteopathic training project, while those from Tulsa and eastern Oklahoma—e.g., Senator James Hamilton of Tulsa—felt that the Tulsa projects should stand separately and should go ahead. The senate established a committee to study the feasibility of creating a nonprofit corporation for operation of University of Oklahoma hospitals and to examine the provision of indigent health care services. A *Daily Oklahoman* editorial on January 27 stated: "Another way the legislature could improve the situation is to stop imposing on the medical center additional programs and responsibilities without accompanying them with adequate appropriations. The Center should not be expanded until it is on a solid financial footing." Governor Hall's committee suggested that the old University Hospital be razed, while Senator George Miller said that the unopened Everett Tower is the "crux of the whole problem. I now consider it a big white elephant. You can't turn it into a hay barn and we can't afford to operate it" *[DO, 3–16–73]*.

The above individuals and organizations were not the only entities concerned with problems at the Health Sciences Center. A bill authored by Senators Stansberry and Hamilton was passed that established a separate governing body for University Hospital. Representative Hannah Atkins, chairperson of the house subcommittee studying the Center, said, "We will not be rushed into piecemeal, premature platitudes about solving this. We may have been guilty of putting up concrete bricks with no plans for operations" *[DO, 3–21–73]*. The Oklahoma Consumer Protection Agency submitted a recommendation to a house subcommittee calling upon private hospitals in the area to stop building additional beds and to take their share of indigent patients. The Oklahoma City Chamber of Commerce recommended an additional $8.1 million appropriation to the Health Sciences Center for 1973–1974. A supplemental appropriation measure calling for $527,626 was passed by the legislature to operate the Center between March and June 1973. On April 16 Speaker Bill Willis said that the house had reached agreement on how to fund the Health Sciences Center without sacrificing the College of

Medicine branch and Osteopathic School at Tulsa through utilization of HERO bond money and appropriating $1.5 million for the Tulsa projects *[DO, 4–17–73]*. In this rarest of actions, legislators seemed prepared to put their money where their mouths had been—if only in insufficient amounts.

On April 25 the House of Representatives passed, by a vote of 84–7, HB 325, which transferred University Hospital to a separate governing board and provided an appropriation of $5.5 million to give a pay raise to employees, add sufficient new positions to open Everett Tower, provide health insurance for employees, and equip the new tower. Representatives Hannah Atkins (Oklahoma City) and David Boren (Seminole) were among seven legislators voting against the measure.

Both SB 325 and SB 316, transferring the Children's Memorial Hospital to the Oklahoma Public Welfare Commission, were on the governor's desk by May 1. On that day he signed the Children's Hospital bill, with an authorization to spend "up to $1.2 million dollars for renovation to bring it up to standards." By May 24 the Public Welfare Commission had authorized the expenditure of $1.3 million for the renovation of Children's Memorial Hospital. Vera Alder, the Welfare Commission secretary, remembered that: "When we got the Children's Hospital, the doctors wouldn't even operate there if they could avoid it. We had to stress the Department's credit and meet with vendors from here to Texas to get things started. I don't know how old Dean Everett had managed to get such incredibly good doctors to work there. We had Webb Thompson, Jolly West, Stewart Wolf . . . lots of them. I think it was just because they felt that they had an obligation to help people."[20]

According to Ms. Alder, who recounted her tale with an inch of cigarette ash bobbing periously at her lower lip, Ms. Dorothy Jones, the head nurse at Children's Hospital:

> was thrilled to death [at the transfer] because they didn't have equipment [needed to do their work]. They didn't have supplies, or even nurses. They were woefully underpaid. Mr. Rader told Miss Jones to go ahead and hire nurses and we'd pay the going rate and everything . . . . She just looked at him a while, and then said, 'Mr. Rader, I don't think you can afford us.' He said, 'We'll manage,' and we did. Mr. Rader also backed up the nurses when one of the residents—the Neonatal Unit was getting real exciting about this time—refused to wash his hands between examining patients. When Miss Jones told him he must, he said he didn't have to, and didn't care what Mr. Rader said. Mr. Rader was taking a group of legislators through the building at the time and this doctor flew

onto him like a dirty shirt, and Mr. Rader said, 'Listen, young man. When Miss Jones tells you to wash your hands, you wash your hands! Or you won't practice in this hospital!' Well, the man lost his residency because he refused to comply with the ordinary rules of sanitation. You know, those little babies just hanging on by a thread, and he didn't see any reason to be sanitary.[21]

Lloyd Rader had named Harris D. "Pete" Riley, M.D., as medical director by this time. Concerning the transfer of the hospital, which occurred in June, Dr. Riley recalled:

Mr. Rader asked me to serve as medical director and chief of staff, which I did. As you know, that caused a lot of hard feelings toward me. In the past, as reflected by the old name—'Crippled Children's Hospital'— much of the activity was surgical and orthopedic. There were references to it being a 'Rader-Riley hospital.' So I suggested to Mr. Rader that the position of medical director and chief of staff be divided into two positions. I recommended three people who were not pediatricians, one of whom—Dr. Donald Halverstadt—was selected. A lot of my time was spent in interpreting to Mr. Rader and his people what an academic medical center was, what it does, and what it can't or shouldn't do.[22]

(When questioned later about his appointment by Lloyd Rader, Dr. Halverstadt did not recall who recommended him, but conjectured that it might have been Mr. Jack Dumas from the Herman Smith organization.[23])

On April 17 President Paul Sharp announced that Dr. Leonard Eliel, vice-president for health sciences, indicated he was resigning, a decision that resulted in great chagrin in a number of quarters. Dr. William Brown, acting vice-president during Dr. Eliel's absence on vacation, said, "He hasn't talked with any of us. I admit I'm very saddened if this is in fact true" *[DO, 4–18–73]*. This announcement followed closely the regents' action in returning more of the responsibility for running the Health Sciences Center to the Norman campus and restricting the duties of the Center vice-president to administering the academic programs of its six colleges. The vice-chair of the regents, Jack H. Santee of Tulsa, in his usual supportive way, stated, "If it [Dr. Eliel's resignation] is true, it would not be difficult to understand why he would leave" *[DO, 4–18–73]*. Upon his return to Oklahoma City at the end of April, Dr. Eliel stated that his reasons for leaving were personal, but that the "problems at the health sciences center have played a significant role" in this personal decision, and that "the preservation of the concept of a health sciences center is in considerable jeopardy." The remaining choices, as he saw them, were to provide for "mediocrity across the board" or to strive for "certain islands of excellence" *[DO, 5–1–73]*. This sentiment echoed the comments of Dr. Stewart Wolf, who believed that the prime responsibility of the Center administration was to strive for excellence. Meanwhile, Senate Pro Tempore President James Hamilton and Senator Phil Smalley of Norman said that, "University of Oklahoma regents are charged with the responsibility of determining priorities. They will not be able to do everything they have been doing. Some programs will have to be eliminated" *[DO, 5–3–73]*. Representative Hannah Atkins, chair of the House Subcommittee on the Health Sciences Center, cautioned that "morale is very low" and that Dr. Eliel's resignation might contribute to lowering it, and further, "the legislature has never adequately supported the medical center. We have not been willing to pay for the jobs we have assigned them to do" *[DO, 4–18– 73]*.

In June, Dr. Jeptha Dalston, administrator of the newly independent University Hospital, summarized the crisis in health care as due to several historical circumstances converging: (1) no effective program for indigent health care needs; (2) an ambitious late-1960s plan for $180,000,000 in capital improvement without provision for the concomitant operational costs; (3) the sharp withdrawal of federal programmatic funds across the nation; (4) inseparable mixing of educational and health delivery costs; (5) lack of understanding and communication between political leadership and administration—i.e., the legislature directing the University to terminate no programs and to increase faculty salaries. (As a result of legislative actions such as this, President Paul Sharp said, "Both OU's main Norman campus and the health sciences center will have to go to minimum programs in some areas to meet commitments" *[DO, 5–24–73]*) and (6) the State Regents for Higher Education fiscal management system.

Doctor Dalston later added: "A continuing and overshadowing characteristic of the whole crisis lies in the sharp schism between the academic/ medical community and the political leadership in the State House. . . . Moreover, an unfortunate dichotomy has existed for years between the University of Oklahoma Regents and the [state's] political leadership. Also playing a role in this whole affair has been a seemingly strained relationship between the University Regents and the State Regents for Higher Education" *[DO, 5–24–73]*.

This strained relationship, continued Dr. Dalston, extended not only to the question of the Tulsa Osteopathic School and College of Medicine, but to the

School of Law, use of bond issue funds, and general operating policies on the Health Sciences Center campus. This commentary by Dr. Dalston summarized many of problems and events of 1972–73. Interestingly, most of the points had been made earlier in 1963 in a confidential memorandum from Mr. Hugh Payne, executive secretary of the Oklahoma Medical Research Foundation, to Dr. DuVal and Foundation Director Leonard Eliel.

Even among the Board of Regents of the University, there was lack of unified support for the integrity of the Health Sciences Center. Some members favored directing private-paying patients to hospitals and physicians outside the University rather than admitting them to the teaching hospitals, while others were protecting developments in Tulsa rather than having the Oklahoma City campus as the primary focus for their loyalty and concern.

In April the regents made two politically significant changes in departmental names in the College of Medicine. First, the Department of Community Health in the Colleges of Medicine, Health, and Dentistry was changed to the Department of Family Practice and Community Health. Secondly, the Department of Laboratory Medicine was dissolved and the faculty and responsibilities of the department were assumed by the Department of Pathology, a return to a more traditional model. This latter action coincided with the departure of Dr. Ben Heller from the University to become president of a private medical foundation in California. Thus ended the long separation of "clinical" or "laboratory" pathology from the discipline of "anatomic" or "surgical" pathology.

In April, operational guidelines for the Tulsa Branch of the College of Medicine were approved. The regents recommended reassignment of HERO bond funds in the amount of $1.6 million for equipping Everett Tower, renovation and new equipment for "Old Main," and renovation and equipment for Children's Hospital. The latter action, when approved by the State Regents, would eliminate funds for Ambulatory Medical Clinics and reduce money for general administrative space and the auditorium at Tulsa.

At the May regents' meeting, a $10 million bond issue for purchase and extension of the Steam and Chilled Water facility was approved and the final reorganization plan for administration at the Health Sciences Center was reviewed and approved. In other actions, the resignation of Dr. Leonard Eliel was accepted, Dr. William E. Brown was appointed acting provost, and Dr. Philip E. Smith was appointed acting dean of the College of Health and Allied Health Professions. These actions followed a meeting called by President Sharp with Health Sciences Center deans at which the president told Dr. Schottstaedt, "You are no longer dean of the College of Health." Dr. Lynn recalled that Dean Bird returned from this meeting in anger and frustration.

At this same May meeting, the regents also discussed Senate Bill 115, which would bring under institutional control most grants and contracts, and Senate Bill 325, which transferred the Center's hospitals to an independent authority. Regent Mack Braly pointed out that Senate Bill 325 did not fulfill a requirement of the regents for transfer—i.e., that the educational subsidy for the hospital from higher education funds should be appropriated through the State Regents and the University Regents. Braly further said that this was an unconstitutional encroachment upon higher education's responsibilities. He moved that legal action be used to determine the constitutionality of the act. The motion failed 1–6. However, the agencies which became the governing bodies of the two hospitals later accepted the concept that the educational subsidy—i.e., payment for services of University clinical faculty within the hospitals, as well as for intern and resident house-staff—would be made directly to the University, which in turn would pay the individuals concerned. In late May, the Senate President Pro Tempore James Hamilton wrote a letter to the regents' chair, Mr. Huston Huffman, asking that "OU suspend any further action on the proposed [heating and chilled water plant and student housing] projects until all agencies and entities who will use the facilities are consulted" *[DO, 6–2–73]*. The reason for this request was not clear, although some believed it had to do with a movement to require natural gas as the energy source for the Center, or to divert the heating/cooling activity to private enterprise, especially to budding cogeneration ventures.

On June 22, salary increases of 5.5 percent were approved for Health Sciences Center faculty subject to funds being available—i.e., from sources other than the state's General or Education budget. Non-academic employees were authorized raises from 6.5 percent to 16 percent by classification, again subject to available funds. A minimum wage of $2.02 per hour was approved for University personnel. Also at the June meeting, Regent Tom Brett reported that the State Regents had allocated over $1 million for establishment of the Tulsa branch of the College of Medicine and first-year operation of the Osteopathic college. Predictions that the operating costs per student would be low ("$8,290," according to the *Daily Oklahoman* of June 23), were wildly optimistic because within two years the cost was over $25,000 per student [FBM, 10–9–74]. Regent Brett reported that the State Regents, meeting in Durant, had approved the Tulsa allocations by a vote of 9–0 and 8–1 respectively, in spite of the fact that he had made an eloquent plea for delay. He said that the presentations in favor were primarily made by the Tulsa Chamber of Commerce, a delegation of physicians from Tulsa, and by osteopathic physicians from throughout the state *[RM, 12298]*.

University Hospital facilities and equipment were officially transferred to the new University Hospital Authority on July 26 and governance of Children's Hospital was moved to the Oklahoma Department of Institutions, Social and Rehabilitative Services. In addition, the regents recognized the signal contributions of past president Nancy Davies to the University and especially to the Health Sciences Center. Her courage in bringing the severity of the fiscal crisis on the Oklahoma City campus to the attention of the regents and the state at large was "exemplary" *[RM, 12294]*.

In midsummer, Dr. William W. Schottstaedt resigned as dean of the College of Health, and the college was combined with the College of Allied Health Professions. Many observers believed that the consolidation of the Colleges of Health and Allied Health under Dean Philip Smith and the forced resignation of Dean Schottstaedt was not primarily a cost-saving measure but punishment for the political activity of students in Schottstaedt's College of Health, who had demonstrated in an attempt to influence the legislature to maintain the integrity and increase annual appropriations for the Health Sciences Center and the College of Health. Contributing to the impetus for this merger was suspicion by legislators and the University administration that the Oklahoma Health Sciences Facilities, Inc. masked fiscal misdeeds of the medical faculty, especially with regard to the real estate transactions entered into by the group. Dean Schottstaedt believed the latter to be the principal cause of the elimination of his college. The Health Sciences and University administrations, however, presented reorganization of the Colleges of Health and Allied Health as "streamlining the administration and changing programs where necessary in order to bring the college within operating funds" *[RM, 12607]*. Dean Bird and Bill Brown were reportedly furious about the closure. Finally in July, Lippert Brothers Construction was awarded the $8.7 million contract for construction of the Biomedical Sciences building, and a bid was accepted by the regents for issuance of Utility System Revenue Bonds.

The University Hospital Board of Trustees authorized immediate occupancy of the new Everett Tower on August 26. The facility had been empty since being accepted from the builders on March 1. Within days, the legislature expressed surprise that occupancy would lead to a new deficit. Senate President Pro Tempore James Hamilton said, "This is absolutely beyond my comprehension; a tremendous increase in personnel will be required to maintain the same number of beds because of the way the new building is designed" *[DO, 8–30–73]*. Rumors that the Department of Institutions, Social and Rehabilitative Services would take over Everett Tower were dispelled by Lloyd Rader, the director, who said, "Nothing could be further from the truth. I cannot, and will not, recommend this to the Welfare Commission or legislature" *[DO, 9–1–73]*. Vera Alder, longtime secretary to the Welfare Commission, recalled that Senator Hamilton wanted the agency to take both hospitals. When Mr. Rader informed her of this, she said, "Lord, if we have to take one of those things, take the kitten; don't take that old cat. But we eventually got the old cat anyway!"[24] Instead, a 10 percent budget reduction was instituted by the University Hospital Board. One casualty of the fiscal axe was the cardiac catheterization program, whose discontinuation severely restricted availability of new and popular diagnostic tools for diagnosis and treatment of cardiac insufficiency. The public outcry at this reduction was considerable.

By September the implications of reductions in the flow of funds to the Health Sciences Center had grabbed the attention of Governor Hall and the legislature. A six-member delegation left for Washington, D.C., to join with House Speaker Carl Albert and meet with Caspar Weinberger, secretary of health, education and welfare, who "danced the customary diplomatic minuet that cabinet officers are expected to perform when accosted by angry state delegations" and, to Albert's plea, "shrugged eloquently—and a little disdainfully" *[DO, 9–19–73]*. Subsequently, both the Senate Finance Committee and the House Ways and Means Committee asked Secretary Weinberger to concur in their proposed compromise on implementation of the new reimbursement rules. Weinberger remained refractory to the suggestions of the senate and house leaders, including Senators Bellmon, Russell Long, and Herman Talmadge *[DO, 9–20–73]*.

In October 1973 action on a proposed Affiliation Agreement with Children's Hospital was deferred because of faculty objections to a clause forbidding staff physicians from admitting any patient under the age of twenty-one to any other hospital without permission of the medical director. A proposal by the clinical faculty of the College of Medicine to form a corporate entity for the practice of medicine was not looked upon with favor by President Sharp, who stated, "We do not . . . believe that the incorporation of individuals is in the best long-range interest of the institution" *[RM, 12496–7]*. Sharp proposed an amendment to the Professional Service Auxiliary document requiring faculty to practice as individuals. The amendment was approved by the regents. An affiliation agreement with the Veterans Administration Hospital setting up a "Dean's Committee" to serve with the hospital director was also approved. Thus, the University of Oklahoma hospitals were among the first "Dean's Committee" hospitals, fully integrating a Veterans Administration Hospital into the educational enterprise.

In late October, Governor Hall announced that he was "prepared to support adequate funding" as well as a January 1 opening for the new Everett Tower *[DO,10–31–73]*. At the same time, the Welfare Department announced that it was embarking on a $2 million expansion of Children's Hospital. Also in October, Professor of Surgery John A. Schilling wrote to President Sharp concerned that the failure to complete University Hospital facilities, including ambulatory care clinics, would negate the dream of creating "the outstanding medical center in the Southwest."[25] In a later summation of accomplishments and goals for the University, Schilling wrote to the president saying, "I was dismayed to note that the separation of the University Hospitals from the University is an accomplishment. In all probability it dooms the Medical College to mediocrity or worse, inferiority in perpetuity. This 'resolution of hundreds of practical problems' sounds more like euthanasia."[26]

Dr. Schilling also wrote to Governor Hall in October reemphasizing his previous pleas to the governor that there were two essential priorities for the Center: first, "completion of the Everett Hospital Tower as a total hospital unit with new pediatric and internal medical facilities; and secondly, improved ambulatory office facilities for the staff, perhaps analogous to a doctors' office building."[27] In an earlier letter to the governor, Schilling had written, "To fail to complete the University Hospital will . . . lead to . . . an ensuing inferior health manpower teaching and training institution. Under these circumstances, in my opinion, it would be better to close the Medical Center forthrightly."[28] In the Surgery departmental minutes for October 29:

> a consensus of the faculty present was that individuals in higher administrative positions who had a role in the creation of the disarray at the Medical Center were beginning to realize the destructive effects of their efforts—be they unintentional or with malice. In historical perspective the Legislature is attacking the Medical School and dismembering it as it had attacked the University in periods gone by. . . . Further, the Regents of the University were continually subject to legislative blackmail into the possible acceptance and implementation of Chancellor Dunlap's game plan of some fifteen years ago. The support of the community leaders and Chamber of Commerce members was specifically mentioned as a progressive step, as was the favorable press that we have recently enjoyed.[29]

Central Billing Issues

Provost Leonard Eliel submitted a recommendation stemming from the administrative reorganization plan that there be a "central billing system for all professional services rendered by faculty physicians." Herman Smith Associates had been asked in June 1973 to devise such a system. By November the firm asked that the agreement be terminated due to "lack of progress in the establishment of the system because of a number of issues that have not been resolved" *[RM, 12572]*. The Smith group suggested that since the regents and the administration desired central billing, the Financial Services Office of the University should develop it. The regents terminated the agreement and charged Financial Services with the task. Behind this issue lay widespread faculty opposition that can be summarized in three statements: first, a fear that the administration would try to control expenditure of private patient income as well as supervise the billing and collecting; second, a concern that central billing would be costly as well as inefficient (later proven to be true) and result in reduced collections; and third, general satisfaction with the collection ratio of the existing system, in most instances departmental billing and collecting.

Regents received a proposal from President Sharp for a revised policy on Outside Employment and Extra Compensation (1972) in November. For full-time faculty, it limited such employment to forty-eight days during any twelve months. For nine-month faculty, no restriction was placed on the remaining three months' employment. "In no case does the University set a limit on the income a faculty or staff member may earn from outside employment" *[DO, 11–7–73]*.

Action by the University Board of Regents on revisions to the Professional Practice Plan was postponed in December because the proposed changes were still being considered by the faculty and "action by the Board at this time on the revised policy would be premature" *[RM, 12601]*. There was considerable faculty suspicion that the document would merely be a subterfuge for the administration to control all practice income. In a letter to Dr. Schilling on September 14 Dr. Ronald C. Elkins had written: "I see no way to accept the concept that we must pay for facility fees, that we must earn our own academic expenses, that we must support our own department, and even more important, that we can be promised an academic base salary but must earn it. I think that until the committee develops a proposed practice plan that has the philosophy to encourage rather than discourage the practice of clinical medicine by the clinical faculty at the University of Oklahoma, we have no hope of success."

At the same December regents meeting, a memorial tribute was adopted recognizing the many contributions of the late Mary Zahasky, who had served the Health Sciences Center and its hospitals for twenty-six years as director of the Department of Dietetics and the Dietetic Intern Program as well as chair of the Department of Nutrition and Dietetics in the College of Allied Health Professions. Zahasky was an articulate, selfless leader who exemplified the growing influence of women faculty members on the various campus colleges.

December also saw changes made in the Department of Family Practice and Community Health. These changes were: (1) transfer of the Physician's Associate Program from that department to the College of Medicine dean's office; (2) transfer of the Family Medicine clinic and all clinical training of residents to the College of Medicine; and (3) transfer of the department itself to the Colleges of Medicine and Dentistry as the joint Department of Family Practice and Community Medicine and Dentistry, effective July 1, 1974. The Departments of Environmental Health and of Human Ecology were merged. Each of these recommendations was approved by the regents without comment.

A complex document dividing hospital-related assets between University Hospital and the University, negotiated by attorney Tom Tucker and the hospital—a document of delicate fabric of such complex negotiations easily torn beyond repair—was also approved in December without comment by the regents. The thorny problem of who would own what assets was finally resolved by this action *[RM, 12639–12641]*. Meanwhile, there were intermittent tensions between the new University Hospital administration and the Children's Memorial Hospital, precipitated by the continued treatment of patients under the age of twenty-one at the adult hospital. Simultaneously, a recurrence of the old habit of the federal government delaying payment to physicians for services rendered in the teaching hospitals, and ultimately paying reluctantly, if at all, caused the Oklahoma City Chamber of Commerce to come to the assistance of the college. The Chamber exerted pressure on Oklahoma's senators and representatives to demand indefinite postponement of the Social Security Administration's plan to reduce physician reimbursement. Stanton Young was a prime mover in this action.

The final action of the year was a mid-December announcement by the regents that the construction of a new five-story, $2.2 million building to house the Dean A. McGee Eye Institute would begin early the following year.

1974

Nineteen seventy-four began with an announcement by University of Oklahoma Regent Bob Mitchell (appointed by newly installed governor David

Boren) that the Health Sciences Planning and Advisory Committee of the regents had established a sub-committee to develop a plan to coordinate activities of the Health Sciences Center's three hospitals—Veterans, Children's, and University—for the purpose of avoiding duplication of services. This sub-committee was composed of Regent Mitchell, Veterans Administration Hospital Director Dan Macer, ex-Regent Ira Monroe, and DISRS Director Llloyd Rader. Mr. Tom Tucker, variously attorney for the University, the Center, and DISRS, stated that the group would look at facilities in the light of program planning to maximize utilization and efficiency on the campus in future construction.

At the same January meeting, a revised Site of Practice policy for the College of Medicine faculty was adopted. Regent Thomas Brett expressed appreciation to Vice-Presidents John Dean and Eugene Nordby, and to University Counsel Tom Tucker, for outstanding work in developing the revision. This policy, which defined the limits of the Health Sciences Center Campus, pointedly did not mention the Presbyterian Hospital, which had been the focus of criticism directed at Health Sciences Center faculty for practicing outside of state and federal hospitals. However, a mechanism for exceptions to the restrictions on location of faculty practice was noted: given the "importance of the contribution of these individuals and their appropriate compensation, certain specific arrangements, that are exceptions . . . can be made" *[RM, 12689]*. This gave the dean flexibility to permit high-earning specialists, who might otherwise leave the university, to continue practicing where they wanted. (See, for example, the issue of Dr. Donald Halverstadt later in this history.)

The University of Oklahoma Board of Regents in March 1974 revised and adopted new guidelines for expenditures from faculty Professional Practice income. Typically, these changes were not well received by a large segment of the faculty. At the same time, a cooperation agreement between the Tulsa campus and the Muskogee Veterans Administration hospital was signed. Thus, the Muskogee hospital was brought into a close affiliation with the Tulsa branch, mirroring the situation in Oklahoma City with Presbyterian Hospital.

Meanwhile, at the February Faculty Board meeting, the recurrent problem of the National Board of Medical Examiners (NBME) exam was again investigated. An ad hoc committee, consisting of Dr. Gordon Deckert, chair, and Dr. Jackie Coalson and Dr. Timothy Coussons, prepared an extensive report on Intramural and Extramural Evaluation and concluded that most institutions perceived a need for a comprehensive examination at the end of the basic science years, and that if the NBME examination was not required, then the institution had a need for an "intramurally developed, comprehensive examination" *[FBM, 2–24–74]*. On March 4 the committee presented to the Faculty Board the recommendation that: (1) the faculty should move as quickly as possible toward the development of an intramurally developed, criterion-referenced comprehensive examination which must be passed to move from the second to the third year; and (2) until that was obtained, the College of Medicine should require students to take extramurally developed certifying examinations. It is of interest to note that although periodic efforts occurred to develop a comprehensive examination where this was a centerpiece of proposed curriculum reform, none was ever developed. Further, it was recommended that the pass-fail honors grading system, adopted in the 1960s in response to student agitation for a non-competitive environment, be replaced with a five-level, A-to-F system and that approximately equal weight should be given the extramural (NBME Parts I and II) and intramural examinations in reference to promotion to the third year *[FBM, 3–4–74]*.

In March, the State Senate held hearings on Senate Bill 245, which would revoke licenses of hospitals that refused to admit patients on the basis of their ability to pay. The hearing was characterized by sharp exchanges between state senator E. Melvin Porter and Jay Henry, president of Baptist Hospital. After two and a half hours of debate, the committee "laid Senate Bill 245 over for future action" *[DO, 3–13–74]*. This action was principally the result of pressure by the State Hospital Association, which was wary of any examination of the charitable status of its members. Curiously, with University Hospital only a few months into its new independent administrative board, Governor Hall, Speaker Willis, and Senate President Pro Tempore Hamilton were meeting to discuss possible transfer of the Hospital to DISRS. This suggestion was abandoned when the degree of unrest engendered by the proposal among hospital employees surfaced and became a topic of conversation.

In April, President Sharp announced the appointment of a search committee for a new Health Sciences Center provost, chaired by Dr. Tom Lynn. At the same time, he and the University of Oklahoma Board of Regents commended Dr. William Brown for his praiseworthy role as interim provost *[RM, 12824]*. The president also announced that the chair in Surgery, established by Dr. John A. Schilling in 1967, now was funded with a $500,000 gift from Dr. Schilling. The regents activated the chair and named it the John A. Schilling Chair in Surgery. These actions coincided with the announcement by the regents that both Dr. Schilling and Dr. Len Eliel would be moving out of state in a few months. At the end of April, Dr. G. Rainey Williams was named interim chair of Surgery, effective May 15, and in July his appointment to the endowed chair was made permanent. Dr. Schilling's title was changed from head of surgery to professor of Surgery.

In a letter dated April 7, 1974, Dr. Schilling shared some of his feelings about his tenure at the Health Sciences Center with his successor, Dr. Williams:

> I have vivid recollections of the period, but then the whole eighteen years was a period of one crisis or another, so I never felt that the 1972–74 era was much different except that it represented the continued struggles of dedicated people to make things better rather than being content with the status quo, or worse, deterioration. But in summary, my basic concerns were . . . first, the politicization of the Regents by Governor Hall; second, the weak position of Paul Sharp as he was more or less ground up in the political arena; third, Len Eliel's uncertain position and inability to communicate effectively, despite his academic stature; fourth, the loss of the University Hospitals to State administration—that, I felt, was catastrophic; fifth, the Regents altered our income plan and installed central collection . . . which could have placed the faculty in a position of indentured servitude; sixth, the stalling of the building plans, with Eliel's accepting the mothballing of the new University Hospital as a viable option—that was unconscionable; and seventh, [Governor] Hall's establishment of an Osteopathic Medical School in Tulsa with a Y Medical School had terrible and predictable consequences and portent for the future. Those schools should be closed. . . . Lloyd Rader did what no governor, college president, dean or provost could do. He put together a remarkable physical complex during the past ten years. [He was] an individual who was fundamentally interested in the development of his State.

G. Rainey Williams

Following the retirement of the nationally known and respected physician and educator John Schilling, a man who would match his accomplishments succeeded him as chair of Surgery. Born in Atlanta in 1926, G. Rainey Williams was a University of Texas graduate who obtained his M.D. degree at Northwestern University in 1948. After an internship and surgical residency as a Halsted fellow at Johns Hopkins University, he completed a residency in thoracic surgery at the same institution, this time as the Blaylock Fellow. Following training, he joined Dr. Schilling's faculty in Surgery at Oklahoma, attaining the rank of professor in 1963. Dr. Williams would serve with distinction as chair of Surgery from 1974 until the time of his death in 1997. On three occasions, he occupied the position of acting or interim dean of the College of Medicine. He received many honors, including the University of Oklahoma's Distinguished Service Citation in 1982 and election to the Oklahoma Hall of Fame in 1986.

Rainey Williams benefitted from—and made extensive use of—his long-standing connections to community, legislative, and social leaders throughout the state. In the words of a prominent Oklahoma physician, the Presbyterian Foundation "turned back flips for him." One colleague believed that Dr. Williams could have used his connections more forcefully to speed University Hospital development—i.e., he could have obtained desperately needed funds or named the individuals who ran the hospital—and could have placed demands on the legislature that they could not have refused, but his personality and inclination did not lead him in this direction. Still another faculty member felt that Dr. Williams: "could, as dean, have been a major figure in enhancing [building] the faculty in other departments. But he was adverse to coercion. He was gentle—a gentleman in the true sense of the word. His quality as a person can certainly be viewed as a 'fingerprint' on the College of Medicine because he was of such high quality."

Another significant "fingerprint" clearly left by Rainey Williams was his heralded skill as a surgeon. Perhaps more than any other surgeon at the Health Sciences Center, he brought renown to his department and to the University with his pioneering approach to the surgical arts. He achieved national prominence in the 1960s when he led a group of Health Sciences Center surgeons in dramatically reattaching the severed arm of Bob Swafford, a basketball player at Oklahoma State University. The arm had been ripped from the 6'10" center when he reached into a spinning clothes dryer to retrieve a uniform before the machine had adequately slowed. Another priceless "fingerprint," as former Dean Lynn described it, was that "there is no questioning the fact that Rainey, by staying on the faculty (with Dr. Ron Elkins) when the department nearly collapsed after the departure of John Schilling, saved the Department of Surgery for all time. I publicly give him full credit for that."[30]

A senior Surgery faculty member recalled Rainey Williams "speaking out strongly" on only two occasions: when he was openly confrontational over Health Sciences Center urologists doing kidney transplants at University Hospital; and in his belief that Dean Donald Kassebaum "had to go." Another, and possibly more influential, stance taken by Dr. William's years earlier, was his outspoken opposition to establishment of the Tulsa College of Medicine, during a time when the Oklahoma City parent institution was in dire financial straights. Dr. William's life and work were greatly aided by his wife Martha, who in her own right contributed immeasurably to the Health Sciences Center in her tireless work with the Breast Health Center and Faculty Wives Club and by cofounding with Alice Everett, the Hospital Volunteer Organization.

Dr. Williams always provided a much needed equanimity for, and occasionally even a restraining hand on, the College of Medicine faculty, especially when there was a precipitous tendency to embark on actions which would be ill received by the legislature or the local business and medical communities. Furthermore, he was an invaluable and critical link with the local centers of financial power. He frequently garnered moral and fiscal support from state leaders for critical Health Sciences Center objectives. Rainey Williams also was a loyal friend ready to provide a willing ear and a word of comfort when fellow faculty members were troubled. In the words of former Dean Tom Lynn, "Rainey Williams was one of the shining stars on the faculty."[31]

In January 1974 Dr. Martin Fitzpatrick, professor of Medicine at Tulsa, was appointed dean of the University of Oklahoma Tulsa Branch of the College of Medicine, at a salary of $78,000. Fitzpatrick was a Notre Dame graduate who studied medicine at Columbia University and later served on the Medicine faculties at Kansas City and New York University before coming to Tulsa as professor of Medicine in 1969. He would serve as dean at Tulsa for slightly more than one year. Leeland Alexander was appointed assistant dean for administration and business manager at the Tulsa branch in February. Alexander would be a key player in the Tulsa operation for many years. At the same meeting, a budget of $457,823 was approved for the Tulsa branch for the period February 20–June 30, 1974.

The Child Study Center

In Oklahoma City in March 1974, the Board of Regents approved a lease for a site at 4020 North Lincoln Boulevard for the Child Development Center (later re-named the Child Study Center). The Center had been located in the old Maclanburg house on North Lincoln for several years and was evicted when the structure was sold as a private home. The building had been used as an evaluation and treatment site since 1963. Following the transfer of the Children's Hospital to the Department of Human Services in 1973, a separate building was built on N.E. 13th Street east of the Children's Hospital. Pending completion of this structure, the Center was temporarily moved to a house at 214 East Madison.

According to Dr. Loy Markland, the Child Study Center had been established in 1958 as a clinic to evaluate "retarded" children under the supervision of Dr. Theodore Pfundt. Shortly after his arrival as the new chair of Pediatrics, Dr. Harris D. Riley established the clinic as an evaluation center, initially directed toward the problem of mental retardation in children. In September 1958, newly arrrived Dr. Sylvia Richardson, an assistant professor of Pediatrics, was named director. Inasmuch as her interest was in the field of learning disorders, the mission of the Child Study Center was broadened to include mental growth and development in children. The unit grew rapidly with the support of NIH funds and the cooperation of the Department of Pediatric Neurology and the National Cancer Institute. Dr. Richardson left in 1965 and was succeeded by Richard Gilmartin (1965–1967), Dr. John Saunders (1967–1969), and Dr. Ella Thomas (1969–1985). Dr. Owen Rennert, the chair of Pediatrics, then directed the Center until Dr. Jack Metcoff was appointed. In 1990 Dr. Harriet Coussons was appointed as director and serves to this date.

The independence of the Child Study Center was essentially unchanged during both the period of ownership by the Department of Human Services and while the Health Sciences Center's hospitals were under the University Hospitals Authority. The scope of its interests was broadened to include, at various times, the visually impaired and a wide variety of central nervous system and neuromuscular disorders. Following merger of the hospitals with Columbia-Presbyterian in 1998, negotiations were undertaken to return direction of the Child Study Center to the Department of Pediatrics in July 1999, with the building leased to the Health Sciences Center at a nominal fee.

Also in March 1974 the legislature "vitalized" the last $18.7 million of the 1968 Bond Issue for Higher Education. This led to a prediction from the State Regents that $45 million more in educational funds would be needed because of new campuses and increased costs. The increased costs were the result of lengthy delays in construction projects anticipated from the 1968 bond issue due to the unavailability of federal matching funds.

The following month, the State Senate appropriated $580,000 from DISRS funds for deficit operations at University Hospital. Governor Hall recommended an increase in higher education funds of only $14 million, while some members of the legislature favored a figure closer to the State Regents' request of nearly $30 million. The Senate ultimately approved the governor's figure. Also in April, the Oklahoma Medical Research Foundation announced the selection of Dr. Clayton S. White as its president and director. Dr. White played only a minor role in Health Sciences Center affairs during his brief tenure.

In May, numerous bequests made through the years to Children's Hospital were transferred by the regents to DISRS. The following month, regents signed a lease with the Oklahoma City School Board for use of the Moon School as an operations building for the Health Sciences Center campus.

Faculty Departures

During the spring and early summer of 1974, a series of faculty resignations shook the confidence of the Health Sciences Center and resulted in widespread reverberations. Several physicians left for positions which clearly were advancements—e.g., Dr. Tom Bruce, professor of Medicine, to become the dean of the School of Medicine at the University of Arkansas, following his mentor, James Dennis, who was now head of the Arkansas Medical Center in Little Rock. Since coming to the University of Oklahoma, Bruce had become not only head of the cardiovascular section in Medicine, but also a leading member of the faculty heavily involved in administration, serving as chair of the Academic Council under Dean Dennis. He would occupy the position of dean at Arkansas until 1985, when he became program director in health for the W. K. Kellogg Foundation. Dr. James Merrill later recalled that Bruce, while dean at Arkansas, invited him as a personnel consultant when a new chair of Obstetrics was to be appointed: "I spent a day and a half studying and making recommendations. In conference, they talked only about one candidate, and when I advised selection of another, I found Tom had already appointed this guy—he'd already decided to select him as chairman! The candidate lasted about a year, and then he ended up being dean at one of the offshore schools. I thought that it was a strange way to operate; it sort of reminded me about how we did the curriculum [at Oklahoma]."[32]

Dr. Douglas Voth, a professor of Medicine, left Oklahoma for personal advancement—as chair of the Department of Medicine at the Wichita State University Medical Branch. However, many other faculty departures reflected disenchantment and exhaustion brought on by the continual struggle for funds for the Center and the persistent lack of interest and faith in the College and its hospitals by the Oklahoma legislature and the state's higher education authorities. For example, Dr. John Schilling, chair of the Department of Surgery, left to become professor of surgery at the University of Washington in Seattle; Dr. Leonard P. Eliel accepted a position with the American Lake Veterans

Administration Hospital in Tacoma, Washington; and former dean William W. Schottstaedt resigned as professor of Family Practice and Community Health to accept a similar position in Texas.

Still other resignations reflected a dissatisfaction with the rancor and bitterness associated with the recent imposition of the faculty private practice directive which classified income to faculty from private patients as "state" money. The resignation of Dr. Robert M. Bird in July to accept an appointment as director of the Lister Hill National Center for Biomedical Communications was one of many resignations caused in part by this directive. Dr. Bird indicated that the "climate at OUHSC was uncongenial to the scholarly education" of medical students and young physicians, saying, "I'm not running away. . . . I have no feelings of failure, just sadness at leaving my home" *[DO, 7–13–74]*. Dr. Harris Riley tried to intervene: "I remember going to talk to Bob to persuade him to continue. It always seemed to me that he made a small problem bigger by jumping ship."[33]

On the other hand, in response to the inquiries of several regents, former dean Thomas Lynn stated that he believed Dr. Bird clearly enjoyed the full support of the faculty, and that the summary firing of Dean Schottstaedt, a close friend of Bird, was principally responsible for his sharp criticism of the regents and the legislature. Lynn recalled that one time the two of them were driving down I-35 and Bird said, "Tom, I want you to do me a favor. If you ever think that my presence as dean is hurting the school, please let me know." Later that summer, just before Bird resigned, Lynn called him and said, "Bob, we are really losing support both at the regents level and in the legislature. I just want you to know, as you asked me to tell you." He said, "Thank you very much." As Dean Lynn recalled these events, a pensive expression clouded his face. "I look back on that and feel very sad about having said it. He was one of those persons you really could believe in."[34]

In July, Dr. James Hartsuck, a cardiovascular surgeon in the Department of Surgery, left the University for private practice in Oklahoma City. His departure also related to the regents' policies regarding faculty practice income. Shortly thereafter, Dr. Lazar Greenfield, head of Surgery at the Veterans Administration Hospital, also resigned. With the departure of these skilled surgeons, six of the nine members of the surgical faculty had departed within a single year! Dr. G. Rainey Williams, the interim chair of the Department, "blasted the medical school's posture of 'not being able to attract and retain top personnel' due to lack of positive leadership at all levels of the administration and in the state legislature" *[DO, 7–9–74]*. Dr. Ronald Elkins recalled that "I knew that it was a sink-or-swim situation.

Rainey was undertaking a gigantic task to maintain the department. I had a lot of loyalty to him and stayed. Plus, I saw an opportunity to assume considerable responsibility. We were the only two surgeons in the department for almost a year and a half!"[35]

The mass defections from the Health Sciences Center caused ripples in areas other than the Oklahoma City campus. In reaction to the numerous faculty departures, the Oklahoma State Medical Association "voted $20,000 in July to finance a campaign to aid the Health Sciences Center by informing legislators, political candidates, and Oklahoma's 2,800 medical doctors about Center needs" *[DO, 7–15–74].*

The Physicians' Practice Plan and the Donald Halverstadt Affair

One of the most controversial matters to reach the regents in 1974 was the resignation in May of Dr. Donald B. Halverstadt, professor of Urology. Dr. Halverstadt resigned subsequent to "considerable attention in the press and from others in the University" *[RM, 12983; DO, 7–14–74]* because of policies regarding Site-of-Practice and the disposition of faculty income as limited by the regents' recently approved Professional Practice Plan for the faculty. This policy was in response to Senate Bill 115 which required that all full-time faculty practice income be deposited directly to the state via a special University agency account. As previously noted, the legislation resulted from the feeling among many legislators that "doctors were getting rich with money which should go to the state," a view that was fueled by the fiscal crisis on the campus, especially the University Hospital funding issues. True to form, these same legislators ignored the real issue, which was inadequate funding of higher education in general, and of the Health Sciences Center in particular. As articulated to the authors by several legislators, many members saw physician earnings as a "free" source of money with which to fund anemic academic programs at the Health Sciences Center, thus releasing other state funds to finance pet "pork barrel" projects elsewhere. The idea by legislators that these restrictions on physician income would unleash a vast sum of money for other purposes was largely illusory, since faculty fees were already being spent primarily for Health Sciences Center and departmental development, not physician enrichment.

Donald Halverstadt had come to the University of Oklahoma in 1967 as the first full-time pediatric urologist, following training at Harvard and Massachusetts General Hospital. He played a prominent role in the teaching hospitals while they were under the control of the Department of Human Services (aka, DISRS) as chief of staff, functioning as the right-hand man of director Lloyd Rader. He was also to serve as interim provost of the Health Sciences Center in 1979–1980. Following his resignation as a full-time member of the faculty in 1974, Dr. Halverstadt applied to the regents in June for "volunteer faculty" status. Regent Santee asked for a motion regarding this volunteer appointment. Regent Mitchell moved that the application be denied. Regent Brett asked that "this matter be given further consideration," with the thought that, perhaps, an accord could be reached with Dr. Halverstadt *[RM, 12983–4]*. Brett realized that Halverstadt's recent appointment by Lloyd Rader as chief of staff at the Children's Memorial Hospital "somewhat complicates the problem." However, the request was denied on a vote of 5–0–1. Regent Santee stated that he hoped that "Dr.Halverstadt finds it possible to assure that he will fully comply with the PPP policies" *[RM, 12983–84]*. The *Daily Oklahoman* on June 14 quoted John Dean, a University of Oklahoma vice-president, as saying that Dr. Halverstadt had possibly violated the mandatory physician's Practice Plan and Site-of-Practice directive requiring that physician fees be collected by the university, and that private patients be admitted only to Health Science Center hospital beds. According to the *Oklahoman*, "the dean said Dr. Halverstadt's letter of resignation in May took him off a list of ten to fifteen physicians at the College of Medicine who are now being investigated to determine if professional income has been withheld from the university" *[DO, 6–14–74]*. Halverstadt had requested in January to be placed on half-time status. This request was denied by President Sharp the following month, who stated that the denial "was essential to the total well-being of the Health Sciences Center" *[DO, 6–14–74]*.

Dr. Halverstadt later recalled that because he had continued to admit patients to Presbyterian Hospital, where he believed the care of Urology patients was superior to that in the University hospitals, he was asked to appear before the regents. The encounter proceeded as follows, in the succinct words of Dr. Halverstadt:

I met with them; Jack Santee was the chairman at the time. He said, 'Doctor, do you know what the Site of Practice policy is?'
I said 'Yes.'
'Doctor, have you broken the Site of Practice policy?'
'Yes, sir, I have.'
'Doctor, do you intend to continue to break it?'

'Yes, sir.'

'Doctor, why is that?'

'Well, Mr. Chairman, the decision whether to admit a patient to a hospital is a medical decision. And I will admit my patients to the hospital where I think they will get the best care. And unfortunately, Mr. Chairman, right now that's not in your hospital.'

To make a long story short, they indicated that I could resign from the faculty or I would be terminated. I opted to resign, and in the process I made a request for a volunteer appointment. They refused the request. The rumor was that they did it to try to make an example out of me so nobody else would do the same thing.[36]

Halverstadt then recalled, "So, anyway, there I am without a faculty appointment. Lloyd Rader loved the underdog, and it strengthened his resolve to work with me [to be reappointed]."[37]

Dr. Halverstadt's appointment as clinical professor of Urology was renewed (without comment by the regents) in January 1975 presumably due to the influence of Lloyd Rader, who reportedly delayed the delivery of several hundred thousand dollars in reimbursement checks to the regents until they granted his demands. When called by president Sharp inquiring where the checks were, Rader replied, "They're right here in my desk. And they'll stay here until you give my boy a volunteer faculty appointment."[38] Regent Julian Rothbaum recalls: "The regents did not cross Lloyd Rader very much. He had a reputation of having marvelous, marvelous contacts. Every time he did a favor for a congressman or representative or state senator, he put it down in his book [the famous 'Rader Rolodex'] so he could come back and call on it. He was a great friend of [Senator] Bob Kerr's. As far as I know, people just let him run his own show. He was very powerful, probably because as an individual he could give jobs to politicians' constituents. Overall, Lloyd Rader was very good for Oklahoma."[39]

Interestingly, in the following month the regents added some language to their Practice Plan document, the purpose of which was to clarify the relationship of faculty to the University and assist in complying with IRS regulations regarding income taxes. "Members of the geographic full-time faculty are, and should be considered as, employees of the University when they are carrying out their academic activities. They are not, and should not be considered as, employees when they are carrying out their professional private practice activities" *[RM, 13062]*. This enabled Health Sciences Center faculty to file Schedule C income tax statements regarding their medical practice income. The policy seemed in direct contradiction to the mandated depositing of faculty patient fee money directly into a state agency account, that was made policy at this same meeting. The regents further voted that "The University shall not possess the right to control or direct the faculty members in the performance of their professional private practice activities, it being understood that whether or not a faculty member conducts professional private practice activities shall be within each faculty member's sole discretion. . .". [*RM, 13063*]. Later, when this statement was rescinded, there was renewed faculty discontent with the Practice Plan.

Another faculty leader, Dr. James Merrill, chair of the Department of Gynecology and Obstetrics, publicly stated that he believed the probe of medical faculty income being conducted under the direction of vice president Eugene Nordby and an auditor, Harold Zollen, was vindictive, and that if "the regents do not stop their harassment, they may find themselves with no College of Medicine at all." He said that the implication there had been a willful mishandling of funds was "totally false." Continued Dr. Merrill, "For years this faculty has generated income and turned it over to the University willingly. The conflict is in having the Practice Plan imposed upon them!" [*DO, 7–19–74*].

Indigent Patient Care and the University Hospital Crisis

In May, Senator E. Melvin Porter (D-Oklahoma City), a longtime supporter of higher state spending for social programs, rekindled the long-standing controversy over payments for medical care to indigents in state hospitals when he said that he had become convinced that "There is some kind of conspiracy to force the closing of University Hospital for the benefit of private hospitals in the Oklahoma City area" [*DO, 5–1–74*]. In spite of the obvious need for upgrading University Hospital and its capital equipment in order to attract the private patients necessary to achieve some semblance of a balanced budget, legislative leaders continued to oppose adequate appropriations. Senate President Pro Tempore Hamilton (D-Poteau) stated that he was firmly opposed to increasing the budget at the Health Sciences Center, while Senator Gene Howard (D-Tulsa), who was slated to succeed Senator Hamilton, insisted that the hospital operate with a $5 million subsidy, stating that "I will personally oppose very vigorously a supplemental appropriation next January" [*DO, 5–1–74*]. Senator Hamilton generally reflected the views of eastern Oklahoma and Tulsa, which often echoed the thoughts of Dr. Donald Brawner, Tulsa Chamber of Commerce president, who maintained that "only central

Oklahoma benefits from the hospital" *[DO, 3–6–74]*. President Sharp criticized reports that the legislature was considering closing University Hospital, pointing out that it "plays a vital role in the education of health care professionals, and its presence is essential" *[DO, 5–2–74]*.

The legislature finally approved a bill appropriating $6,685,033 to the hospital and a $14.6 million increase in funds for higher education on May 6. Simultaneously, the Hospital Board of University Hospital asked regents to provide $1.59 million as an educational subsidy. As a result, the hospital and the University created a joint task force to explore solutions to the Center's continuing fiscal dilemma. On May 23 Governor Hall publicly pledged that he would not allow University Hospital to close its doors. Meanwhile, Children's Hospital was prospering under the umbrella of the Oklahoma Public Welfare Commission, which authorized a $17 million expansion of facilities and equipment *[DO, 6–5–74]*.

The long-standing debate over whether Oklahoma City's private hospitals were carrying their share of indigent patient care, or whether they were using University Hospital as a dumping ground for those who could not pay, continued through the summer of 1974. The Oklahoma Consumer Protection Agency proposed that nonprofit hospitals should be placed on the county tax roles because, by refusing indigent patients, they violated the tax exemption law. As reported by the *Daily Oklahoman*, the agency was referring to a law which stated specifically that "Facilities are required to accept patients without discrimination as to race, color or creed and regardless of the ability to pay" *[DO, 3–12–74]*. Meanwhile, a group of newly graduated physicians criticized local private hospitals for not accepting a greater load of medically indigent patients. At a press conference, Dr. Michael Nichols, the group spokesperson, said: "One thing needs to be made clear about University Hospital: it is not a charity hospital, but a referral center for complex cases and a teaching hospital. Sharing of the medically indigent load must be accomplished in the Oklahoma City Area. Many of us would like to remain in Oklahoma but feel that we cannot do so as long as this uncertainty at University remains the same. University has been twisting slowly in the wind all the years that we have been here. The situation must be satisfactorily resolved before we will return to the state" *[DO, 6–11–74]*.

The graduating physicians recommended that the legislature must: "(1) be responsible for establishing an accountable mechanism for the financing of indigent care; (2) direct the attorney general to enforce the provisions of the state's charitable tax exemption laws; and (3) establish a mechanism for the development of an urban-rural preceptorship program at OU to encourage the rational distribution of health professionals throughout the state" *[DO, 6–11–74]*. Horror stories about seriously ill indigent patients being turned away from private hospital emergency rooms because they could not pay appeared in several state newspapers in the days following this account.

Throughout the spring of 1974 University Hospital administrators had worried about diversion of paying patients to Presbyterian Hospital through too many exceptions to the regents' Site of Practice policy. The University Hospital administrator, Dr. Jephtha Dalston, predicted such practices could cost University Hospital $1 million in revenue in the current fiscal year. The other side of the practice policy disagreement was stated by state Senator Richard Stansberry, who said that "The 'tight' affiliation agreement on patient placement between the College of Medicine and the University Hospital severely hurts the chances of survival of the new Presbyterian Hospital" *[DO, 10–10–74]*.

Controversy over the financing and role of University Hospital continued into the fall as regents did not see why educational funds should be used to underwrite deficits at the hospital. The legislature did not wish to appropriate additional money to assure viability of the hospital, nor did it assume any responsibility for financing medical care for indigents. (In the past, the legislature had decreed that each county was responsible for its own medical care of indigents, but failed to provide enforcement or a mechanism for reimbursing University Hospital). Increasingly, private hospitals sought to limit the amount of unreimbursed care which they provided. However, the alternative, creating a quasi-private public trust to run the hospitals, as advocated by University Hospital director Jephtha Dalston, was resisted by the legislature. Said Dr. Dalston, "The hospital primarily needs front end capital which would assure long-term support for patient care and medical education in the state" *[DO, 10–11–74]*.

In late summer, Senator E. Melvin Porter continued to see a "raid" on private patients by other hospitals, particularly Presbyterian, while the latter's president, Stanton Young, said, "I share Senator Porter's desire to see University Hospital become the major referral hospital in the state" *[DO, 7–23–74]*. An Oklahoma Health Planning Advisory Council report suggested various ways in which tax exempt hospitals might appropriately share in the costs of care of indigent patients, including: (1) relating amount of charity care to the amount of annual tax relief from federal sources and from freedom from ad valorem taxation; (2) abolishing pre–admission deposits to hospitals; (3) a hospital pool of funds for indigent care; (4) assessment of an "in-lieu of" ad valorem tax; and (5) institution of a bed tax *[DO, 10–8–74]*. Needless to say, none of these proposals would see the light of day, although the Joint Interim Legislative Study Committee on Health Care Delivery considered pushing for legislation aimed at requiring individual counties to reimburse University Hospital for treating the medically indigent.

By October, there was a positive omen when the Democratic candidate for governor, David Boren, told citizens, "It is a tragedy if in a state with a budget of $1.5 billion we can't make sure to have enough money to operate this health center" *[DO, 10–15–74]*. The University Hospital board of trustees grew more optimistic about the future as its chair, Julius Bankoff of Tulsa, observed in November that with a modest subsidy, within a few years the hospital "will earn its own way" *[DO, 11–18–74]*.

Thomas N. Lynn, Jr.

In the summer of 1974, Dr. Thomas N. Lynn was named acting dean of the College of Medicine, a decision that was to point the Health Sciences Center in a new direction. Two years later, he would be appointed permanent dean by President Sharp. Mark Allen Everett, chair of the Faculty Board as well as the Department of Dermatology, recalls that:

> President Sharp had spoken to each of us [Lynn and himself] about the possibility of becoming the acting Dean. One morning Dr. Sharp called me and said, 'Mark, you're a fine faculty member, and an administrator with a national reputation as a dermatologist, as well as director of a highly regarded training program, but we have decided to go along with an emphasis on family medicine, rather than specialization, so we have decided to go along with Tom Lynn and Family Practice. When I went to Dr. Lynn the next morning to congratulate him, he replied that he had heard nothing from Dr. Sharp. Interestingly, Tom was not called by the president for over a week, which proved personally embarrassing for him.[40]

Dr. Tom Lynn was a 1955 graduate of the University of Oklahoma College of Medicine who trained at Barnes Hospital in St. Louis, served at the National Heart Institute from 1957–1959, then came to Oklahoma as chief resident in Medicine from 1959 to 1961. He served as professor and chair of the Department of Family Practice, Community Medicine, and Dentistry from 1969 to

1980. As dean, he was respected as a friendly interface between the faculty and the administration. Dr. Merrill recalls that:

> I seldom had the feeling that I would not be supported by Tom Lynn if I really wanted to do something One way or another, the department [Obstetrics-Gynecology] would be able to do what it wanted to do. We didn't hide things; it was just that it was easy to get approval if we needed to do something. . . . I remember when a state salary increase was proposed for all departments by Lynn, and [Provost] Thurman went to the Board of Regents and said that OB–GYN was a bad-behaving department and should receive no faculty raises. Lynn at least tried to get them for us, but, as he put it, 'The president was unable to do anything about it.' Lynn later recalled that the reason Merrill usually gained approval for his plans, was that "they usually were well thought out and benefitted the campus as a whole, and not just his department."[41]

One of the immediate consequences of Tom Lynn's appointment as interim dean was that his position as chair of the search committee for the new provost was terminated. He was replaced by Dr. Oscar Parsons of the Department of Psychiatry. Lynn would serve as acting dean for two years and then as dean until 1980. Meanwhile, Dr. Parsons, whose Ph.D. was from Duke University, came to the University from a post as research psychologist at the Worcester State Hospital in Massachusetts. He served as director of research and vice chair of the Department of Psychiatry for many years, and was a prominent participant on many campus committees and boards.

In July, Dr. G. Rainey Williams was named permanent chair of the Department of Surgery, while Dr. Don H. O'Donoghue, professor emeritus of Ortho-pedic Surgery and Fractures, was appointed chief of the newly created Division of Sports Medicine in his department. President Sharp stated that he hoped that these three appointments—Lynn, Williams, and O'Donoghue—would reassure those who were concerned about leadership and direction at the Health Sciences Center, "particularly at the College of Medicine" *[RM, 13058]*. Sharp also recommended that the name of the College of Health and Allied Health Professions be changed to the College of Health, thus completing the obliteration of the college once headed by Dr. Schottstaedt. Shortly thereafter, Dr. Phillip E. Smith was named permanent dean of the College of Health.

The federal government announced a $3 million grant for construction of the new library on the Health Sciences Center campus in August 1974. At the same time, the Administrative Service Center for the medical complex moved into the old Moon Junior High School at 1100 N. Lindsay.

After several months of study, a faculty committee consisting of Dr. Oscar Parsons, chair, and Dr. Timothy Coussons, Dr. Mark Allen Everett, Dr. Andrea Bircher, and Dr. Donald Counihan recommended the adoption of a Faculty Senate and a Faculty Charter for the Health Sciences Center. Within weeks the proposal was approved by the regents. Dr. Parsons was elected the first chair of the Health Sciences Center Faculty Senate.

On October 25, groundbreaking for the Dean A. McGee Eye Institute was held. The Institute, formed by a group of practicing ophthalmologists (led by Dr. Tullos O. Coston) and community leaders (including Dean McGee), was conceived as an independent but University-related center for ophthalmologic research and patient care, modeled somewhat on the Oklahoma Medical Research Foundation. However, the central concept was that the Institute should also house one of the related departments of the College of Medicine, but be administratively and fiscally independent of the University. This model—a department housed in an institute with its own board of governors, completely separate from the University, but incorporating University departmental funds—was distinctly different from the setting when the Department of Dermatology built a clinic in 1969–1970 using a similar concept but one in which the free-standing facility continued as a full departmental component of the University both for administrative and fiscal management. Although Dr. Mark Allen Everett, head of Dermatology and principal donor of the building, consciously decided to maintain the full University link upon construction of his new building, he later believed that the Eye Institute model lent more fiscal stability and self-determination, while permitting more flexibility and virtually full participation with the University in clinical care and research.

Also in October, a budget for the Health Sciences Center was finally approved by the regents. Dr. Sharp commended associate vice-president Eugene Nordby and auditor Harold Zallen, and acting provost Dr. William Brown "for the time and effort they . . . invested in putting this budget together this year" *[RM, 13153]*. When informed of this commendation, a Health Sciences Center senior faculty member rebutted the praise for the two Norman-campus vice-presidents by stating that: "Nordby and Zallen were very unpleasant characters. Kind of autocratic people who kept saying bad things about the [medical] faculty. I remember Nordby at a meeting saying 'You know, you have had it easy here. . . . You've been able to do whatever you want. . . . That's come to an end now. . . . Henceforth, you'll do what we tell you to do, or you'll be gone.' I remember that very well. He was anti-Medical Center right from the get-go."

October brought about significant changes in administrative personnel at the Health Sciences Center. Due to serious concern and unrest among the deans and faculty of the College of Medicine over what they perceived as lack of appropriate management, Harold Zallen, associate vice-president for administration and finance, and William Jordan, director of financial services and comptroller, were re-assigned by Vice-President Nordby to the Norman Campus. Gary Smith, director of internal audits at the Norman campus, was promoted to chief financial officer at the Health Sciences Center (later changed to vice-president for administrative affairs). During his tenure (1974– 1988), computer technology was introduced to budgetary/financial management systems, and the first investment program for faculty practice funds, whereby proceeds remained within the departments, was implemented. Smith played a critical role in the University's (and later the State Regents') endowed chairs program. Highly effective with an ever-suspicious medical faculty, he came to be highly regarded and well respected because of his expertise and innovative management. In 1988 Smith became executive vice-chancellor and chief operating officer for the state higher education system, but continued to be a strong advocate for the Health Sciences Center.

November saw the Joint Policy Board of University Hospital replace Dr. Robert Bird with Dr. Tom Lynn, and Harold Zollen with hospital administrator Gary Smith. Gary Smith came from the auditor's office on the Norman campus, where he had worked from 1968 to 1974. He served diligently and with distinction for many years when he joined the office of the chancellor for higher education as vice-chancellor for fiscal affairs in 1986. Always effective with an ever-suspicious faculty at the Health Sciences Center, Smith came to be regarded as a faithful colleague in dealing with the Norman campus. His efforts were crucial in the development of the University's endowed chairs program, both at the Health Sciences Center and later from the chancellor's office.

Also in November, the Board of Regents accepted the role of successor trustee of the R. J. Edwards Rural Medicine Trust, and thanked Mr. Archibald C. Edwards, Oklahoma City, for transferring the assets of the Trust to the regents. The approximately 3400 shares of stock in various companies had furnished income for various medical charitable activities of the Edwards family for several years.

In December, the regents approved creation of three new departments at the Health Sciences Center branch in Tulsa: Medicine, Family Practice, and

Psychiatry. A decision on a source for funding these departments was put off until later. The regents completed the year arguing—to the point of impasse—over who should pay for extensions and change orders in the steam and chilled water tunnels on the Oklahoma City campus, especially as they related to the extension of services to Presbyterian Hospital. The question before the Board of Regents was: Should the expense be borne by University Hospital or by Presbyterian Hospital? President Sharp recommended that the University pay for the changes, but the regents defeated his motion. After a period of some-times rancorous debate, Regent Santee declared the voting deadlocked. The matter was ultimately referred to the Facilities Planning Commission.

December 1, 1974, witnessed the long-anticipated opening of Presbyterian Hospital at the southeast corner of N. E. 13th and Lincoln Boulevard in Oklahoma City. As part of the opening, more than 100 patients were transferred from the old, still-handsome hospital that had sat for decades among massive, spreading elms in a largely residential neighborhood at 300 N. W. 12th Street. Combined with the newly opened Everett Tower of University Hospital, the future course of the Health Sciences Center appeared optimistic and bright at this point in its history.

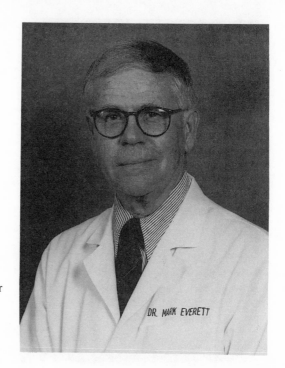

Mark Allen Everett, M.D.,
Regents Professor of
Dermatology, long-time Chair
of the Faculty Board, Chair
of the Department of
Dermatology, and Chief of
Staff of University Hospital.
(AAE)

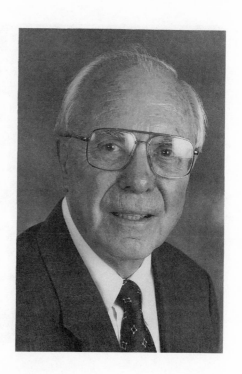

Paul Sharp, Ph.D., President of the
University of Oklahoma. (OUPA)

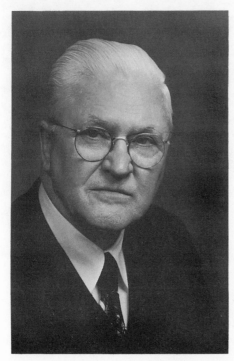

Lloyd Rader, J.S., Director of the
Department of Human Services.
(AAE)

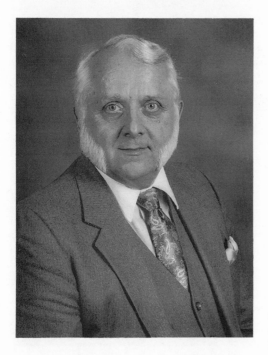

Gordon Deckert, M.D., Chair
of the Department of
Psychiatry. (OUHSC)

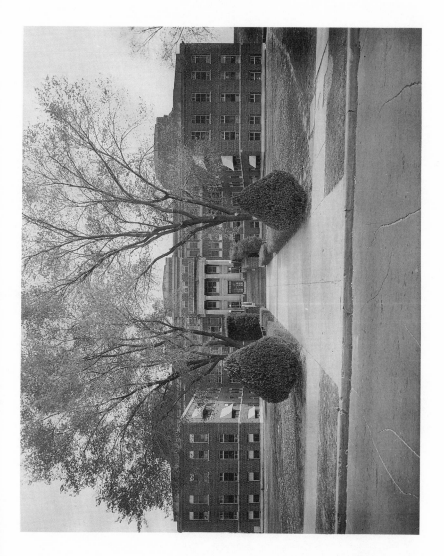

The old Children's Hospital
prior to its transfer to the
Department of Institutions,
Social and Rehabilitative
Services. (DHS)

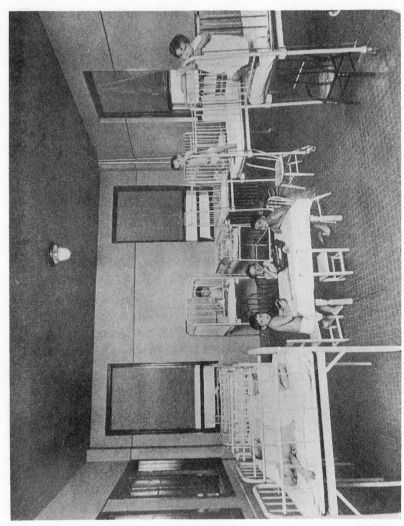

A ward in the old Children's Hospital, ca. 1945. (DHS)

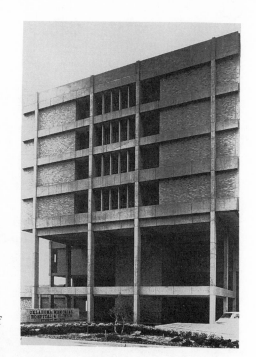

Oklahoma Memorial Hospital and Clinics, Everett Tower, at the time of transfer to an independent Board of Governors. (DHS)

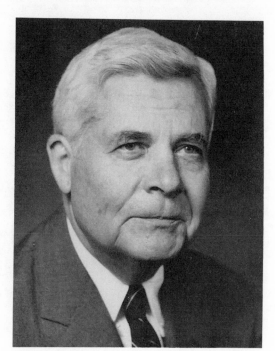

G. Rainey Williams, M.D., Schilling Professor of Surgery, Chair of the Department of Surgery, and frequent Interim Dean of the College of Medicine. (OUHSC)

The Child Study Center, 1973. (DHS)

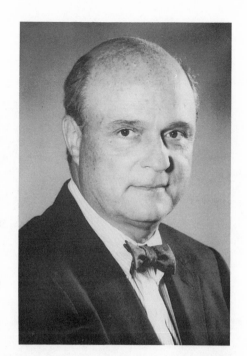

Donald Halverstadt, M.D., Professor of Pediatric Urology, Executive Chief of Staff of the Oklahoma Teaching Hospitals, and member of the University and State Boards of Regents. (OUHSC)

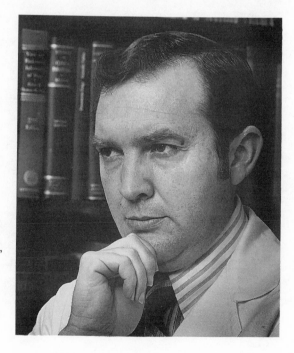

Thomas N. Lynn, Jr., M.D., Professor of Preventive Medicine, Chair of the Department of Family Medicine, and Dean of the College of Medicine. (OUHSC)

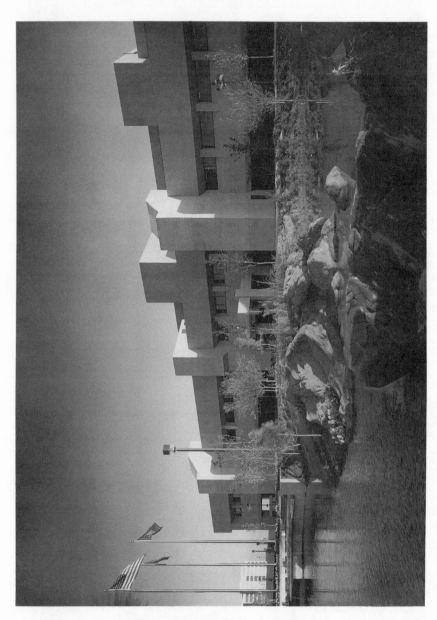

The new Presbyterian Hospital. (OUHSC)

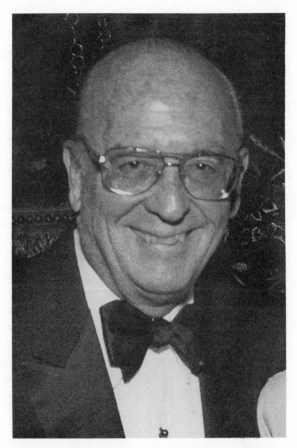

Stanton Young, President of the Presbyterian Foundation.
(OUHSC)

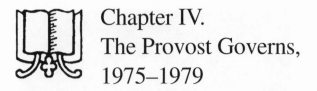

Chapter IV.
The Provost Governs,
1975–1979

 If governance of the University of Oklahoma Health Sciences Center hospitals and the ultimate structure of the faculty's Professional Practice Plan dominated the first half of the decade of the 1970s, a variety of more academic issues monopolized the second half. First among these was the question of the role of the examinations of the National Board of Medical Examiners in the evaluation and promotion of students from the second to the third year of Medical School. Second was the degree-granting controversy of 1977–79 in which the provost approved graduation status for two students who were not recommended by the faculty for the M.D. degree. Third was the issue of national accreditation of the College of Medicine by the Liaison Committee on Medical Education following establishment of a Tulsa College of Medicine.

1975

As nineteen seventy-five dawned, no new emergencies appeared on the University of Oklahoma's agenda. On January 9 Regent Jack Santee acknowledged a communication from Mr. James Monroe, chair of the University Hospital and Clinics Board of Trustees, commending Dr. Tom Lynn's performance since accepting the deanship of the College of Medicine. Monroe also praised Dr. G. Rainey Williams' service as chief of the medical staff for effectively dealing with some very difficult problems at the cash-strapped institution *[RM, 13285]*. Regent Santee verbally agreed with these proclamations and then, in a sudden switching of gears, suggested to the regents that it would be "appropriate to adopt a resolution commending the coaching staff and the 1974 football team for their attainment of the No.1 position in the Associated Press college football poll" *[RM, 13286]*. This resolution was adopted unanimously. Throughout the University's history, few actions were taken by its Board of Regents with more obvious glee, pleasure, and hail-good-fellow-well-met camaraderie than acknowledging the success of its powerful football team. In a motion advanced with somewhat less enthusiasm on the same date, space for the Ophthalmology Clinic was leased from the Oklahoma Medical Research Foundation in the Rogers Building in Oklahoma City.

Also in January, in a matter of considerable importance to University Hospital, the Areawide Health Planning Organization, citing lower cost and faster implementation, voted six to one to locate a controversial "burn center" at Baptist Hospital. The decision was made in spite of the recommendation by its own executive committee and the local health planning agency that University Hospital was the more logical site for the facility. The recommendation was forwarded to the Oklahoma Health Planning Commission, where Baptist Hospital finally won the struggle in a unanimous vote *[DO, 2–27–75]*. Burn centers, like trauma centers, were expensive, money-losing, operations. Since there would be a need for only one such center in any major city, the institution that was awarded a center acquired a certain prestige. Many hospital officials, however, thought that the prestige accruing from a burn center was not great enough to justify the cost of the facility. They invariably lost money, in part because so many indigents were hospitalized in them.

William G. Thurman: "Chairman of the Board"

On April 1, 1975, Dr. William G. Thurman arrived on the University of Oklahoma Health Sciences Center campus and began his duties as provost. Thurman was a graduate of the University of North Carolina, where he played blocking back for Charlie "Choo-choo" Justice. He received his M.D. degree from McGill University Medical School, and served on the faculty at Emory, Tulane, and Cornell Universities. He was former chair of Pediatrics at the University of Virginia, and served as dean at Tulane just prior to his appointment as provost at Oklahoma. His nearly five-year tenure at the Health Sciences Center was characterized by strong, directive leadership, in addition to full utilization of the interest and support of Lloyd Rader, the powerful director of the Department of Human Services.

During Dr. Thurman's administration, fewer campus controversies were reported in the news media and at regents' meetings than under previous administrations, despite his tendency to make major decisions that affected the faculty without consulting them. The lack of public protest to this administrative style was due, in part, to his not avoiding, but accepting, or even seeking, direct confrontation with faculty who opposed his decisions, arguing with them and defusing their impulse to more visible action.

Dr. Thurman attributed the decreased adverse publicity on campus to the fact that: "in 1975 we had three of the regents coming to Oklahoma City for meetings and defusing things before they came up in open meetings. These sessions [of the Medical Center Committee] were very helpful from the standpoint of educating the regents about what was going on here—i.e., why there were some problems with the State Regents. We all agreed that these problems wouldn't make it to the official meetings unless it was a personnel action, which, by state law, *had* to be acted on by the regents. That was why there was officially so little going on in 1975. They gave me plenty of running room in those first eight months."[1]

An additional factor in what, on the surface at least, was decreased controversy at the Health Sciences Center, was the greatly increased stability of the Center's hospitals resulting from the strong support of Lloyd Rader and the Oklahoma Public Welfare Commission, the governing body of the Department of Institutions, Social and Rehabilitative Services. Despite this lack of "problems" reaching the press or the regents, and the positive decisions made by Provost Thurman, tension between the College of Medicine faculty and the provost reached new heights and remained throughout his tenure.

The College of Medicine and the
Oklahoma Medical Research Foundation

From February through April 1975 the Faculty Board, through both a temporary task force and in deliberations during regular meetings, discussed the relationship of the College of Medicine to the Oklahoma Medical Research Foundation, and the need for a formal affiliation agreement between the College and the Foundation. There was a general feeling among the majority of the faculty and College administration that the Foundation was getting much more out of the relationship with the College than the reverse.

The Oklahoma Medical Research Foundation (OMRF) had originated from discussions of members of the School of Medicine faculty and the Medical Alumni Association, including Drs. John Lamb, Onis Hazel, Fred Woodson, and Dean Mark R. Everett, with suggestions by University President George Cross, about the need for alumni support to the College of Medicine. In June 1946 they incorporated the OMRF with a board of directors, consisting of twelve members from the alumni association and eight members from the business community, with the purpose and intent of "cooperating with the School of Medicine of the University of Oklahoma to the fullest extent for the mutual benefit of such School and this Corporation."[2] The bylaws established as ex-officio directors, the president of the University, the president of the Alumni Association, the dean of the School of Medicine, the director of the Research Institute, the chairman of the School Research Committee, and the "superintendents of any affiliated hospitals."[3]

On December 6, 1951, the Executive Committee of the Board of Directors of the OMRF established the policy that "20 percent of net undesignated funds" would be available for research by the general faculty.[4] Fifteen years later in 1965, an aggressive minority of the Board of Directors managed to have the bylaws of the organization amended so that all ex-officio positions on the Board were eliminated, in essence disassociating the OMRF from the School of Medicine. Since 1969 the Faculty Board had been concerned that there was no agreement of affiliation between what were now two dissimilar organizations; instead there was only a limited agreement regarding in-patient beds (the OMRF had a small in-patient oncology unit at the time). Instead of cooperation, there was frequently indifference and/or animosity between the OMRF and the full-time faculty of the College of Medicine *[FBM, 10–16–75]*. Contributing to this animosity were the rules for faculty appointments of OMRF scientists, problems in Biochemistry (operating as a joint department, but one in which an OMRF employee functioned as chair), an obvious emphasis on developing the OMRF section while neglecting the College of Medicine faculty and its teaching function, the handling of overhead money from grants and contracts to faculty, and faculty reimbursement policies.

On February 14 Acting Provost William E. Brown directed the College of Medicine to prepare, with representatives from the OMRF, an appropriate and comprehensive agreement. An ad hoc Faculty Board committee concluded that: (1) the academic stature of OMRF staff was dependent on College affiliation; (2) the movement from competitive grants to contracts was regarded as unfavorable scientifically; and (3) administrative arrangements vis-a-vis academic responsibilities were unsatisfactory from Board to employee level.

By April 1975 Dr. Brown's successor, Dr. William Thurman, had arrived. He was not anxious to formalize an affiliation agreement quickly, even though a recent LCME accreditation report had criticized the lack of such a document. In March 1976 Thurman resisted closure on the issue until a "consultant report commissioned by the Executive Committee of the OMRF" had been received, ignoring the fact that as provost he was responsible for assuring that there was an affiliation agreement with the OMRF, as with all institutions on the campus at which faculty and/or students worked.[5] Finally, in August, Dr. Thurman directed Dean Lynn to prepare personnel "change of status" papers for all OMRF faculty with less than 50 percent of their salaries from the University, modifying their titles with the prefix "research." (The Dean, as part of a general effort to "straighten out the whole business of tenure, adjunct appointments, and what you could and could not use state funds for," had already ordered "volunteer" titles for Drs. Tang, Carubelli, Carpenter, Bradford, and Alaupovic on April 22.) However, Dr. Thurman then stated, "It would be my intention not to forward it for regential action" until "we can develop an adequate affiliation agreement" *[FBM, 8–14–75]*. It seemed that he wanted to use these title changes as leverage in the negotiations! Turmoil over this issue continued on both the OMRF staff and the University of Oklahoma faculty for more than a year. In August 1976 an affiliation agreement was still unsigned. The most pressing issue of whether overhead payments on grants and contracts would be shared, and if not, in which institution they would be placed, was one which was never resolved.

In March 1975, there seemed to be an excessive number of students in Health Sciences Center graduate programs applying for admission to the College of Medicine. The Faculty Board approved a policy of "encouraging completion of the graduate degree program, and that it will not normally consider students currently enrolled in a graduate program on the HSC campus for admission to the College of Medicine unless the degree towards which they are working will be awarded by the end of the academic year in which they apply" *[FBM, 3–11–75]*. This action was largely in response to basic science department concerns that there would be attrition of their graduate programs if such students could be admitted to Medical School prior to completion of their graduate degrees.

In March the University of Oklahoma Board of Regents approved the issue of $6.5 million in Utility System Revenue Bonds, as well as the design and plans for both the College of Nursing building and the new Health Sciences Center Library. They also gave emeritus status to three retired volunteer faculty members who provided devoted and long-term service as professors in the College of Medicine: Forrest M. Lingenfelter, Surgery; Gerald Rogers, Gynecology and Obstetrics; and Harry Wilkins, Neurosurgery.

Also in March, a revision of the bylaws of the faculty of the College of Medicine was approved. The major change was placement of the Curriculum Committee and the Curriculum Implementation Committee under the Academic Council. The Academic Council was a new faculty organization conceived by Dean Dennis who, upon its creation, appointed Dr. Tom Bruce as chair. Bruce was an internist faculty member recruited by Dr. Dennis who later followed him to Arkansas when he served as dean of that Medical School. The new bylaws also incorporated the Site of Practice and disposition-of-income rules of the regents *[RM, 13333–6]*. Subsequently, the provost announced that the regents had withdrawn approval of the bylaws, saying that since they were merely internal rules of governance, they did not need to be approved by the regents, and hence appropriately should be subjected to "withdrawal of regential approval." This decision precipitated another conflict between the provost and faculty of the College of Medicine. In a letter to Dr. Mark Everett, Thurman explained that the "withdrawal" phrase "merely means that the Regents will not approve such documents in the future." This was, according to Thurman, because "some of them were not adequate documents and some were in conflict with overall university policy. If anyone has interpreted it (withdrawal of approval) as Machiavellian in intent, I would merely reassure them that he has been dead for many years."[6] Nonetheless, the University regents, on many occasions, were very concerned with the exact wording of passages in the bylaws of the medical faculty, especially with regard to Site-of-Practice, Professional Practice Plan funds, and fiscal oversight. In fact, the regents reworded and revised the bylaws on many subsequent occasions.

Tulsa, Again

Regent Jack Santee announced in March that the mayor of Tulsa had written him urging construction of facilities for the Tulsa branch of the College of Medicine near the Children's Medical Center. This proposal regarding facilities, like those related to faculty, student selection, etc., all reflected a general view held by the Tulsa medical community that the entire Tulsa operation was in essence a free-standing and independent institution. In fact, when the initial administrative appointment was made at Tulsa, Martin Fitzpatrick was named dean of the College of Medicine in Tulsa, and it was assumed that he was in no way subordinate to the dean in Oklahoma City. This had been affirmed at the Faculty Board meeting of September 17, 1974, following a vigorous debate in which Dr. James Merrill advocated that the Oklahoma City campus have no relationship with the Tulsa operation, and urged that the school apply as an independent institution for full, free-standing accreditation.[7] By January 1975 five Tulsa branch departments had been established: Medicine, Surgery, Pediatrics, Family Medicine, Obstetrics and Gynecology; and Psychiatry, through recommendation of the Tulsa administration and concurrence by the Faculty Board. A Department of Obstetrics came after prolonged faculty debate and strong opposition by Dr. Merrill. The Faculty Board recommended to the president and to the regents that other disciplines be subordinate to their corresponding departments in Oklahoma City, as well as the rules for selection (admission) of candidates who would attend the Tulsa branch *[FBM, 1–29–75]*. President Sharp responded to the continued pressure for construction of a facility in Tulsa by emphasizing that the establishment of the Tulsa branch was only conceived as a low-cost method of increasing the number of physicians, and that submission of a request for federal matching funds for construction of a facility was not "an alternative which we as a University can consider unless all construction and land acquisition costs can be paid from resources outside higher education" *[RM, 13365]*. The regents voted to include the Tulsa facility in the Capital Construction Plan under these circumstances, with Regent Braly repeating that a request for federal matching funds could be withdrawn by the regents at any time.

The Tulsa actions were taken at what was Regent Santee's last meeting. President Sharp congratulated him on his service, especially for the "time, energy, and leadership [he] devoted to the Health Sciences Center during the troubled times on that campus" *[RM, 13366]*. The consensus on the Oklahoma City campus was that Mr. Santee had worked primarily for the establishment and expansion of an independent Tulsa operation. He was a leader in the development and enforcement of the faculty Practice Plan and the Site of Practice policy, because of his belief that any private practice by faculty physicians was intrinsically bad, especially if physician income was enhanced thereby. Neither of these "examples of leadership" endeared him to the faculty in Oklahoma City. Dr. Thurman recalled that when he was interviewed for the job of provost, Santee expressed the need for a "strong provost who could bring the faculty under control."[8] Santee was reputed to never change his mind about a subject once he had come to a conclusion. He believed that the faculty needed firm direction, especially following what he perceived as a series of weak administrators on the Oklahoma City campus.

In April the Facilities Planning Committee under Regent Tom Brett recommended that the construction grant application for Tulsa be withdrawn. Regent Braly announced that the State Senate and the House of Representatives had passed a resolution asking that the application be withdrawn, and he moved for approval. The motion failed, with Braly and Bell voting yes, and Brett, Mitchell, and Bailey voting no *[RM, 13400]*. That same month, the State Regents for Higher Education included construction of the Tulsa Facility as priority three in the Capital Improvements Plan, if federal funds were available "to underwrite the major portion of the cost of construction and other non-state funds being required for matching the federal funds" *[RM, 13411]*. Governor Boren strongly opposed the building of any facility for medicine in Tulsa, pointing out that the institution had only twenty students and that over a million dollars in state funds was being sought. This issue of "independence" would come to a head later in the year when the Liaison Committee for Medical Education (the accrediting authority for medical schools) made it clear, on a pre-accreditation visit, that: (1) there was no such thing as a free-standing "clinical years only" medical school; (2) the dean in Oklahoma City must be responsible for the facilities and programs in both Oklahoma City and in Tulsa; and (3) the dean in Tulsa must report through the dean in Oklahoma City. Clearly the Tulsa College of Medicine was to be a branch of the Oklahoma City College. The issue regarding control of individual departments in Tulsa was not settled until the Faculty Board, acting on the recommendations of an ad hoc committee chaired by Dr. R. T. Coussons, approved a plan that set down several guidelines, including provisions that: (1) although separate departments in the six major clinical disciplines would be established and would report through the Tulsa dean, the other disciplines would, "in concert" with the Tulsa dean, report through their respective heads in Oklahoma City; and (2) a vice chair for Tulsa would be appointed *[FBM, 1–6–75]*. These actions settled once and for all the issue of independence for the Tulsa College of Medicine, which now would be a branch of the College in Oklahoma City.

Meanwhile, at the April 1975 Faculty Board meeting, there was general dissatisfaction with the concept of "conjoint" departments with the College of Dentistry in the basic science disciplines. A task force led by Dr. Solomon Papper, distinguished professor of Medicine, recommended to the Faculty Board that the issue be reconsidered and that basic science departments reside exclusively in the College of Medicine, reporting only to its dean. It recommended that instead of joint departments, the basic science departments, through the dean, develop contracts with the Dental College for whatever educational services to dentistry were needed in the basic sciences.[9]

The Admissions Board

In May a change in the composition of the Medical School Admissions Board was adopted at the recommendation of the College of Medicine faculty and administration. This was in response to Senate Resolution 22, which specified that Admissions Board membership should be apportioned among the state's congressional districts. This bill was stimulated by the continued distrust of some practicing physicians around the state regarding the admissions decisions made by full-time faculty. At the March 11 Faculty Board meeting, a decision had been made to computerize all cognitive data regarding applicants (MCAT scores, college grades, interview scores, etc), and following the interview, rank-order all students using the computerized numerical data, rather than merely employing subjective impressions in selecting students. The full Admissions Board would then receive a printout of the numerical values. Also, the presence of students as voting members on the Board had been the subject of complaints from some practicing physician members who maintained that there was no point in having students participate in the interview process, especially if they reflected immature and unpopular values.

At the May regents' meeting, following consideration of Senate Resolution 22 and after a heated discussion, it was voted to increase the number of Oklahoma State Medical Society nominees from twelve to twenty-four. The newly constituted Admissions Board consisted of ten full-time faculty, ten volunteer faculty, ten student members, and twenty-four members selected from throughout the state, four from each of the six congressional districts. This proved to be an unwieldy and relatively nonfunctional group, with little more than propaganda value, since, except for the full-time faculty members, few physicians were willing or able to devote the many hours required during working days to the interview process. As a result, selections were made by an executive or "steering" committee. The full Board only reviewed the steering committee's actions, and then voted to extend or to deny a place in the incoming class to those who had been recommended to the Board.

Throughout the history of the College of Medicine, an additional irritant regarding admissions was continual pressure on the dean, as well as on members of its Admissions Board, to admit friends and relatives of politicians and prominent citizens. Dr. Rainey Williams acknowledged this problem when, years later, he stated, "You can't separate the selection of medical students from politics, and for that reason, the elaborate process that makes certain that no one gets in *just* because of political pressure is probably necessary. I don't like it. I think we waste a fair amount of a medical practitioner's time going back and forth to meetings—but we have gone as far as it's reasonable to go to insure fairness in the admissions process.[10]

An affiliation agreement with the Tulsa area hospitals was also passed by the Board of Regents in May. Institutions included in the agreement were

Hillcrest, St. John's, St Francis, and later, the Children's Medical Center *[RM, 13466]*. The document of affiliation carefully catered to all the various sensitivities involved. An additional agreement with Griffin Memorial Hospital in Norman was made for provision of resident medical staff in Medicine, Radiology, and Surgery, an action that would partially insulate the University hospitals from a continual procession of criminals to the Health Sciences Center, since the Griffin medical unit was designated as the site of first consultation for Department of Correction patients.

In College of Medicine Faculty Board actions in May, the Curriculum Design Committee was removed from the jurisdiction of the Academic Council, which had rejected almost all its proposals. The Curriculum Committee was restored to the Faculty Board which, as the executive body of the faculty, was charged with supervision of the curriculum, setting of admission standards, and establishing the criteria for graduation.

The new University Hospital throughout the spring and summer of 1975 had experienced capacity admissions to its wards, especially to the special care units. This had led to the hospital frequently being on "divert" status, forcing ambulances wishing to bring patients—usually indigent—to the University Hospital to take them instead to other area hospitals. On July 23 partly in response to the February request of the University Hospital Board of Trustees to consider county ad valorem tax collections as a source for indigent care dollars, yet another examination was undertaken of the funding problem for indigent health care by the Legislative Committee on Health Care Delivery, headed by Senator Al Terrill of Lawton. A recommendation to use 10 percent of federal revenue sharing funds for charity care was made. Needless to say, this proposal would not see the light of day in the subsequent session. In addition, the increasing amount of uncompensated care to inmates of the state correctional system placed an intolerable burden on University Hospital— i.e., costs estimated at over $435,000 per year. A proposal to force the Department of Corrections to pay for the health care of its inmates also failed to receive support in the legislature.

University Hospital Administrator Dr. Jephtha Dalston resigned his position in May, effective September 1, to become director of the University of Michigan Hospitals. In reviewing his tenure as administrator at Oklahoma, he indicated that the major accomplishment during his administration was the creation of an independent board of trustees for University Hospital, partly stimulated by the need to "keep the hospital functioning" during the 1973–74 period of insolvency. According to Dalton, the of lack of reimbursement for indigent patients, combined with legislative scrutiny that was often adversarial and intrusive, were two elements that unfavorably marked his years in Oklahoma City *[DO, 5–26–75]*.

Appointments at University Hospital dominated regents' meetings during the summer of 1975. Dr. Stanley Deutsch succeeded Dr. G. Rainey Williams as chief of staff, and Dr. Don O'Donoghue became president of the hospital's Board of Trustees in June. The following month, Donald L. Brown was named acting administrator of the Hospital. In August, the appointment of a new University Hospital administrator, Mr. Bruce Perry, a pharmacist and administrator from Columbus Medical Center in Columbus, Georgia, was announced.

A drive by University Hospital and its Radiology Department to be the first in the state to acquire a linear accelerator for treatment of cancer gained support of the legislature for an additional $1.9 million in appropriated funds for this purpose, following intense lobbying by the Radiology faculty at the capitol during the spring and summer. This coup was not without controversy, however, as Representative Jerry Smith of Tulsa alleged that "the hospital administration and trustees have put a $550,000 ceiling on the amount they will spend on the building and plan to divert $200,000 for other capital improvements" *[DO, 8–6–75]*. Don Brown, now ensconced as acting hospital administrator, denied the charges. The accusation by Smith was another example of legislative misinformation and micromanagement of the Health Sciences Center, but the successful achievement of the accelerator by the facility demonstrated the power and effectiveness of faculty lobbying when everyone acted in concert.

In July Provost William Thurman received notification by the Liason Committee for Medical Education that the University of Oklahoma College of Medicine had received full accreditation following the recent survey visit. At the same time, a search for a dean of the College of Nursing came to a close when Gloria Smith, a highly regarded faculty member who had served as interim dean of the College, was named the Health Sciences Center's first Black dean. She would later fill the important post of director of the welfare department in the state of Michigan.

The search for a dean of the College of Medicine also ended in July when the names of three candidates were forwarded to the provost by a search committee under chair Dr. Richard T. Coussons. From these names, Dr. Thomas N. Lynn, the acting dean since the previous July, was selected as permanent dean. Also in July, the regents named Dr. Timothy Coussons to replace W. O. Smith as vice chair of the Department of Medicine, while Dr. Martha Ferretti was named acting chair of Physical Therapy, with the rank of instructor *[RM, 13524]*. At the same time, various leases were approved to house activities for which facilities were not yet completed on the campus—i.e., Family Counseling and the Child Development Center, Financial Services, and Shipping and Receiving *[RM, 13532]*. Also in July the Board of Regents commended Dr. George Garrison, retiring as Secretary of the faculty board, for his many decades of service to the Health Sciences Center. The regents also placed the Psychology Intern Program in the graduate programs of the College of Medicine.

The Faculty Board was busy at this time debating the position of a proposed director of Emergency Services for University Hospital, and going on record with a recommendation that the director should be responsible to a College of Medicine department rather than to the hospital administrator. The Board also voted that Dr. George Garrison be made a permanent ex-officio member. In a final action, Dean Lynn thanked the Faculty Board chair, Dr. Mark Allen Everett, and vice-chair, Dr. James Merrill, for "helping him through an exceedingly trying academic year" *[FBM, 7–1–75]*.

For many years, the Health Sciences Center administration had sought a pedestrian concourse over busy N.E. 13th Street in Oklahoma City to protect personnel, patients, and family members intent on going from Children's or University Hospital to the Veterans Administration Hospital on the north side of the busy, four-lane road. Senator Henry Bellmon announced in August that he had successfully obtained much of the federal funding for the concourse. When architectural plans for the project were made public, several faculty members commented favorably on the attractive, glass-covered design that would prove a welcome contrast to the white, metal-encased tubes that crisscrossed the campus and looked for all the world like passenger cars on a speeding train. The structure was one of several walkways that would be built during the heyday of Lloyd Rader to connect the Center's hospitals and other buildings.

In early September 1975 Dr. William J. Felts retired as chair of the Department of Anatomy. Later the same month, Dr. Robert A. Patnode relinquished the acting chair of the Department of Microbiology and Immunology, which he had held while the permanent chair, L. Vernon Scott, was in New Zealand *[RM, 13577]*.

During October, the University Board of Regents discussed the possibility of modifying plans for the Biomedical Sciences building to reduce the space (the entire fourth floor) allocated to the Department of Pathology, permitting them to retain some space in the old College of Medicine building, and devoting

7,000 square feet of the floor space to the Department of Psychiatry and Behavioral Sciences. President Sharp and the Facilities Planning Committee recommended the plan, and Regent Tom Brett moved for approval. Dr. Robert O'Neal, chair of Pathology, asked to address the regents and stated that such action would be "disastrous" for the department. Provost Thurman pointed out that a discussion of the project had been going on for some time, and if the changes would cause "irreparable" damage, he would ask the regents for a change in the plan. The regents then approved preparation of plans for the change *[RM, 13610]*. As it turned out, Psychiatry did not occupy the fourth-floor space, but accepted a much smaller area on a lower floor, and that for a period of only two years.[11]

On a simple tenure recommendation in October, regents voted against tenure for an assistant professor of nursing, not because of the performance of the individual, but because of regent "dissatisfaction with the current tenure format, its inadequate screening process, and its total absence of post-tenure review" *[RM, 13616]*. Regent Dee Replogle articulated the view that tenure in the modern age should incorporate post-tenure review and renewal. Until such changes were adopted, he opposed granting tenure to anybody. President Sharp spoke in favor of tenure as currently understood in all major universities in the United States. Regent Neustadt indicated that the administration should bring forward recommendations for strengthening the tenure process as soon as possible *[RM, 13618]*. Throughout the period covered in this history, tenure was a recurrent subject. Some of the faculty and many administrators and legislators thought that the practice was inappropriate in the modern age, while most faculty regarded tenure not as a license for inaction and laziness, but a protection for unpopular views. At Oklahoma, there were frequent references to Vernon Parrington, the first English professor and football coach who was forced out because of his political views and personal behavior, although he was a distinguished, indeed nationally famous, writer.

Also in October, final plans for the campus Library and Learning Center were approved, and the regents, upon recommendation of President Sharp, approved a reorganization of the Health Sciences Center administration, whereby the budgetary and fiscal supervisory functions of the vice president for administration and finance were transferred to the office of the provost. Included were Operations, Budget, Purchasing, Personnel, and Computing Services for the Health Sciences Center campus. For all of these functions, the provost would report directly to the president, as did all the vice presidents for their respective areas. The regents approved the motion unanimously. In effect, the provost now had the same powers and responsibility as he had prior to the fiscal crisis of 1972–1973, when the position was that of executive vice president for health science affairs, but now without the title *[RM, 13629]*. A week later on October 23 the faculty expressed its appreciation to President Sharp for the confidence he exhibited in the Health Sciences Center administration that this reorganization implied.

In November Governor David Boren questioned whether the meetings of the University of Oklahoma Board of Regents were completely in accord with the "open meeting laws of the State," and emphasized that executive sessions that were closed to the public "will be permitted only for the purposes of discussing the employment, hiring, appointment, promotion, demotion, disciplining or resignation of any public officer or employee" *[RM, 13649]*. The regents determined that the discussion in executive session on October 16 concerning the appointment of Dr. Gordon Atkinson as dean of the Graduate College met the requirements of this law. President Sharp said, "Within the current climate of our society, it may not be possible to hold an executive session within the law without bringing forth some public criticism. There are simply too many groups with too many causes to have everyone agree" *[RM, 13651]*.

Also in November, the Departments of Medical Technology and Cytotechnology were combined within the College of Allied Health Professions (later, during a time of fiscal austerity, both departments would be abolished) and a "two-plus-two" program—two years at Norman and two in Oklahoma City—in Medical Technology was approved by the State Regents for Higher Education. At the same time, the financial agreement with the Oklahoma Medical Research Foundation was amended to provide that all money paid to University employees would be paid to the University and then transmitted to the employees, not unlike the Professional Practice agreements implemented the previous year *[RM, 13660]*.

In December the University discontinued all day care operations at the Health Sciences Center, primarily because (1) the newly mandated minimum wage scale far exceeded the salary scales in effect at other day care centers, and (2) far too many of the children at the day care center were under the age of two years, greatly increasing the costs of providing care.

Also in December, Dr. Martin Fitzpatrick completed his tenure as dean of the Tulsa Medical College. In a final December action, at a ceremony attended by Oklahoma City business and Health Sciences Center leaders, the Dean A. McGee Eye Institute was formally opened. President Sharp welcomed the new institution to the "University Family" as another important step in the creation of "the most comprehensive health sciences center in the United States" *[DO, 12–5–75]*.

1976

The new year dawned, not surprisingly, in the midst of another fiscal crisis, as the University of Oklahoma Board of Regents, in an "impromptu, unannounced meeting" on January 31 approved a plan to request tuition hikes if the funding needs of the University were not met by legislative appropriations. The *Daily Oklahoman* criticized "the lack of an appropriate announcement for the meeting as provided by State statute" *[DO, 2–8–76]*. At the same impromptu meeting, the Health Sciences Center's Regional Medical Program was renewed for another year.

At their regular January meeting, the regents purchased property east of the Dermatology building on N.E. 13th Street for "future purposes," specifically one of the following: (1) use by the Department of Dermatology for a parking lot or future building expansion, (2) functions at the "provost's residence," including parking, just north of Dermatology on N.E. 14th Street, or (3) use by the Faculty House as parking space. The purchase was finalized in March, at a cost of $135,000, through the University of Oklahoma Development Authority. The property had been owned by a state agency head with lofty plans for developing a facility to function as a health maintenance organization. The official, whose plan might well have succeeded ten years later, encountered financial difficulties which forced him to sell the property to the highest bidder.

Also in January, Dr. Irwin Brown resigned as director of Postgraduate Education, while Mr. Dan Macer, recently retired administrator of the Veterans Administration Hospital, was hired as a full-time faculty member for medical administration in the Department of Family Practice and Community Medicine and Dentistry. Meanwhile, in Tulsa, the fourth and fifth floors of the Midway Office Building were leased for use by the Tulsa Medical College.

Local newspapers reported in early February that the Federal Bureau of Investigation was completing a background check on former University of Oklahoma Department of Psychiatry Chair Louis J. "Jolly" West, who had examined heiress Patty Hearst in Los Angeles in preparation for her criminal trial *[DO, 2–1–76]*. The "kidnapping" of the daughter of the heir to the Hearst family fortune, and her subsequent involvement with the Black Panther movement, including participation in a bank robbery, would prove to be the major news story of the year.

The February meeting of the Board of Regents saw responsibility for the Health Sciences Center's preceptorship program moved from the office of the dean to the Department of Family Practice at the request of Dean Thomas

Lynn, who had been head of the Family Practice program since 1972. At this same time, Dr. Lynn, who had served as interim dean of the College of Medicine, was welcomed as the new permanent dean. Also in February, regents approved renovation plans of the College of Medicine to house the $3.2 million grant received by Dr. Fletcher Taylor from the National Heart and Lung Institute to conduct studies on thrombosis and related blood disorders. Simultaneously, renovation of quarters in the old "A" wing of University Hospital for the Thrombosis-Coagulation Laboratories was approved. This program project grant under Dr. Taylor and others would be a centerpiece of the College's research effort until the mid-1980s when the program was transferred to the Oklahoma Medical Research Foundation.

In March, a contract for construction of the Library and Learning Resources Center was let by regents for $5.1 million. The board also approved the move of the Breast Cancer Detection Center from leased space in the Oklahoma Medical Research Foundation to the nearby Presbyterian Office Building. In a final March action, regents adopted a new clinical curriculum for students that had been approved by the Faculty Board the previous month. Additionally, a required third-year rotation in Family Medicine as part of a fifteen-week ambulatory care experience was initiated for the first time.

The College Budget and Tuition

A petition from first- and second-year medical students objecting to proposed tuition increases initiated a prolonged discussion of fees at the April Board of Regents meeting. As Regent Mack Braly stated in a letter directed to the State Regents for Higher Education, "I am sure that you and other members of your Board are aware . . . of the inescapable fact that the relative quality of the instructional programs available to students at the University has deteriorated during the last fifteen years when compared to other major state-supported universities across the country." He defended the proposed tuition raise as an attempt to permit a "stand-still" budget and prevent further erosion of program quality. It was also proposed that one percent of the "E & G" budget (i.e., appropriated state funds) should be allotted for scholarships. "The total cost of educating a medical or dental student at the Health Sciences Center," declared the regents, "is in excess of $11,500 per year . . . and is quite modest compared with the national average cost of $19,000." (At the same time, a Faculty Board study showed that the cost of educating a student on the Tulsa campus was nearly $23,000 per year.) "We must assume from the fact that Oklahoma is providing the second lowest state appropriation per student in the nation, that the people intend for the students to bear a greater portion of our educational costs," concluded the regents' statement *[RM, 13866–7]*.

At the same April meeting, two other actions were taken by the regents: Dr. Wilson D. Steen was named acting head of the Department of Family Practice and Community Medicine and Dentistry, and a new Equal Employment Opportunity policy was adopted for the University to conform with federal guidelines *[RM, 13891]*. In an April 16 decision by the Health Sciences Center Faculty Board, it was decreed that all "promotion actions" for the Tulsa branch must come through the College of Medicine Promotions Committee. To ensure that Tulsa was represented on the committee, a faculty member from the Tulsa campus would be appointed in the future.

Regents Challenge the Chancellor

By May, the serious underfunding at the University of Oklahoma and the Health Sciences Center during the previous fiscal year had been frequently commented on by the Board of Regents. As though to make matters worse, E. T. Dunlap, chancellor of the State Regents for Higher Education, announced that he planned to fund selectively, at a higher cost per student, several of the state's small colleges. The purpose of this action, in the words of the chancellor, was "to make them better" *[RM, 13916]*. The two comprehensive universities with graduate programs were to receive less funding in order for the chancellor to accomplish his stated goals (goals, apparently, that could be achieved only by the small institutions, or at least requiring the assistance of the state senators and representatives within whose constituencies these schools resided). The University regents and President Sharp challenged this policy, to the great chagrin of Chancellor Dunlap, who always expected "his" institutions to fall in line when he issued a pronouncement. At the May meeting of the University of Oklahoma Regents, President Sharp expressed dismay at the severe constriction of the Health Sciences Center budget caused by the chancellor's policy, as well as the overall poor funding prospects for the University in general for the 1976–1977 fiscal year. Regent Dee Replogle issued a detailed statement about the inadequate funding of the University and suggested that there were ways to fund it at a level which would provide Oklahomans with the educational opportunities that were already available to citizens in Kansas, Colorado, Missouri, and the other schools in the Big 8 Conference. In Replogle's opinion, it was the responsibility of the Board of Regents to attain this goal.

Following Regent Replogle's statement, President Sharp said, "The current legislature and Governor Boren appear prepared to give higher education its largest appropriation increase in history" but not enough to correct the "appallingly low level in comparison to those of other states." After a dramatic pause, he continued:

> It is important to note that the Chancellor, E. T. Dunlap, has not historically shared this commitment. . . . Rather than programming gradients of quality into the State system of higher education, the Chancellor has pursued a course of educational socialism through which he has sought the arbitrary equating of the caliber of instruction at all state institutions. As in the case of most efforts at egalitarianism, the result has not been to raise all institutions to a uniform standard of excellence, but rather to pressure universities and colleges to move towards a common mediocrity. . . . It is frustrating indeed to attempt to upgrade programs, particularly in vital fields such as health care, only to have those efforts frustrated by an individual such as the Chancellor, who shows neither sympathy, nor apparent understanding, for any program dedicated to quality" *[RM, 13917]*.

The *Daily Oklahoman* reported that an annoyed Dunlap replied: "The writer of this statement, whoever he or she is, obviously is not familiar with [my] record of development of higher education in the last 15 years" *[DO, 5-14-76]*. Many Oklahomans who agreed with the criticisms of the University of Oklahoma regents and its president believed that it was a mistake to openly attack the chancellor because, in the words of Provost William Thurman years later, "you never won with Dunlap. You had to out-calm him, and out-smooth him, and make him lose *his* temper." In Thurman's opinion, "Paul Sharp wanted Oklahoma to be the equivalent of [the University of] North Carolina—the flagship of the state. He couldn't see that he would never overcome the E. T. Dunlap hurdle in Oklahoma. And he never did. Dunlap beat him out, in the final sense."[12]

At their June meeting, Dunlap's State Regents for Higher Education approved fee and tuition increases averaging 17 percent system-wide. And in a peculiar wrench of logic, he garnered a measure of revenge over the University of Oklahoma by increasing tuition for medical and dental students by some 74 percent—a dollar figure of $1,200 per student! *[DO, 6–11–76]*.

While these political shenanigans were playing out at the state level, the Health Sciences Center Faculty Board on May 25 ended the long-term confusion regarding authority of the Academic Council and its committees by adopting the report of an ad hoc committee, chaired by Dr. Gordon Deckert, which recommended that all committees and boards of the faculty report directly to the Faculty Board. This included the Graduate and Undergraduate Education Committees, and, upon motion of Dr. George Garrison, secretary of the Faculty Board, the Academic Council as well. A poll of all Health Sciences Center departments resulted in a unanimous verdict that the Council should be reduced from forty to no more than nine members. Several departments felt that the Council was superfluous and should be eliminated altogether. Simultaneously, an ad hoc committee composed of Drs. Deckert, Traub, and Weiss advised the Faculty Board that there was also unanimous agreement that, considering the size of the faculty, student enrollment, and budget of the college, representation of the College of Medicine on the Faculty Senate was too small *[FBM, 5–25–76]*. The provost and deans however, considered the Faculty Senate to be just that—i.e., equal numbers of representatives from each of the colleges, regardless of their size and influence.

At the June regents meeting, the retirement of Raymond D. Crews, longtime director of operations at the Health Sciences Center, was announced, effective October 1. Also retiring was Professor of Biochemistry Alton C. Kurtz, who had for over thirty years walked daily from his home near Shepard Mall to the Health Sciences Center campus, a distance of more than three miles! In other June actions, Oscar Parsons, professor and frequent vice chair of Psychiatry, was named a George Lynn Cross Research Professor, while Mr. Walter Neustadt Jr. completed his 1969–1976 term as a regent, including one year as president of the Board. He was given a well deserved accolade by the Board and the University administration. The regents also adopted an Affirmative Action Plan dedicated to increasing employment of women and minorities at the University as well as at the Health Sciences Center.

On June 19 the *Daily Oklahoman* reported that the Oklahoma State Bureau of Investigation was investigating expenditure of University Hospital funds for private purposes by its director, Bruce Perry. This report reflected the lack of trust between Perry, who worked for the independent Hospital Authority, and the Department of Human Services and its director, Lloyd Rader. As a result, Perry resigned and exercised a long-term offer of a position with Harry Near at Presbyterian Hospital.

Also in June, a decision by University Hospital Trustees to except the chemo-therapy program from the Site of Practice agreement, permitting its physicians to utilize facilities at Presbyterian Hospital, was criticized on the House floor by Representative Hanna Atkins *[DO, 6–28–76]*. Atkins also found fault with Health Sciences Center reports that the availability of minorities in nearly all fields of specialized medicine was highly limited, which would make reaching proposed faculty hiring goals extremely difficult. In spite of the widely publi-cized preference of qualified minorities for medical institutions such as Harvard and Johns Hopkins, which maintained large financial reserves for such pur-poses, the representative felt that the Center could do a better job in its minority recruitment efforts. In a final June action, the regents accepted from contractors the completed Biomedical Sciences building.

In July, the Board of Regents approved an expanded TIAA/CREF benefit plan for the Health Sciences Center campus effective July 1976, with the expec-tation that the benefit structure would equal that of the Norman campus by 1981. This 401k retirement program formed the core of the benefit plan for faculty of the University of Oklahoma and most other colleges and universities in the United States.

September 1976 witnessed the installation of the 40-million volt linear accelerator in its new home in a building adjacent to Everett Tower on the Health Sciences Center campus. Also in September, the Board of Regents approved a "professional Practice in Family Medicine Clinics Plan" to permit a "salary" to be provided to part-time faculty in Family Medicine in lieu of Practice Plan reimbursement. Regents then approved several leases, one for space for the Enid Family Medicine Clinic and another for the office space and equipment of Dr. Frank A. Clingan in Tulsa. Clingan, a practicing surgeon and volunteer faculty member in Tulsa, had served as head of the surgery training program at the Tulsa branch for several years. September also witnessed an extraordinary number of terminations in the Department of Psychiatry: Drs. Peter Abuisi, Barbara Allen, Edward Collins, Rheba Edwards, Kenneth Leveque, Moorman Prosser, Herschel Randolph, Kenneth Shewmaker, and Vernon Sisney. The changes resulted primarily from the unwillingness or inability of these faculty members to devote a sufficient number of teaching hours to warrant their retention as titled volunteer faculty in the department.[13]

During the spring of 1976, the Health Sciences Center Faculty Board had initiated a policy of departmental external reviews and audits, with each depart-ment to be visited by outside experts every eighth year. The purposes of this policy were to evaluate: (1) the status and contribution of the department on a national basis; (2) status and contribution of the department to the Medical

School; (3) the growth and development of the department over time; and (4) the leadership provided by the chair of the department. Particular attention was to be paid to research, pre- and postdoctoral education programs, residency programs, and, in clinical departments, clinical care. A combination of internal and external reviews was planned. In the 1976–77 academic year, Biochemistry, Gynecology–Obstetrics, Dermatology, and Medicine were scheduled. Later, Orthopedics, scheduled for the second year, was moved to the first year. Also, Family Practice, scheduled for 1981–82, was moved to 1977 because of a perceived need for revitalization of that department.

Several construction projects were completed in July, including space in the old School of Medicine building, which was being remodeled to accommodate Pathology professor Fletcher Taylor's large federal program/project grant for the study of coagulation. Funds from the grant were used to construct facilities for his study. Also completed were Phases III and IV of the Steam and Chilled Water Plant, with revenue bonds as the source of funding.

On August 31 the Faculty Board reincarnated the Academic Council as the "Pre-Doctoral Education Committee." At the same time, a student resolution asking for retraction of the provost's decree that the Basic Science Education Building be closed each evening to conserve electricity and save money was favorably endorsed by the Faculty Board.

On October 12 the Board of Trustees of the University Hospitals and Clinics presented a plan to the legislature's Interim Committee on Health Care Delivery Systems (chaired by Senator Al Terrill, D. Lawton) requesting $30 million for renovations, replacements, and improvements at the Hospital. The reaction of the committee was less than enthusiastic, which led to the University of Oklahoma announcing a plan to raise $49 million in funds from private donors during the spring of 1977 for the same purpose. Also in October, the Oklahoma Medical Research Foundation announced a $2.5 million building and expansion program [DO, 8–28–76].

The Dean A. McGee Eye Institute announced construction of a new $1.5 million Eye Research Center in November, to be built with funds honoring Paul and Cora Snetcher. In other November actions, the Tulsa branch's agreement with the Midway Building was amended to increase the lease from $29,000 to $48,000 per year, plus $32,000 for renovations; an agreement was signed with the Tulsa County Medical Society to move its library from Hillcrest Hospital to the Tulsa Medical College building; regents approved plans to remodel the auditorium in the old School of Medicine building for the College of Health; and, in a sad note, John W. Keys, founding member of the Speech and Hearing Clinic, as well as of the academic programs in Speech

Pathology, died on November 6. The Speech and Hearing clinic would be named after him in December *[RM, 14239]*.

On November 23 Dean Lynn presented his views on a broad variety of Health Sciences Center issues to the Faculty Board. He emphasized the inadequate financial support from the state legislature, which continued to be a perplexing problem; the need for private donations to the College to compensate for lack of state support; the importance of aligning funding to the College's mission; the need to emphasize recruiting of American graduates from other medical centers to faculty positions at Oklahoma; the importance of affirmative action at the Health Sciences Center; the importance of a period of curriculum stability during which careful evaluation could take place; the need for a proper perspective for research in the College, one that contributes to the educational mission and is not competitive with education; an emphasis on continuing education needs for faculty; making clear the correlation between medical care and the Center's educational programs; the need to turn the Center into a regional referral hub; the need for clinical department heads to be widely recognized as outstanding clinicians; the desirability of making Presbyterian Hospital a full member of the Center's educational team; and the need to guarantee that any relationship with another institution should clearly augment the Center's ability to educate *[FBM, 11–23–76]*. At the same meeting, the Faculty Board, in response to an interest expressed by the legislature, approved guidelines for admitting applicants from foreign medical schools who were citizens of Oklahoma. This was yet another example of legislative meddling in the internal affairs of the College of Medicine as a result of pressure from legislators' constituents.

In early December, Provost William Thurman announced the formation of a task force to prepare the move of the various colleges into new campus buildings. Also in December, Dr. Gordon Deckert, professor and chair of Psychiatry and Behavioral Sciences, was given the additional title of clinical professor of Psychiatry, Tulsa branch.

1977

The new year began with a typical flurry of actions at the Board of Regents meeting in Norman. The board approved the establishment of a program in Family Practice in Lawton at the Ft. Sill Reynolds Army Hospital in January. Dr. Mark Allen Everett, in the year's first faculty action, was given the additional title of adjunct professor of Pathology, effective January 1, and adjunct professor of Anatomy, effective February 1. Regents also voted to approve the tuition fee increases that had been a topic of discussion and bone of contention in 1976. However, medical students attending the meeting, supplemented by Norman campus students, objected to the fee increases, and a final vote on the proposal was postponed "for further discussion." Later, at a special meeting on February 21, regents determined that "the matter of medical and dental fee increases would not be pursued this year" *[RM, 14298]*.

Also in February, Dr. Boyd K. Lester, professor of Psychiatry, and Dr. Gordon K. Jimerson, associate professor of Gynecology and Obstetrics, resigned from the faculty. These men had served as teachers of distinction and were lauded with near-universal approval by their students. Their departure was a significant loss to the Health Sciences Center, for great teachers were becoming less and less common at Oklahoma, as, indeed, elsewhere.

At the March meeting of the University of Oklahoma Board of Regents, President Matt Braly was replaced by Thomas Brett for a one year term at the helm of that body. Barbara James was re-elected as secretary to the board. Additional business included approval of a faculty practice plan for the College of Pharmacy. It was noted that principal faculty members at the Dean A. McGee Eye Institute continued with the rank of clinical professor, assuring that their income would not be governed by the University's Professional Practice Plan. This in part accounted for the fact that faculty turnover at the Eye Institute was much lower than for any other component of the Health Sciences Center. At the Oklahoma Medical Research Foundation, which continued its faculty title anomaly, the scientists held unmodified titles, even though their income was not regulated by the College.

By the spring of 1977, faculty salaries at the Health Sciences Center had increased only marginally over those paid in 1972. The base salaries for full professors averaged $32,500; for associate professor, $27,700; and for assistant professors, $24,300. A summary of the College of Medicine Budget through the five-year period 1973–1978 appears in Table 1.

The figures in this chart, which appear in the dean's Annual Report to the LCME (1973–1977), illustrate the increasing dependence of the Center on its clinical practice income. One element the chart does not illustrate is the considerable tension between the Faculty Board and the Health Sciences Center provost over the fact that the College of Medicine, which contained the overwhelming majority of faculty and students, was receiving only 32 percent of new instructional (E&G) funding at the Center.[14] The faculty naturally felt that with over half of the faculty and budget, the College should receive at least half of the new state-funded dollars.

TABLE 1.   COLLEGE OF MEDICINE BUDGET (IN MILLIONS OF DOLLARS), 1973–78

Source	1973–74	1974–75	1975–76	1976–77	1977–78
State (prorata share)*	4.0	5.5	6.5	8.6	10.9
State (direct funds)**	3.6	3.7	4.4	5.4	6.8
Federal Grants	3.0	4.1	4.2	4.3	4.5
Faculty Practice Plan	3.6	4.4	6.8	7.5	7.8
Other	3.5	4.3	5.4	6.2	6.2

*   Includes prorata share of Administration, Operations, Physical Plant, and Library.
** Includes direct funds to the College of Medicine.

Affirmative Action

Early in March 1977 the Oklahoma State Regents for Higher Education "criticized college presidents . . . for the slow pace of their desegregation efforts" *[DO, 3–1–77]*. Surprisingly, and somewhat ironically, the *Daily Oklahoman* would point out in July that the "least progress" in desegregation was being made at the state's only predominantly Black college, Langston University in Guthrie. "The effort to boost White enrollment at Langston was a notable failure," said a higher regents' report several months later *[DO, 6–6–77]*.

The Health Sciences Center's Faculty Board had grappled for several years with mechanisms to increase the number of qualified minority candidates applying to the College of Medicine. The most successful effort was in relation to the American Indian population, of which Oklahoma boasted the largest number of citizens in the country. Professors Harris D. Riley and Joseph Ferretti had initiated programs for Oklahoma Indians earlier (op. cit.), and in April 1975, the Faculty Board had approved a comprehensive program for recruitment, training, and mentoring of American Indian students in Oklahoma high schools and colleges. The Faculty Board and the dean applied for support of these efforts to both the Institute of American Indian Medicine and the federal Indian Health Service in 1976 *[FBM, 6–26–76]*. A summer teaching program to "increase basic skills" of minority students in the College was initiated by the Faculty Board in July 1976. That autumn, the senior class included two American Indians, six Hispanics, one Asian American, and one Black.

The 1977 senior medical class included six American Indians, one Asian American, and eight Blacks. Four of the latter were on academic probation, however. A year later, in 1978, the senior class would include one Black, one Asian American and six American Indians, reflecting the positive effects of the programs to recruit the latter category of student.[15] In April 1978 Provost

Thurman would write to Dr. Mark Everett, chair of the Faculty Board, emphasizing the need for a comprehensive plan for minority participation in the admissions process because of the "Adams Case" settlement between the state of Oklahoma and the United Stated government, which had mandated that the affirmative action programs be implemented by the regents. He would say, "To me, it is critical that we begin now to plan an approach and discuss it with all involved. If we do not formulate a plan, we will be presented with one, and that is unacceptable."[16]

In the spring of 1977, three of five Black applicants were accepted into the College of Medicine freshman class. By comparison, approximately one of every twenty white candidates was admitted. This disproportion reflected the University's response to a federal court directive regarding higher education in Oklahoma (see page 323). The efforts of the College to recruit qualified Black candidates was limited by the lack of scholarship funds for minority students. As a result, most highly qualified Black students from Oklahoma colleges were immediately offered full four-year scholarships at prestigious private schools in the East or North, and they understandably accepted the offers.

In addition to complaints about the slow pace of affirmative action at state colleges and universities, the Regents for Higher Education also questioned the admissions policies at the University of Oklahoma Health Sciences Center in March 1977. Several members of that body wondered if decisions on the admission of students to the Center were being made by persons "without any accountability to any state agency" *[DO, 3–1–77]*. This was a reference to the previously mentioned reorganization of the Admissions Board of the College of Medicine to include a large number of practicing physicians from around the state. In trying to placate the state medical community, the Center had now riled the higher regents!

Throughout 1977 and 1978, there was much faculty discussion at the Health Sciences Center regarding the low attendance rate of students at lectures. It was concluded that several factors contributed to this situation: (1) too many hours of lecture; (2) an erroneous sense on the part of students that it was neither necessary nor useful to attend certain lectures; (3) a contention by students that many of the lectures were "irrelevant" to their impending specialties; and (4) a feeling that the lecture format was not conducive to maximum performance on examinations. At the same time, there was a student request to eliminate class ranking.[17] The following year, Dean Lynn wrote to the department heads that: "We have already been though a pass-fail-honors system and, as a faculty, we decided to return to a graded (A B C D F) format. It doesn't seem to me that either going back to an ungraded system, or using a system where grading is kept secret from the students, is appropriate. Life is competitive and I do not feel that taking away [competition] gets at the problem [of class attendance]."[18]

In April 1977 Ronald H. White, M.D., became a regent of the University. At his first meeting, the regents unanimously approved a policy whereby there would be community representation on search committees for endowed chairs, especially "where significant outside funding has been given" *[RM, 14349]*. In addition, endowed chair committees would have to include two departmental representatives, two outside individuals appointed by the president, and the dean of the relevant college or his designee.

April also saw the faculty of the College of Medicine renew its endorsement of the requirement that the Part I examination of the National Board of Medical Examiners be prerequisite to promotion and graduation. This requirement was first affirmed on December 9, 1970, and again on June 16, 1971. "This means," said the Faculty Board, "that none of the eight current junior students who have failed to complete Part I will be recommended for promotion to, nor be permitted to enroll in, the fourth year until such time as each has successfully passed" *[FBM, 4–15–77]*.

The Hammarsten Affair

In May, the witch's brew of dissension between the Health Sciences Center faculty and the provost was stirred once again when the chair of Medicine, Dr. James Francis Hammarsten, was requested by the provost to resign his position, after Dean Lynn had refused to terminate his appointment. Years later, in a 1999 interview with the author, Dean Lynn recalled, "Thurman fully expected me to resign over the Hammarsten removal; he was disappointed that I did not. But at that point, he did not have enough other reasons to ask me to resign. Bill later told me, 'You know, you have a unique ability to compromise.' I thought that I would be doing the school a disservice to resign. I think the [Hammarsten] firing was requested by some of the town internists."[19]

James Hammarsten was a University of Minnesota graduate who had served as chief of the Medical Service at the Veterans Administration Hospital in Oklahoma City from 1953 to 1962. During the years 1962–66 he served as chief of medicine at the St. Paul-Ramsey Hospital in St. Paul, Minnesota, following which he returned to Oklahoma as vice chair of the Department of Medicine. He became chair in 1967 following the departure of Dr. Stewart Wolf. Dr. Hammarsten was a gruff but gentle and scholarly man who had served his department and the College of Medicine diligently. A resolution from the Medicine faculty, dated May 10, criticized the "sources, . . . information, . . . and data that led to a negative assessment by the provost of Dr. Hammarsten's role as chair. This assessment is in conflict with the recent external review of the Department." Continued the resolution, "We believe that this episode has broader implications for the future stability and growth of the College of Medicine, the Health Sciences Center, and the University of Oklahoma at large." An in-person explanation by the provost and dean was requested by the Department of Medicine. At the Faculty Board meeting of May 17 the resolution was endorsed unanimously. Additionally, the chair named a committee of Dr. G. Rainey Williams, Dr. Warren Crosby, and Dr. Gordon Deckert to prepare an additional response regarding this issue *[FBM, 5–17–77]*. Like most of the conflicts between the provost and the College of Medicine faculty, this demand for an explanation was met with a barrage of verbiage that obscured the issues raised, while the decision in question remained in force.

The reign of Dr. William Thurman as provost was not one an objective observer would label a period of collegial government; rather, it was an essentially autocratic one. It was unfortunate that although many of the actions of the provost challenged by the faculty were ultimately proven to be appropriate or even beneficial to the Center, the dissatisfaction produced by the methods used in making the decisions, and the way the decisions were imposed (through edict rather than through consultation with faculty) led, in the long run, to unhealthy morale among many of the faculty and staff.

Following the resignation of Dr. Hammarsten in the summer of 1977, Dr. Solomon Papper was named the chair of the Department of Medicine by Dean Lynn, who believed that this action was essential for the health of the department. The dean also requested that the provost provide at least six new faculty positions for Medicine. Dean Lynn felt that Dr. Papper's recruiting ability was good, but that his judgment about whom to recruit was less so. Papper served as chair from 1977 to 1984, and overall was a distinguished leader. Dr. R. Timothy Coussons, who served as vice chair under Papper, as well as acting chair during the fall of 1983, viewed Dr. Papper as a unique man with a good participatory leadership style. His dedication to scholarship led him to be one of the early supporters of the M.D./Ph.D. program at the Center. Dean Lynn also appointed Owen M. Rennart as professor and head of Pediatrics, effective July 1, 1977, following the recommendation of a search committee formed to identify a replacement for Dr. Harris D. Riley.

In May 1977 the administration of the Department of Institutions, Social and Rehabilitative Services (DISRS) agreed to build a pedestrian walkway connecting University Hospital and the Children's Memorial Hospital. This walkway, built at the insistence of Lloyd Rader with funds provided by DISRS, as well as through Veterans Administration funds obtained through the office of Senator Henry Bellmon, would be extended over 13th Street to connect with the Veterans Hospital concourse constructed earlier.

In mid-1977 it was calculated that on the Health Sciences Center campus, the annual costs of educating students were: first year, $8,500; second year, $9,200; third year, $11,000; and fourth year, $14.000. Tulsa branch costs for the third and fourth year were considerably higher, exceeding $20,000 per year per student *[FBM, 7–12–77]*. These higher costs in Tulsa were due to the costs of faculty salaries for the core clinical faculties and the small number of students assigned to the program. The costs of educating these professional students were always used as ammunition for attempts to increase tuition fees to students who, in Oklahoma, were charged only a small fraction of the total cost of their education.

At their July meeting, the Board of Regents presented an analysis of how the University of Oklahoma's 1976–77 budget stacked up in comparison to other universities in the Big Eight Conference. Oklahoma ranked last in state appropriations, while it ranked third in student credit hours taught by its faculty, seventh in money spent on organized research, and last in library expenditures! *[RM, 14653]*. At the same meeting, an agreement was struck by the regents with the Oklahoma Medical Research Foundation whereby the latter would provide funds for use of the new library building in return for unlimited access to its facilities for their staff. In return for this access, the Foundation would make four payments of $112,500 per year from 1977 through 1980.

In August, Peggy Culver of the Health Sciences Center Student Council wrote a letter to Dean Lynn requesting that the faculty modify its rule that students in the second year must pass the Part II examination of the NBME in order to proceed into the third year class. She requested that students be permitted to continue into the third year, take a reexamination in September, and, if they pass, not lose a year.[20] This perennial request was not acted upon by the board. Also in August, the Faculty Board, practicing the ancient adage that if you want something done, give it to somebody who is already overwhelmed with work, approved the name of Dr. James Merrill as chair of the Postdoctoral Education Committee.[21] In a final August action, the regents accepted as complete the recently constructed College of Nursing building.

October saw the Board of Regents recommending tuition increases to provide much-needed operating funds for the University. These recommendations were then forwarded to the State Regents, who received them with a distinct lack of warmth. Included were increases in medical and dental tuition for in-state students from $600 to $900 per semester and for non-residents from $1,396.50 to $1,3996.50 per semester *[RM, 14633]*. At a joint meeting with the State Regents on October 24, it was revealed that with the Oklahoma Corporation Commission eliminating the institutional rate for electricity, charges by OG&E would increase utility costs by $150,000 per year on the Oklahoma City campus alone! The State Regents eschewed reacting to such economic data and instead concentrated on discovering whether there was favoritism for certain University of Oklahoma students in admission to the professional schools and whether the University was making progress in the racial makeup of its classes *[RM, 14680–82]*.

The Patterson Case

At the same October 1977 State Regents meeting, Chancellor Dunlap queried University regents about "the Patterson case" *[RM, 14682]*. This concerned a third-year medical student who had challenged a College of Medicine faculty decision requiring him to repeat the third year (because of poor performance on clinical rotations). Patterson petitioned the president, the regents, the provost, and others to overturn the faculty decision. His scattergun approach worked. Provost Thurman overruled his faculty and permitted the student to enroll in the fourth year on probation. In December, at the request of Regent Replogle, the Patterson case would be reopened and discussed because the student had written to President Sharp again contesting his probationary status and the Faculty Board's decisions *[RM, 14732]*. The regents would conclude that the student had received more than fair consideration and refused to hear another complaint regarding this same matter. Nonetheless, Dr. Thurman's decision regarding Patterson would later lead to a crisis between him and the faculty when the latter would refuse to recommend Patterson for graduation (vide infra).

Also at the October regents meeting, in response to a question from Regent Richard Bell, Provost Thurman stated that he believed that the Tulsa branch program so far had been "highly successful" and that the problems there were "political rather than educational." He then made a plea for the state's two medical education facilities in Tulsa (the Tulsa branch of the Health Sciences Center and the Osteopathic College) to work together. He said that Evangelist Oral Roberts' plans to open the Oral Roberts Medical School would complicate problems that already exist. "There is no reason a two-year program could not be built to serve both the Tulsa branch of the OU Medical School, which is for third- and fourth-year students, and the four-year osteopathic school. We keep skirting around it," he said, referring to the problems of cooperation *[RM, 14683]*. Following a lengthy discussion, Scott E. Orbison, a state regent from Tulsa, warned that political leaders would not allow either Tulsa institution to be closed, nor would osteopathic forces allow a merger of the two institutions, with its president reduced to the role of a dean *[DO, 10–25–77]*.

The University Board of Regents chose December to amend, and gain tighter control over, the Health Sciences Center faculty Practice Plan, stating that "The University will not recognize individual or departmental corporations."[22] A special meeting of the regents was held on December 22, supposedly to approve plans for the proposed parking structures on the Health Sciences Center campus, with additional student, staff, and service space, since the Attorney General had recently rendered an opinion that issuance of such bonds was appropriate if the regents found that such were "necessary for the comfort, convenience and welfare of the students" *[RM, 14768]*. The regents voted that the issuance of the bonds was necessary.

At the same December meeting, regents approved a $7.7 million revenue bond issue for the Health Sciences Center Parking System, to be operated by University Hospital. The proposed system, approved by Governor Boren and legislative leaders, would include an 1100-car garage for the University and a 400-car garage for University Hospital, both to be owned by the University, with the smaller facility leased by the Hospital *[DO, 1–8–78]*. On a split 5–2 vote, the regents selected Blevins and Spitz, Inc. as architects of the 1100-car garage. The December meeting concluded with an announcement that the State Regents had approved a revision in the MCAT admission requirements to the College of Medicine necessitated by the change in the MCAT examination, the scores of which were now reported in a different numerical system. Furthermore, the State Regents also announced that they had cut by one-half the amount of the tuition increase the University and regents had previously requested for medical and dental students.

1978

Nineteen seventy-eight began with disturbing news for the University Board of Regents. At the January meeting, President Paul Sharp announced that because of the stroke he suffered on November 5, he was "asking the Regents of the University to authorize my retirement from administrative duties to take up new responsibilities as a professor of higher education. I have had a timely warning and I intend to heed it," the 60-year-old Sharp said *[RM, 14771; DO, 1–10–78]*. The regents expressed regret and praise, complimenting the president on his "integrity, perseverance, loyalty, and dependability, and for the favorable image you have created for the University throughout the State and the Nation" *[RM, 14773]*. Dr. Sharp would serve as a professor of History at the University until his retirement, and following that, both he and his wife Rose would participate in campus activities through the 1990s.

Tulsa: A Branch College

In February, Provost William Thurman was given the additional title of executive dean, College of Medicine for a one-year period. This change was in response to a recommendation of the recent visit of a site committee of the Liaison Committee for Medical Education (LCME) which criticized the parallel, rather than subordinate, position of Dean Fitzpatrick in Tulsa vis-a-vis Dean Lynn in Oklahoma City. Upon receipt of the report, Dean Lynn drove to Tulsa and informed Fitzpatrick that "'This is the way it is going to be.' I was reasonably certain, however, that this would be unacceptable to the Tulsa medical community. Giving the title 'Executive Dean' to the provost was Thurman's solution. He told me that, 'No, it will be this way. It is a regents' appointment.' Bill was a charming man, but he made some decisions which I thought were inappropriate. I spent many sleepless nights over this Tulsa affair."[23]

The LCME task force recommended that the Tulsa dean must report through the Oklahoma City Dean. Giving the title executive dean to the provost was, in effect, a face-saving gesture to the Tulsa campus, which temporarily avoided the mandated subordination of the Tulsa dean to the dean in Oklahoma City. However, the LCME report stated: "Prolonged involvement of the Provost in the position of acting dean, supposedly reporting through the Dean of the College of Medicine, to himself as Provost, presents an intolerable administrative situation which should be changed immediately."[24]

On April 20 in reply to a query from Dr. Mark Everett as to whether this action did in fact carry out the LCME mandate, Provost Thurman stated that "The appointment . . . to the position of Executive Dean is a one-year appointment. In that interim . . . I would hope that we can clarify many of the issues that arise."[25] On April 20 the University legal counsel, Kurt F. Ockershauser, rendered the opinion that "There is one college of medicine with a branch program located at Tulsa, and named the Tulsa Medical College" *[RM, 14828]*.

Professor of Pathology Walter Joel died in February 1978. He was a German immigrant who had fled Germany, gone to Egypt in the 1930s, and came to the United States when Hitler's troops overran North Africa during World War II. He was an accomplished teacher and pianist, with a particular fondness for the music of Johann Bach. His fractured English endeared him to both students and faculty. On one occasion, while discussing the contents of his under-equipped pathology laboratory, he told this author, "At one time, I had the 'ureene' of three kings in my laboratory!" Students invariably were amused when he proclaimed, in reference to an unusual occurrence of this or that phenomenon, that it was a "seldom bird."

In March, there were charges within the College of Nursing that "at least one-fourth of the entire student body is involved" in cheating on examinations. Dean Gloria Smith said that a key test had disappeared in February, which prompted the accusations and subsequent inquiry. "You can't just accuse someone," Dean Smith said, "You almost have to catch them in the act of cheating" *[DO, 3–10–78]*.

At the April regents meeting, the appointment of James F. Hammarsten as professor of Medicine was terminated, in anticipation of his move to the Veterans Administration Hospital in Idaho. At the same time, development of a new series of bonds for expansion of the Steam and Chilled Water System was also authorized.

In May, the architectural firm of Shaw Associates challenged the designation of Blevins and Spitz as architects for the 1100-car parking garage at the Health Sciences Center, charging irregularities in the selection process. By a split vote of 4–2–1, the regents reaffirmed their choice, citing the State Consultant Act which stated that "If qualifications of competing firms are found to be equal, the contract shall be awarded to the firm which has had the least State business within the last five years." Concluded the regents, "The Board of Affairs has now certified that Blevins and Spitz has performed no State work in the past five years and that all other firms have performed State work within that time frame" *[RM, 14981]*.

The Degree Granting Controversy: Part I

On May 31 the general faculty of the College of Medicine approved "for graduation and awarding of the M.D. degree" those students recommended by the Faculty Board who had completed satisfactorily all of the requirements for the M.D. degree. The names of two students in the senior class were omitted from the list because of poor academic and professional performance, and they were not recommended to receive a degree. The students had been on probationary status throughout much of their time in medical school. It had been recommended by the Third-Year Promotions Committee that one of the students be dropped altogether from the college.[26] This student subsequently initiated a letter writing campaign to numerous state and university officials. Both students appealed to the provost to overrule the faculty. The provost apparently found the students' laments persuasive, and indicated to Dr. Mark Everett, chair of the Faculty Board, that he would recommend to the regents that the two students be awarded the M.D. degree.[27] Between Provost Thurman's decision and graduation day, Dr. Everett attempted to reach the University legal counsel, who failed to return calls and did not reply to a written communication. Upon advice of the president of the Faculty Senate, Dr. Everett then called President Sharp, reviewing the events with him and expressing the faculty opinion that to award degrees to these two students would be a grave mistake. Sharp replied that although he had been unaware of the issue, he would have it discussed at the next regents' meeting. On June 2 the provost called Dr. Everett and informed him that the regents had decided to award the degrees, although Regent Replogle had indicated that the regents would look with favor upon a "friendly [law]suit" by the faculty, and accordingly, Dr. Everett indicated that a public protest by faculty at the graduation ceremony would be avoided, although he himself, as head of the faculty, would not attend the event.[28] Dean Lynn recalled that Dr. Thurman did not use the traditional wording that "the faculty recommends this student for the M.D. degree" during the ceremony.[29]

On Sunday June 4 degrees were awarded to the entire Medical School senior class, including the two students who had not been recommended. On June 5 the Faculty Board met and moved that their chair, with the advice of the Executive Committee, seek an independent counsel—Oklahoma City attorney F. C. Love—as well as the assistance of the legal firm of Couch and Hendrickson. Love had been general counsel for the Kerr-McGee corporation, and upon retirement from that organization joined the powerful legal firm of Crow, Dunlevy, Thweat, Swinford, and Johnson.

The next act in the "graduation drama" occurred on June 19 when the provost forwarded to the president the faculty-approved list of graduates and, in addition, the names of two additional candidates for the degree, which were awarded "by action of the regents of the University of Oklahoma." Provost Thurman's letter said, "The list is now complete and ready for submission to the Oklahoma State Regents for Higher Education."[30] A week later, the faculty approved a resolution, to be transmitted to the provost, president, and board of regents, requesting that they meet with the Executive Committee of the Faculty Board at the earliest possible date. On that day, the Executive Committee requested that Dr. Everett contact the State Board of Medical Examiners and the Surgeon General of the United States, informing them of the "irregular" awarding of degrees at the University of Oklahoma. Nine days later, on June 28, Dr. Everett received a letter from the State Board of Medical Examiners indicating that they would utilize the faculty's list of proposed graduates in issuing licenses. That same day, the Executive Committee met with the provost, and it was agreed that a general faculty meeting would be called for July 5 to discuss the issue and outline the sequence of events. At the meeting, Dr. Everett said,

> The [provost's] stated reason for graduating the students was that criteria for graduation as outlined by the faculty had not been approved by the Oklahoma State Regents for Higher Education. . . . The provost contends that the requirement for passage of Parts I and II [of the NBME] is invalid because the requirement has not been approved by the State Regents. The Faculty believes however, that under common law, as well as by statute and the rules of the University, the M.D. degree can be given only upon recommendation by the Faculty. An M.D. degree has never been awarded without recommendation of the faculty of the College of Medicine *[FBM, 6–28–78]*.

Dr. Gordon Deckert stated that "this is a critical issue. There is a moral and perhaps a legal issue involved in the granting of the degrees without faculty recommendation" *[FBM, 6–28–78]*. Dr. James Merrill concurred, saying, "The prerogative of the faculty is to insure that qualified students are graduated and sent out to practice in the state of Oklahoma. That prerogative has been usurped. Is the faculty going to let the regents and provost graduate students and decide who is adequately prepared to go into practice?" *[FBM, 6–28–78]*. At the conclusion of the meeting, the faculty passed the following resolution proposed by Dr. Merrill and seconded by Dr. Robert Patnode: "We the Faculty of the College of Medicine request an audience with the President of the University and the University of Oklahoma Regents to discuss an item of paramount importance that urgently needs attention and resolution" *[FBM, 6–28–78]*.

On July 25 President Sharp met with members of the Medical School faculty to discuss the M.D. degrees that had been awarded to two students whom the faculty had not recommended as suitable candidates. The students were identified by local newspapers as "John Patterson and Dwayne Henry Atwell" *[DO, 7–21–78; Oklahoma Daily, 7–21–78]*. Provost Thurman had overruled the decisions of the Faculty Board, the general faculty, the Appeals Committee, and the dean. Dr. Mark Everett, speaking for the faculty, pointed out that the issue was not whether each criterion utilized by the faculty in making a recommendation had been specifically approved by the State Regents, but the fact that University policy specifies that the faculty of the College of Medicine is the group which recommends individuals as qualified or not for award of the M.D. degree *[FBM, 7–20–78]*. Faculty members had contributed money to a "war chest" to assure proper legal advice regarding this matter. The faculty attorney, F. C. Love, determined that the faculty position "may well have as much legal merit as that which Thurman has attributed to the State Regents" *[Oklahoma Daily 7–19–78]*. Provost Thurman later announced that President Sharp recommended that the opinion of the University's legal counsel be obtained. "There was general agreement that the matter should be settled within the College," Thurman said *[Oklahoma Daily, 7–19–78]*. Dr. Everett felt that the controversy boiled down to two key issues: (1) whether the faculty determines—through its system of educational standards, course offerings, and grades—who will graduate from Medical School; or (2) whether the State Regents have the authority to grant the M.D. degree without faculty recommendation. Provost Thurman avoided the first issue by suggesting that any criterion which had not been specifically approved by the State Regents was invalid, and as a consequence the issue was not moot. This was a typically tricky end run by the provost, who had mastered the art of avoiding the big, disruptive discussion in favor of a small sidebar on it.

The battle was joined, and the faculty were determined that, unlike the struggle over faculty practice income, they would not lose this one. They met head-on the provost's "technical" agenda, which was twofold: (1) should an external comprehensive examination such as NBME I and II be a decisive element in faculty decisions regarding graduation (many, including the provost, thought it should not); and (2) had the faculty criteria for graduation been approved by the State Regents. Just as important, the faculty felt, was the "philosophical" agenda, which was more complex and involved issues such as faculty authority, student grades, lenient criteria for minority admission and graduation, etc. After a series of meetings, the Faculty Board on August 9 approved and sent to Provost Thurman and the University administration the following proposal: "Successful completion of standard referenced comprehensive examinations are requirements for advancement and graduation. Until internal collegiate examinations fulfilling this description have been perfected, this means that passage of Part I of NBME is a requirement for promotion from the second to the third year, and passage of Part II is a requirement for graduation" *[FBM, 8–9–78]*.

Although the provost met with the Faculty Board on September 26, at which time the resolution was reaffirmed, and with the general faculty on September 27, no official action was taken. The faculty, through a letter by Dr. Everett, requested on October 17 that the president and the chair of the Board of Regents place the resolution on the agenda of their meeting of October 19. The president replied, "Provost Thurman did discuss with the Regents the recommendation of the Faculty Board. They asked that he discuss their reaction with the Faculty Board."[31] A letter from the president of the Board of Regents, Robert G. Mitchell, M.D., indicated that the resolution had not been discussed at the regents' meeting, but only by the Health Sciences Center Committee of the regents. (Submitting issues only to this committee was another of the techniques used by the provost to avoid bringing issues to the full Board of Regents where they would be a matter of public record.) Mitchell suggested that "If our recommendations are acceptable to the Dean and the Faculty Board, the entire matter will be presented to the full Board of Regents of the University."[32] On the same date, Provost Thurman's Machiavellian strategy was made clear in a letter to Dr. Everett in which he stated:

I write to inform you that the Health Sciences Center Sub-Committee of the Regents of the University approved making Part I and Part II of the National Board Examinations mandatory for promotion to the Third Year and Graduation respectively if: 'In any given year two or more students do not perform satisfactorily in an academic department category on either Part I or Part II of the National Board, that Department will have its entire teaching function and tenure responsibilities of its Faculty scrutinized by an ad hoc Committee of the Board of Regents of the University of Oklahoma. . . . If that performance is repeated in the subsequent year, termination or abrogation of tenure of all faculty involved will be considered.'[33]

Provost Thurman cynically added, "I trust this meets with your approval."

At an electrified Faculty Board meeting the same day, responses to Dr. Thurman were predictable, just as was his attacking mode of defense:

Dr. Wizenberg: "This paragraph has nothing to do whatsoever with what we have asked the regents to decide, or with the improvement in performance of our students."

Dr. Thurman: "Everyone must pay the price. If a student fails the course, don't let him take Part I [of the NBME]."

Dr. Merrill: "This is a punitive response which I resent enormously."

Dr. Thurman: "Jim, you've resented everything about this process."

Dr. Kopta: "Don't single out Dr. Merrill; there are other members of the Faculty Board who resent this response."

Thurman's only support came from Dean Lynn, who tried to calm the waters by suggesting that, in his view, "It is appropriate that the performance of departments be looked at" *[FBM, 10–31–78]*.

In spite of this encounter and the rapid exchange of letters, no specific action was taken, and the matter was referred to the Faculty Board Executive Committee. Upon review, the Committee rejected the Thurman proposal and asked that the regents' Health Sciences Center Subcommittee consider the resolution of August 28 on its own merits. On the same date, Dean Lynn suggested a less punitive trigger for evaluation of teaching functions be initiated: when the NBME in any one section "of all or a substantial majority of a class falls one standard deviation below the national mean of non-candidates for that section, an enquiry into the causes . . . shall be conducted by the Dean . . . with results reported to the University Administration." He requested permission to present this proposal to the full Board of Regents in mid-December *[FBM, 11–7–78]*.[34]

On February 23, 1979, Provost Thurman wrote to Dr. Everett stating that "The regents have voted not to make PartI/II requirements for promotion/ graduation."[35] Finally, on April 13, 1979, University President William Banowsky forwarded to the State Regents revised promotion and graduation requirements passed by the University Board of Regents on April 12. These requirements watered down academic criteria and made passing of Part I a non-requirement for any student with a 3.0 grade average over the first two years. Additionally, Provost Thurman agreed that he would not again recommend the awarding of degrees to students unless they had been proposed by the faculty. The issue soon became moot because in March 1979, Thurman announced his resignation effective July 1. After all the fireworks and bitter recriminations, this was the rather anticlimactic resolution of a crisis in University of Oklahoma faculty-administration relationships. It did, however, produce a residual distrust of administration among faculty for years to come.

And in a final counterpoint to Provost Thurman's actions, it was reported years later that neither of the two students who initiated the controversy and received the disputed degree was ever licensed to practice medicine.

Dr. Joseph Kopta, chair of the Department of Orthopedic Surgery, recalls that some of his biggest battles were with Provost Thurman. Perhaps the biggest, most cantankerous, and most public was Kopta's decision to withdraw orthopedic residents from private hospitals in Oklahoma City. Over several years, Kopta had gradually decreased the number of residents assigned to such hospitals. He accomplished this in part by reducing the total number of residents in his department from five per year to four, making fewer residents available after filling University services. When the ratio of private hospital residents to University residents fell below 50/50, there was an outcry from the hospitals. Community orthopedists complained to Dean Lynn, who informed them that Dr. Kopta was chair and could run his department as he saw fit. Orthopedic surgeons from these private hospitals then went to Provost Thurman, who directed Dean Lynn to order the chair to restore the 50/50 ratio. Dr. Kopta refused to comply with the order. At the next Faculty Board meeting, Dr. Merrill sided with Dr. Kopta, proclaiming that "If Thurman wants more bodies in the private hospitals, let Thurman go there as a resident!" The provost told Dr. Lynn that his options were to fire Kopta or resign his position as Dean. Although he fully expected to be fired, Lynn did neither, and within a few days the provost backed off his position regarding both men.[36]

Joseph Kopta came to the University of Oklahoma in 1974 as chair of Orthopedic Surgery after a stint as chair of the same department at the University of Illinois, replacing Dr. Marvin Margo. He served as chair at the University of Oklahoma until 1992, then remained as a professor until 1997, at which time he initiated a private practice in Norman. When asked why he gave up his prestigious chairmanship, Dr. Kopta ruefully observed that managing the financial and personnel components of a major department "was no longer fun," whereas surgery and patient care certainly were. Consequently, he returned to the latter.[37]

At the May 31, 1978, meeting of the University Board of Regents, Dr. Don O'Donoghue was honored for his many years of dedicated service to the College of Medicine. In reviewing his career at the University of Oklahoma Health Sciences Center, Dr. O'Donoghue stated, "There has never been a year in the fifty years I have been here when we had any money. We have always been broke; but look what has been done without any money!"[38]

On June 2 a special meeting of the regents was held in Tulsa, where the 1978–79 Health Sciences Center budget was approved. Later that month, a contract with the Oklahoma City Zoo for construction and operation of a Laboratory Animal Research Center was approved, professor Jaqueline J. Coalson, Ph.D., was named interim head of Pathology, and Katherine Hudson, professor of Psychiatry and Behavioral Sciences, retired. The regents also approved a June proposal to permit individuals in the College of Dentistry Professional Practice Plan to incorporate.

Money matters for Family Medicine and other departments dominated regent discussions during July, as a lease agreement for a clinic in Shawnee was renewed for $20,400 per year, while a building at 50th and Lincoln in Oklahoma City was purchased for that department for $400,000, using unspecified funds *[RM, 15120–15124]*. Facility costs, personnel costs, and hence the entire Family Medicine program at the Health Sciences Center—as well as at its off-campus facilities in Oklahoma City, Wakita, Enid, Tulsa, and Bartlesville—were never included in the departmental budget, so that accounting for the total resources of the College of Medicine devoted to the Family Medicine program was never readily identified. Nevertheless, much more extra departmental funding was devoted to Family Medicine than to any other departments, and these were garnered from a variety of sources—i.e., the Physicians Manpower Agency, bond issues, the College of Medicine budget, and the Health Sciences Center general budget. As a result, the cost of educating physicians in Family Medicine was heavily subsidized, since infrastructure costs of education were not attributed to the department, disguising the true cost per resident. These funding mechanisms attest to the fact that the college was committed to the development of family medicine from an early date, in spite of the frequent complaints by citizens alleging the contrary.

In July, the regents continued planning for 30,000 square feet of student service space in the east end of the 1100-car parking garage. Harmon Construction company was the low bidder for this project at a base bid of $4.7 million, which was $800,000 over the estimate. The 434-car garage project, on the other hand, included space for the emergency room, clinical laboratories, and expansion space at an estimated cost of $1.7 million.

The New President

Throughout the summer of 1978 the search for a new president for the University of Oklahoma accelerated following the announced resignation of Paul Sharp. On August 9 the *Daily Oklahoman* reported that the leading candidate, Dr. William S. Banowsky, president of Pepperdine University in

California, had withdrawn his name from consideration, possibly because he learned that he had the support of only four of the seven University regents. Among the remaining candidates, it was widely assumed that Provost William G. Thurman, focus of the degree-granting controversy throughout the May-November period, had the greatest amount of political support. On August 14, however, at a Board of Regents Executive Session called to discuss presidential candidates and possible selection of a president, the regents met with Dr. Thurman, who announced that he wished to withdraw his name from consideration for the position. As a result, the regents felt that "Dr. Banowsky should be called to see if he would reconsider the action he took last week in withdrawing his name." By telephone, Banowsky stated that he "would accept the presidency if an offer was made" *[RM, 15163]*. Asking Dr. Banowsky to remain on the line, the regents then voted unanimously to offer the position to him effective September 15, 1978. Banowsky accepted the appointment at the conclusion of the vote *[DO, 8–15– 78]*. It was generally understood that Dr. Thurman withdrew his name from consideration primarily for personal reasons which he did not wish to have aired in the media. When the new president was named, Thurman undoubtedly knew that his tenure as a relatively independent provost, answerable essentially to no one, would come to an end. Furthermore, said Dr. Donald Halverstadt later, "as all good administrators realize, Thurman saw that he had accomplished the most that he was likely to accomplish [at the Health Sciences Center], and knew that it was time to move on. He had accomplished an enormous amount."[39] Dr. Thurman would leave the Health Sciences Center in November of 1979.

The *Daily Oklahoman*, in an August 14 article reviewing the status of the University and its choice of a new president, contrasted the "liberal" atmosphere in Norman with the political mood in Stillwater, that "quiet peaceful town . . . where wholesomeness and goodness thrive." The *Oklahoman* depicted the University of Oklahoma's image as a negative one "in the minds of the basically conservative state residents and its legislators, who control the higher education dollar." The board of regents, said the paper, "in recent years has come under fire for a lack of forward-looking leadership and candor. . . . Regents were accused of forcing the resignation of Paige Mulhollan, former Dean of Arts and Sciences and [they were also] criticized for the way they handled an alleged plagiarism incident." To counteract this generally negative view, the newspaper said, the new president of the University must be "a dynamic, energized person" with power to have complete control over the University of Oklahoma Foundation and the Athletic Department, as well as the full backing of the regents *[DO, 8–14–78]*. William F. Banowsky was selected, by unanimous vote of the regents, as that "dynamic, energized person" best able to change the University's negative imagine held by many citizens of Oklahoma. He would commence his term as president on August 14, 1978.

At the September regents meeting, Dr. J. R. Morris served as acting president of the University. Dr. F. Daniel Duffy, chair of Medicine at the Tulsa branch, resigned his title of assistant dean of student affairs, as well as that of acting medical director of the educational program for medical students at the Veterans Hospital in Muskogee. He would later become the chair of the Tulsa Department of Medicine. The regents also adopted a Financial Emergency Policy for the Health Sciences Center, the chief purpose of which was to outline the steps needed to terminate faculty, employees, and students. Alternatives to termination were early retirement, fractional appointments, and salary reductions.

In October, President William Banowsky presided over his initial University of Oklahoma Board of Regents meeting. The first issue he confronted was the suggested recognition of the Gay People's Union by the Student Congress as an official student organization *[RM, 15225]*. Although he was from California, Banowsky reflected the conservative political attitudes of his adopted state by stating that "granting official institutional license to any campus homosexual organization is not in the best interest, long term or short term, of the University of Oklahoma" *[RM, 15229]*. Following a brief discussion, the regents voted unanimously to reverse the Student Congress decision.

Also in October, regents accepted the completed Health Sciences Center Library building. In addition, a change in the Children's Hospital Affiliation Agreement, which would permit physicians who were not faculty members to become members of the medical staff if they were recommended by a joint Department of Human Services-Health Sciences Center Committee, was also approved. This change was urged by the DHS director, Lloyd Rader, probably because of the problem he experienced when Dr. Halverstadt resigned from the University faculty but remained at Children's Hospital. Also, a provision that the medical director/chief of staff should be chair of the Department of Pediatrics was deleted, and the two positions were separated *[RM, 15250]*. Dr. Harris Riley later stated that this was done to decrease the perception that only he was running the hospital.

In December, regents voted to sell an additional three properties belonging to the Oklahoma Health Sciences Facility, Inc. Because of zoning restrictions imposed by the MedCap Zoning Commission and the resistance of nearby Lincoln Terrace home owners to "commerical" (i.e., University) use of the buildings, properties at 607, 615, and 619 N.E. 15th Street were offered for sale *[RM, 15302]*. Also in December, Charles B. McCall, professor of Medicine in Tulsa, was named interim associate dean at the Tulsa branch. At the same meeting, regents adopted a new "Program Discontinuance Policy" in an effort to facilitate changes they might wish to make on the Norman or Oklahoma City campus.

1979

Typically at the beginning of a new year, much of the regents' time was devoted to a harried study of contracts, construction change orders, purchase orders, and vendor agreements, not to mention personnel problems and political considerations. Although 1979 was to see the departure of embattled Provost William Thurman and the ascension of Dr. Donald Halverstadt (once considered a "renegade" by the regents) as interim provost, the new year dawned in relative tranquility on the Health Sciences Center campus. Only three significant construction projects were underway in January: the usual additions to the Steam and Chilled Water Plant, the 1100-car parking structure, and the 434-car parking structure. The long-promised student housing project had once again been abandoned to the vagaries of the state budget. Other projects—specifically, the College of Pharmacy building, the Emergency Room-Surge space for University Hospital, and the Student Activities Building—were put on "hold" pending identification of funds. A revised Professional Practice Plan was adopted for the College of Medicine which incorporated recently approved changes and specified certain exceptions for Family Medicine *[RM, 15383–93]*.

In February, a special campus-wide meeting to identify examples of Health Sciences Center sex discrimination, as defined by federal Title IX, was scheduled for February 20 at noon in the Basic Sciences Education Building. Surprisingly, no one attended! Even more surprisingly, no one complained! *[Oklahoma Daily, 2–21–79]*.

Turmoil in Otorhinolaryngology

Another important clinical department at the Health Sciences Center, Otorhinolaryngology, was in turmoil and disarray throughout much of 1978 and 1979. It had struggled since the departure of its nationally known chair, Dr. James Snow, and matters deteriorated when the new chair, Dr. Willard Moran, also resigned effective January 1979. Dr. Moran was succeeded by Dr. Robert Keim a few months later *[FBM, 12–12–78]*.

The turmoil in Otorhinolaryngology related to the issue of control over audiology services in the University hospitals—an income as well as a "turf" issue. The Department of Communication Disorders, in the Allied Health (Health Related Professions) College, under the direction of the energetic Donald Counihan, Ph.D., documented that it had an insufficient number of patients to maintain the graduate program in Audiology. The department therefore proposed that audiology services at the Children's Hospital be assigned to them. The Department of Otorhinolaryngology countered with a proposal that the Department of Communication Disorders be made a division of Otorhinolaryngology in the College of Medicine. Provost Thurman proposed dual control of the clinic. An argument then ensued regarding the appointments of return patients: should they go to the clinic in the Keyes Speech and Hearing Building or to the Children's Hospital Clinic? Dr. Keim asked the Faculty Board to support his position of assigning all audiology activities to his department at the December 1978 meeting of the Board of Regents. On December 14 the provost said in a letter to Dr. Mark Everett, "It has come to my attention that the situation in reference to the Speech and Hearing Educational Programs on this Campus of the University was discussed at the December meeting of the Faculty Board. This is an area in which I have detected a lot of misinformation as well as misunderstanding."[40] He asked to be present at the next Faculty Board meeting.

On January 11 the provost wrote to Dr. Keim, declaring that "there will be no further delay in resolving the issue. . . . It is obvious that I cannot accept the recommendations proposed [by your faculty] inasmuch as they are inappropriate in reference to the university and college structure."[41] At the January 30, 1979, Faculty Board meeting, Provost Thurman stated that there had been on-going discussions of the problem since three weeks after his arrival at the University: "The two deans, the two department chairs, and my office have been working on this problem for three years and ten months. . . . When no solution for the benefit of the educational programs could be derived to the satisfaction of everyone, it then became necessary for me to enter the discussions. . . . We don't need any more heat in the controversy than exists. It has been taken to the level of the legislature. Our business is really our business and doesn't need to be carried any further. We seriously damage everyone. It is totally unrealistic" *[FBM, 1–30–79]*.

A rancorous exchange between the provost and Dr. Keim ensued. The chair said, "You are mandating a line of referral for patients!" Thurman replied, "I am totally impartial in this matter. Your faculty went to the legislature, not to the Department of Communication Disorders people. You are totally inaccurate and incorrect" *[FBM, 1–30–79]*. Noting the rising temperature in the room, Dr. Everett suggested that since this debate could serve no useful purpose, it should be terminated, and a solution sought through the deans and heads of the two departments concerned. Six months later, still no satisfactory resolution to the problem had been found. Then suddenly, in early July 1979, Dr. Robert Keim, who had served as interim head of the department since November, also resigned. In addition, four of the department's six residents failed to renew their contracts in June because all the department's faculty members had resigned!

At the July regents' meeting, Mr. Dee Replogle was named chair of a committee to recommend a solution for the problems in Otorhinolarngology, but there is no subsequent record of a recommendation. Dean Thomas Lynn recalled that although he went to Norman to discuss the situation with President Banowsky, who said, "We cannot have a medical school without a vigorous Otorhinolarngology Department," and, "I will have a talk with Dr. Counihan,"[42] there was never a solution. The department closed. Dr. Joseph Leonard, a member of the volunteer faculty, served as a "caretaker" of clinical activities in the University's hospitals. He also took the responsibility of contacting the Residency Review Committee for Otorhinolaryngology and extracted a commitment that they would view the episode without prejudice when application was made for a newly approved residency program. Leonard was instrumental in recruiting the subsequent chair, Dr. Gail Nealy.

In March, the Board of Regents named Edward J. Tomsovic as dean of the College of Medicine, Tulsa branch, effective April 1, 1979. Dean Tomsovic came from the University of California Medical Center at Irvine where he was medical director and adjunct professor of Pediatrics. Also in March, the experiment of combined departments between the Colleges of Medicine and Dentistry was modified, when the Department of Family Practice and Community Medicine and Dentistry was divided into two departments, one in each college. The regents also voted that "the West Annex Building (used as the nurses' residence and subsequently for college programs such as Biostatistics) be demolished and the land be turned into a park" *[RM, 15428]*. It is of interest to note that the building was still standing in 1995!

The March regents' meeting also witnessed a prolonged disagreement over acceptance of bids for construction of the Health Sciences Center's Steam and Chilled Water Plant, to be paid from the $7.06 million dollar bond issue of 1979. The primary stumbling block was the concern of Attorney General

Cartwright regarding the issuance of tax-exempt revenue bonds for a project that would serve some private as well as several public institutions, even though the private institutions were tax-exempt. This resulted in rancorous interchanges with several of the initial five bidders on the project, especially the First National Bank of Tulsa and Liberty National Bank of Oklahoma City. After several delays over a twenty-four-hour period, the bid of the First National Bank of Tulsa was accepted on a four to one vote. When this action was finally concluded, the regents swiftly voted to join with the University Hospitals and Clinics in a $350,000 project to construct a Coronary Care Unit, as well as to purchase from the Urban Renewal Authority the remaining land between N.E. 8th, N.E. 10th, Phillips, and Lincoln Blvd *[RM, 15464]*.

In April, Tulsa oilman Julian J. Rothbaum was named to a second seven-year term on the University of Oklahoma Board of Regents by Governor George Nigh, replacing Dr. Robert Mitchell. Julian Rothbaum had previously served under Governor J. Howard Edmonson from 1959–1966. At their April meeting, the regents concurred in the establishment of the Associates Program of the University, conceived by President Banowsky, which began with 267 founding members, each giving $1,000 for University development *[RM, 15467]*. In other April actions, an affiliation agreement between the Health Sciences Center and the Claremore Indian Health Facility and the Shawnee Mission Hill Memorial Hospital was signed, while the name of the Department of Orthopaedic Surgery and Fractures was changed to Orthopaedic Surgery and Rehabilitation.

By spring 1979 the approved base salaries for College of Medicine faculty serving as chairs ranged from $35,000 to $68,000, with the long-tenured Mark Everett in Dermatology and G. Rainey Williams in Surgery having the lowest salaries at $35,000 and $38,000 respectively. Some departmental section heads had salaries ranging up to $60,000. The provost was paid $75,000; the dean of Medicine $50,000; the dean of Public Health and the assistant dean of Medicine $45,000. At the Tulsa branch, salaries of chairs ranged from $46,000 to $65,000 *[RM, 15485–15510]*.

Bids for construction of the Coronary Care Units and the 434-car parking garage—with the emergency service, clinical laboratory, and surge spaces for University Hospital—were also let in the spring. By July 1 the Health Sciences Center Library building was completed and turned over to the regents.

At the May 10 regents' meeting, Professor Jacqueline J. Coalson was relieved of her title of interim head, Department of Pathology, and Professor Mark A. Everett was installed as interim head of Pathology effective April 2, 1979. The following month, the title of Willie Vern Bryan of the College of Health was changed from special assistant to the provost for minority affairs to assistant provost for student affairs. At the same meeting, three interim chairs were made permanent: F. Daniel Duffy, chair of Medicine in Tulsa; Solomon Papper, chair of Medicine in Oklahoma City; and Martha J. Ferretti, chair of Physical Therapy *[RM, 15576]*.

Family Practice

For some time there had been groups of physicians at the Health Sciences Center, as well as statewide, exerting pressure in an attempt to influence who would be named as head of the Department of Family Practice. At the July 1979 regents' meeting, Dr. Jack Walker Parish was proposed as head of the department for one year. Regent Dee Replogle moved that if his appointment was approved, it should be without tenure. His motion carried on a 4–0–2 vote, but final action was deferred while other personnel decisions were made. Finally, Replogle again asked for approval of his motion to appoint Parish without tenure. Regent Richard Bell recommended that the board go into executive session to discuss Replogle's motion. The board turned the motion down by a vote of 2–4 *[RM, 15638, 15643–4]*. An "executive session," by state law, allows boards and commissions to discuss delicate personnel matters without revealing their contents to the public or including them in the official minutes of meetings.

Whatever the content of this session, it clearly influenced the regents' subsequent decision to divide the Department of Family Practice and Community Medicine into two separate departments: a Department of Family Practice and a Department of Community Medicine. In addition, the Physician's Associate Program was moved to the office of the dean, College of Medicine, where it had been housed originally. Dr. Jack Parish ultimately became head of the truncated Family Medicine program, a post he held for little more than a year.

Also in July, Dr. Charles B. McCall was named interim associate dean of Medicine, Tulsa branch; Janet Key resigned as assistant director of the Professional Practice Plan, a post she would later return to in a similar capacity; and Dr. Rodman Seeley, professor of Pediatrics, resigned from Pediatrics and from Biochemistry. Finally, Regents Professor Emeritus Ernst Lachman was approved to continue his active role as medical director of Radiography in the Department of Radiologic Technology.

In September, selection of an architect for a proposed $3 million Health Sciences Physical Fitness Center was approved by the regents *[Oklahoma*

Daily, 9–7–79]. The effort to build such a facility ("to be completed by October 1980") would be long, arduous, and, based on grand expectations, ultimately futile. Not until 1996, under the guidance of University President David Boren, would a fitness facility built by Presbyterian Hospital, and a Student Center without the proposed "commercial space, a cafeteria, a faculty house, and a food court" be completed, by the University, in greatly truncated form *[Oklahoma Daily, 10–27–79].*

Other September actions included approval of criteria for admission, promotion, and graduation in the Physician's Associate Program, as well as an extended discussion regarding the establishment of the Oklahoma Blood Institute on the Health Sciences Center campus. The death of Ernest Lachman, Regents Professor Emeritus, was reported on September 21, 1979. Later in the month, on September 25, a special meeting of the regents was held, at which plans for a $12 million expansion of the University of Oklahoma Bizzell Memorial Library on the Norman campus were approved.

William Thurman Resigns

Provost William G. Thurman announced his resignation as provost to accept the position of president of the Oklahoma Medical Research Foundation. The regents accepted the resignation with a resolution commending him for his vigorous leadership in steering the Health Sciences Center through the perilous waters of the 1970s. President Banowsky said, "Bill Thurman has put his stamp indelibly upon this Campus, and for decades to come . . . all will benefit from his great leadership over the past four years" *[RM, 15477–8].*

The William Thurman years were characterized by fearless decision making and decisive action. Unfortunately, actions of great import to the faculty of the College of Medicine were sometimes taken by the provost without consultation of the faculty involved. Dr. Thurman took over in an era when faculty governance, through the Faculty Board and its chair, extended to administrative decisions, through default of action by previous deans and provosts. Following his appointment, the confinement of administrative decision-making to the provost's office inevitably led to friction between himself and the faculty leadership. Many of the faculty were unhappy with Provost Thurman's administrative style, especially his failure to consult with those affected by his decisions, and his tendency to prevent any disagreement from extending beyond the College—i.e., to the regents or to the general public. Dean Lynn, who served four years with Provost Thurman, recalled him as "personally charming, a delightful person to converse with. But the relation-ship between him as provost and me as dean was sometimes uncomfortable. It was absolutely maddening when you wondered where he was getting the facts used to bolster his pronouncements."[43] In spite of opinions such as this, Dr. Thurman's tenure was marked by the solution of many persistent problems, and hence there was general approval of his decisions and actions by the regents, state business community, the legislature, and ultimately, the majority of faculty. (See Epilogue.)

Donald Halverstadt Selected Interim Provost

A special meeting of the University of Oklahoma Board of Regents was held on October 1, at which President Banowsky reported that the search com-mittee for the new provost of the Health Sciences Center had forwarded to him a list of five qualified candidates, each of whom would be returning to the campus for interviews. Inasmuch as Provost Thurman would be leaving his position on November 1, the president recommended the appointment of Dr. Donald B. Halverstadt, clinical professor of Urology and chief of staff at Oklahoma Children's Memorial Hospital, as interim provost at a salary of $50,000 for twelve months for 80 percent time, until such time as a permanent provost was found. Regent Replogle asked about the Professional Practice Plan relationship between the University and Halverstadt. President Banowsky stated that if appointed, Dr. Halverstadt's 20 percent time for clinical practice would not be governed by the Practice Plan. Dr. Thurman pointed out that questions had been asked about whether or not Dr. Halverstadt was a candi-date for the permanent position of provost, and that the urologist had assured both himself and the president that he was not *[RM, 15715–6]*. Regent Julian Rothbaum remembered that "there was a big row over the appointment. It was a real fight. It was about doctors having private patients and keeping the money"[44]

Autumn and winter 1979 witnessed a flurry of activity at the Health Sciences Center, including numerous resignations and reassignments. Carlos A. Garcia-Moral resigned as associate professor of Orthopaedic Surgery and Rehabilitation to enter private practice, while Joseph E. Leonard was named interim head, Department of Otorhinolaryngology. The title of William Thurman was changed from provost to professor of Pediatrics, Oklahoma Medical Research Foundation. Solomon Papper, head of the Department of Medicine, and Jack Metcoff, the George Lynn Cross professor of research pediatrics, were given sabbaticals for six months. Walter H. Whitcomb, professor of Medicine and assistant dean for Veterans Administration Affairs, resigned October 16 to become director of Clinical Management Systems at the national Veterans Administration headquarters. In November, Interim Provost Halverstadt was given the title of clinical professor of Pediatrics, an exception to the usual confinement of "clinical" titles to nonsalaried volunteer physicians. And in December, J. Rodman Sealy and Logan Wright, both members of the Department of Pediatrics, resigned as full-time faculty to enter private practice.

It was announced at the November Board of Regents meeting that the State Regents had, in July, allocated the $23.4 million made available by the legislature for modernization and repair at institutions of higher education. To almost no one's surprise, not a penny of it had been allocated to the Health Sciences Center! Chancellor Dunlap stated that only one project was approved for the Oklahoma City campus, but it was not funded. He said that all other requests from the Center had been turned down. This was a further example of the general animosity of the chancellor toward the Health Sciences Center. The regents then approved and forwarded a list of current capital needs to the State Regents for their consideration. This list included the renovation of many buildings on the Oklahoma City campus as well as projected construction costs of the College of Pharmacy, the Physical Fitness Center, and the Faculty/Clinical Care Building *[RM, 15760–61]*.

Clayton Rich

Upon recommendation of President Banowsky, the regents approved the appointment of Clayton Rich, M.D., as provost of the Health Sciences Center, as well as executive dean of the College of Medicine, at a yearly salary of $92,500, effective March 1, 1980. Rich, who was also appointed professor of Medicine with tenure, was a graduate of Swarthmore College and the Cornell College of Medicine, an internist who had served on the faculty of Rockefeller, Washington, and Stanford Universities, and the chief executive officer of the Stanford University hospitals prior to coming to Oklahoma. He was to serve as executive dean and provost from 1980–83 and then as provost until 1990.

The use of physician practice funds for the purpose of establishing and funding endowed chairs for the College of Medicine was approved by the Board of Regents in December as "a positive investment for and contribution to the educational and research programs of the Health Sciences Center" *[RM,*

15796]. There was also an optimistic discussion of leasing retail space in the "Will it ever be built?" physical fitness center. Representatives from the Department of Human Services indicated a willingness to build a parking structure adjacent to the College of Dentistry for $1.3 million, which the University would repay over time. Thus, the year closed on a hopeful note, with a new provost appointed, a visionary plan to fund endowed chairs from the Practice Plan, and a strong atmosphere of cooperation between the Department of Human Services and the University.

Physician Regents

The role of physicians serving on the University of Oklahoma Board of Regents has seldom been commented upon. According to former Regent Julian Rothbaum, "To this day, the regents think carefully before they do anything about the Medical School. And if there is a doctor on the board, they give him preference [in medical matters]—even if he knows very little about the school. He's a doctor, and they think he *should* know something. You just kinda go along. You're not looking for a fight with a doctor; you might need his vote next time. And [with regard to medical issues] why take on something you don't know anything about?"[45]

There were six physicians on the University of Oklahoma Board of Regents during the three decades covered in this history. Each had his own point of view about the Health Sciences Center, as well as his own special interests. None was disinterested in the goings on at the Center, or without his own biases and prejudices. Like the others with whom he served, each enjoyed the "perks" of being a regent: the public deference, the power to influence educational policy, the proximity to a prestigious football program (which, for some regents, was the most important perk of all!).

Dr. Mark Johnson was the first physician/regent. A University of Oklahoma graduate, he was an internist practicing in Oklahoma City. He was a highly political person, interested in all aspects of the Medical School. He served during 1964–1967, a period characterized by much suspicion on the part of community physicians regarding the influx of full-time clinical faculty at the Medical Center. Subsequently he headed the Ambulatory Medicine teaching program in the Department of Medicine when Dr. Solomon Papper was chair.

In 1970, Governor Bartlett appointed Dr. Vernon M. Lockhard of Bartlesville during the Herbert Hollomon presidency. He served only two years on the Board. His principal role was as a swing vote in the struggle between the various political factions. Governor Hall replaced him with Dr. Robert G. Mitchell, a general practitioner from Poteau, in 1972. Mitchell served until 1979 and was primarily interested in enhancing the influence of non-faculty physicians in the selection of medical students and other operational matters. Mitchell was thought by some to have little or no interest in medical education or academic excellence.

In 1977 Dr. Ronald White, a cardiologist from Oklahoma City, was appointed by Governor Boren. He served until 1991. A man of good judgment who was sincerely interested in higher education, his ties to Baptist Hospital occasionally influenced his decision making. For example, he encouraged the selection of orthopedic surgeons affiliated with Baptist Hospital as "team physicians" for the University football team, rather than the assignment of the University's own Orthopedic service to this activity following the long tenure of Dr. O'Donoghue in the key position. Dr. White served two full terms on the board and hence had a particularly strong influence over a long period of time. (Other two-term regents during this period were Julian Rothbaum and G. T. Blankenship Jr.)

In 1991 Governor Walters appointed Dr. Victor Williams of Lawton, a major contributor to his campaign for office. Some political observers suggested that Victor Williams had, together with Ron Yordy (later prominent as director of the Parking Authority), been the candidate's biggest contributors.

Doctor Williams died prematurely and was replaced on the board by another Walters appointee, Dr. Donald B. Halverstadt of Oklahoma City (1993). Don Halverstadt was an effective political operator as well as an excellent pediatric urologist. He was appointed despite the 1970s conflict with the regents over the Site of Practice policy, presumably because of his strong political interests, as well as influence deriving from having been chief medical advisor to Lloyd Rader and the Department of Human Services. It was felt by some that Dr. Halverstadt too closely protected the interests of Presbyterian Hospital.

Individuals appointed to the Board of Regents were often contibutors to governors' political campaigns. Physicians were no exception. This selection method never guaranteed candidates with a serious interest in higher education, or with impartial and effective leadership ability. In fact, it often assured the opposite. Fortunately, several political contributors appointed as regents throughout this period were sincerely interested in improving higher education without attempting to micromanage the institution they were assigned to, or to grind personal axes.

By the end of the decade of the 1970s, the College of Medicine had increased the size of the entering class to more than 180 students, compared to 75 in the class of 1951. But by 1980, no longer was there a national or state clamor for more physicians. Consequently, the federal fiscal incentive for bigger classes was gone, and the cry was for more "primary care" physicians. The new theme was: "fewer physicians but more general practitioners." General Internal Medicine, Pediatrics, and Family Practice were declared to be "primary care" specialties. Departments of Obstetrics and Gynecology mounted a national drive to be declared "primary care physicians for women," but early expectations for success at the federal level were disappointing. In Oklahoma, the emphasis was on increasing the number of resident positions in primary care to over 50 percent of the total number of house staff trainees. At the same time, the size of the entering class would diminish from a high of 184 in 1988 to a low of 133 in 1993. The class size was officially reduced in 1989 to 150, and even this number was not accepted until 1990.[46] More importantly the era of independent departmental chairs who were primarily in charge of their own destinies had ended with the subordination of the Professional Practice Plan and its revenues to University administration. Simultaneously, the new age of strong administration from the provost's office was well underway.

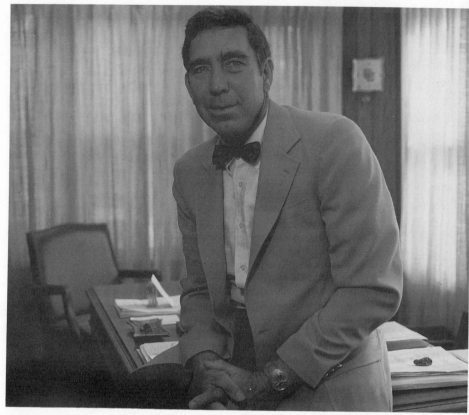

William G. Thurman, M.D., Professor of Pediatrics, Executive Dean of the College of Medicine in
Oklahoma City and Tulsa, and Provost of the Health Sciences Center. (OUHSC)

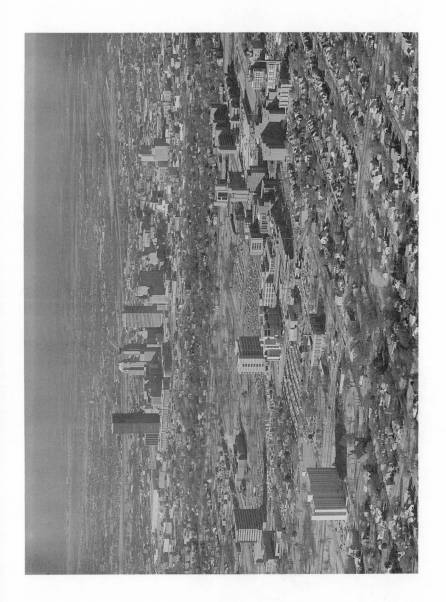

Aerial view of the University of Oklahoma Health Sciences Center campus, 1975. (OUHSC)

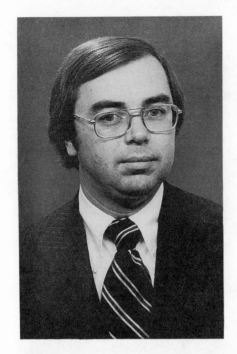

Dee Replogle, Jr., Regent of the
University of Oklahoma. (OUPA)

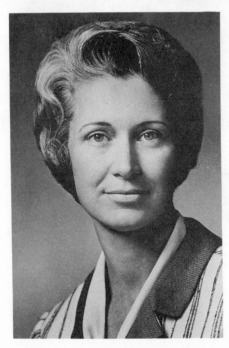

Nancy Davies, Regent of the University
of Oklahoma. (OUPA)

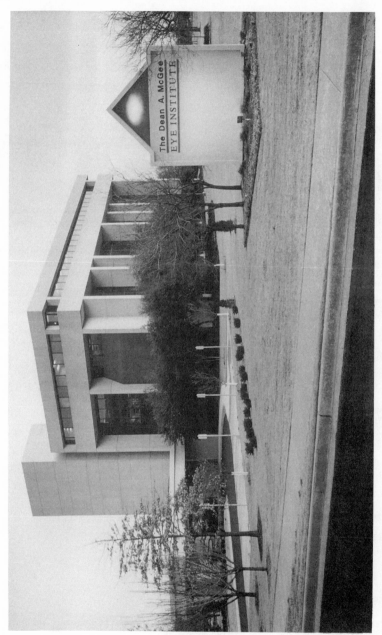

The Dean A. McGee Eye Institute, an independent institution on the Health Sciences Center campus. (OUHSC)

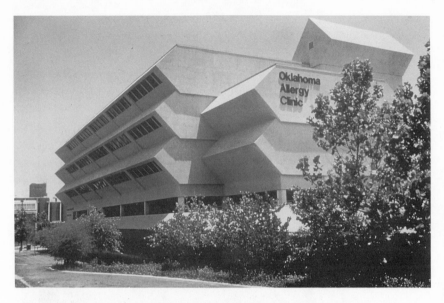

The Oklahoma Asthma and Allergy Clinic, another independent institution on the
Health Sciences Center campus. (OUHSC)

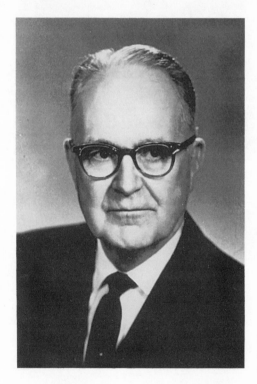

Don H. O'Donoghue, M.D., first
Chairman of the Faculty Board.
(OUHSC)

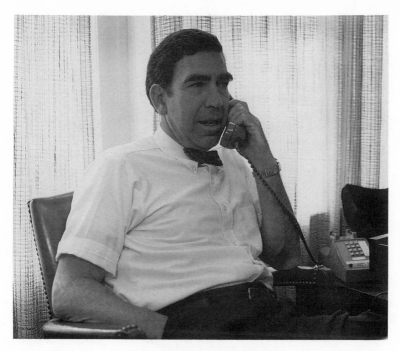

William Thurman, M.D., Provost in charge. (OUHSC)

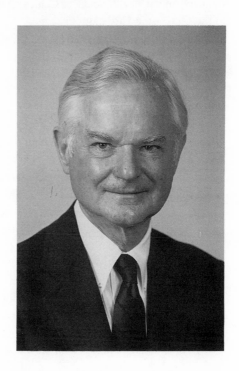

Clayton Rich, M.D., Provost of the
University of Oklahoma Health
Sciences Center. (OUHSC)

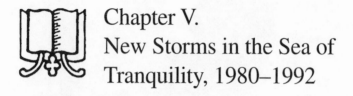

Chapter V.
New Storms in the Sea of
Tranquility, 1980–1992

 The appointment of Dr. Donald Halverstadt to the post of interim provost of the University of Oklahoma Health Sciences Center was a propitious one for the times because of his position as chief of staff of Children's Hospital and his influence with, and high regard by, Lloyd Rader, director of the Department of Institutions, Social and Rehabilitative Services (DISRS—later to be named the Department of Human Services). The collapse of federal funding for an expanded Health Sciences Center precipitated, once again, a fiscal crisis on the Oklahoma City campus, especially for the free-standing University Hospital. This led to a concerted effort by Governor Nigh, the Board of Regents, and many legislators to transfer the hospitals to DISRS, which had so successfully rejuvenated Children's Hospital.

At the January 17, 1980, meeting of the Board of Regents, Richard Bell stated:

> The Regents . . . have observed with great interest discussions surrounding the possible transfer of governance of the University Hospital and Clinics . . . an invaluable teaching facility for our educational activities in all fields of the health professions. . . . The Oklahoma Public Welfare Commission has been the governing body of Oklahoma Children's Memorial Hospital since 1973. Our relationship with the Welfare Commission relative to our educational programs at the Children's has been exceedingly productive. . . . It is the opinion of the University of Oklahoma Board of Regents that a similar relationship at the University Hospital would provide the best situation for educational programs at that institution. It is the unanimous recommendation of all Regents present here today that every consideration be given to a transfer of the University Hospital and Clinics (with the exception of the 1,100-car parking

garage) to the Oklahoma Public Welfare Commission as its governing body *[RM, 15822].*

The regents urged President Banowsky to convey these sentiments to the governor.

The suspicions associated with the original involvement of the Oklahoma Public Welfare Commission in the operation of the Health Sciences Center hospitals had by this time dissipated due to the dedication and strong financial and administrative support of Director Lloyd Rader and the members of the Commission in the operation of Children's Hospital since 1973. On February 20 the House of Representatives voted 61 to 36 in favor of a transfer of University Hospital to DISRS *[Oklahoma Daily, 2–21–80].* One of Dr. John Schilling's worst fears thus was realized. But time and necessity had reversed the opinion of nearly all who had originally opposed the separation of the hospitals from the University. Instead of fear and suspicion, there was now expectation and hope.

At this time, Dr. Donald Halverstadt recalled his eight months of service as interim provost as:

> . . . the most exciting, happiest, perhaps single most productive time of my entire professional career. How I got there is another story; but the University family went out of its way to try to make me comfortable. The regents were very supportive. President Banowsky put no restrictions on me. He said, 'The only thing I'll ask is that you don't embarrass me.' I decided to attack that job as if I were the permanent provost, not interim. I came to know everybody connected to the University and the Health Sciences Center. It changed my life a great deal—just the fact of being there, and having the credibility of being a part of the University, especially after having been separated from it."[1]

The early part of Dr. Halverstadt's eight months was devoted primarily to problems at the Tulsa branch of the College of Medicine. The biggest concern was the extreme overcrowding in the Midway Building. There was an urgent need for more space because clinics were scattered, crowded, and inadequate. To meet this need, the regents authorized a lease of the Eastwood Baptist Church campus for consolidation and expansion of the various Tulsa branch operations. In May the Board requested that the Tulsa Industrial Authority issue five million dollars in bonds for acquisition and improvement of the facilities at 2808 South Sheridan and lease of the property to the regents for use by the Tulsa branch. In June the regents provided a detailed assessment of the Tulsa program, with extensive justification for the proposed lease of the Eastwood Baptist property, in response to a critical evaluation by the State Regents for Higher Education at their meeting of April 28, 1980. Said the State Regents' report:

> At the present time, approximately 60,000 square feet of space is occupied in five different locations in Tulsa. The Midway building . . . has become totally inadequate . . . and the existing leases are the subject of an ongoing lawsuit. . . . The University of Oklahoma concurs with the conclusions reached in discussions with the State Regents staff relative to the Tulsa Medical College program size and content. It is felt that there should be no further proliferation of these programs. However, in order to effectively discharge current programs, adequate resources must be provided. The planned move to the Eastwood facilities will provide the necessary space to support quality educational programs. . . . The current size of the Tulsa Medical College program is appropriate and should be supported, but the program should not be expanded *[RM, 15988–93]*.

Nearly all of the medical disciplines without departments at the Tulsa branch had by this time designated a vice chair in appropriate Oklahoma City campus departments.

"We also got a lot done with the Practice Plan during my stint," added Interim Provost Halverstadt. "I ended up decentralizing the thing, which over the years has turned around and gone the other way, for better or worse."[2] Following the appointment of his permanent successor, Clayton Rich, Dr. Halverstadt's title was changed from interim provost to special assistant to the president for hospital affairs effective July 1, 1980. Thirty days later, on July 31, Dr. Clayton Rich succeeded Halverstadt.

At this time, there was much public speculation concerning the political ambitions of University of Oklahoma President Bill Banowsky. A state senate resolution demanded that Banowsky announce his plans regarding a possible run for the U. S. Senate seat being vacated by Henry Bellmon. This action annoyed Regent Kenneth. Bailey, who suggested that the senate was meddling in an area that should be off limits to political considerations *[Oklahoma Daily, 2–15–80]*.

Also at this time, one of the primary concerns of the Board of Regents, as well as the University administration, was paying competitive faculty salaries—

within the severe limitations placed on them by a consistently penurious Oklahoma legislature—on both the Norman and Oklahoma City campuses. Salaries at the Health Sciences Center in 1980 had increased considerably over those of the early 1970s:

TABLE 2. SALARIES OF INSTRUCTIONAL STAFF, HEALTH SCIENCES CENTER, 1980

Academic Rank	Title	Salary	Title	Salary
Professor	M.D.	$45,000 to $70,000	Ph.D.	$45,000 to $70,000
Associate Professor	M.D.	$30,000 to $60,000	Ph.D.	$28,000 to $32,000
Assistant Professor	M.D.	$30,000 to $45,000	Ph.D.	$25,000 to $30,000

Faculty members might, in addition to these state salaries, earn supplemental clinical and other income as great as $70,000 to $96,000, depending upon faculty rank *[RM, 15,952]*.

FACILITIES AND CONSTRUCTION

Construction of previously planned Oklahoma City campus facilities was virtually complete by the spring of 1980, except for one parking garage and the emergency and laboratory addition to University Hospital, and each of these was 50 percent finished. In addition, there were always the ongoing, endless additions to the Steam and Chilled Water System. Only the Pharmacy building and the Student Center-Recreational Facility were still planned but unfunded. An addition to the Dermatology building was authorized, with a budget of $250,000, to be amortized from patient care fees. A contract was let to Charles M. Dunning Company in June. The project was completed in June of 1981 and accepted by the regents at their meeting of July 22, 1981.

In June 1980 the regents transferred their interest and responsibility for the 1,100-car parking garage contract to the Department of Human Services because its director, Lloyd Rader, was willing and able to furnish funds for the project. Also in June, Regents President Richard Bell, a Norman worker's compensation and personal injury attorney appointed by Governor David Hall, announced that an anonymous donor had provided funds for a clock tower and a plaza associated with the new Neustadt Library addition on the Norman campus. The donor stipulated that "the clock tower and surrounding plaza be named in honor of longtime state educator E. T. Dunlap" *[Oklahoma Daily, 6–12–80]*. Many observers considered this a strangely ironic conclusion to the long and frequently bitter feud between the University of Oklahoma Board of Regents, several of its presidents, and the chancellor of higher education!

June also saw a non-tenure track for Health Sciences Center faculty established by the regents as "renewable, consecutive term appointments" wherein such faculty "may, at any time after the third year elect to be placed in the tenure track, in which case all University policies relating to tenure shall apply." Once election had been made, said the regents, "Faculty members eligible for tenure may not elect a change to a renewable term appointment" *[RM, 15949–50]*.

Leases with the Oklahoma Health Science Facility, Inc. (OHSF) for eight properties on N. E. 14th Street, one on N. E. 15th Street, and the Family Medicine Clinic on N. E. 50th Street were renewed by the regents through June 30, 1981. The seven directors of OHSF were appointed by, and served at the pleasure of, the University of Oklahoma Board of Regents *[RM, 16238]*.

OKLAHOMA MEDICAL RESEARCH FOUNDATION

On July 30 the University of Oklahoma Board of Regents finally approved, by unanimous vote, an affiliation agreement with the Oklahoma Medical Research Foundation which clarified the issue of faculty titles for personnel at that institution. There were to be two types of titles: (1) "volunteer" faculty, with titles prefixed by "clinical," "adjunct," "research," or "special"; and (2) "OMRF faculty" devoting at least 25 percent of their time to teaching or patient care programs of the University. None would be considered for tenure nor considered part of the "general faculty" of the University *[RM, 16045–16048]*. This action led to a storm of complaints from OMRF investigators and, as a result, for the most part the new policy on titles was never implemented!

Personnel actions in June included the retirement of Dr. William George McCreight, clinical professor of Dermatology and one of the early Mayo graduates in Oklahoma City. The title of Gary L. Smith was changed from director of administration and finance to vice provost for administration and finance, effective June 1. This was part of the reorganization proposed by Dr. Halverstadt as he left office. Halverstadt and David Walters, associate provost, had outlined "what we thought would be a reasonable administrative working arrangement for what was then three different hospitals and the university."[3]

In July, Lloyd Rader and the Oklahoma Public Welfare Commission implemented a proposal for an umbrella organization in which there would be a central administration to coordinate all of the public Health Sciences Center hospitals. Following Commission approval, said Dr. Halverstadt, "Mr. Rader turned around and asked me if I would be the CEO of that umbrella organization. That was when Bill Thurman accepted the appointment to O'Donoghue, and you [Dr. Mark Everett] the appointment [as chief of staff] at University Hospital."[4]

Late in July, the regents approved three complex agreements with the Department of Human Services which defined the use, responsibility for, and the exact boundaries of all hospital-related facilities, parking structures, and financial documents. On August 28 at a special meeting, the regents met with Mr. Rader and Dr. Halverstadt, at which time covenants were approved regarding: (1) assignment of all architectural and construction contracts on the 1,100- and 434-car parking garages to the Department of Human Services; (2) conveying use of the "research" building on Northeast 13th Street to the University; and (3) conveying land south of the 1,100-car garage, and on the south side of Stanton Young Boulevard as sites for construction by the regents of the new Biomedical Research Tower (finally built in 1997) and the site of the Family Medicine facility *[RM, 16109–12]*. These agreements, finalized at the September 12 regents' regular meeting, ushered in a long period of friction-free cooperation between these two constitutional bodies *[RM, 16057–64]*. One casualty of the agreement was abandonment of the concept of retail space in the addition to the parking garages. A negotiated settlement was struck with the architectural engineering firm of Barbour and Short, which was to have completed the retail space, and Ratcliffe's Book Store was given space in the Health Sciences Center Library building *[RM, 16178–9]*.

Later in the year, a new addition to the campus began operation: the Oklahoma Allergy and Asthma Clinic at Lindsay and Northeast 13th Street. The building was a modern structure housing internist and pediatrician allergists, laboratories, and technicians.

During August and September 1980 there was a lengthy discussion among regents and the Health Sciences Center administration about leadership and direction in the Department of Family Practice. A report was received from Provost Rich regarding an "investigation of financial issues raised by audits of August 1979 and 1980, as well as with the organization, financing, management, and academic leadership of the Department" *[RM, 16114]*. On September 12 the board approved the reappointment of Dr. Parrish as chair for one year, without tenure. "The reason Dr. Parrish has not been granted tenure, and there is no salary increase for him, is because of the continuing concerns that the regents have for the department and his administration" *[RM, 16115]*. One year later, in May 1981 Dr. Parrish resigned as head of the department, along with Dr. Dixon and Dr. Nasr. Interim Dean G. Rainey Williams asked Dr. Thomas C. Coniglione to serve as interim head of the Department of Family Practice. Dr. Tim Coussons was named chair of the search committee for a new permanent head of the department.

On July 29 Kelly M. West, M.D., George Lynn Cross research professor of Biostatistics and Epidemiology, and clinical professor of Medicine, died. He was the son of the long-term professor and chair of Orthopedics, Willis K. West, and grandson of Archa West, an early head of Internal Medicine. Following study at the Joslin Clinic in Boston, Kelly West spent a year in Ann Arbor, Michigan, with several prominent national figures in research and treatment of diabetes mellitus. Following this, he returned home and pursued a distinguished career in the investigation of diabetes in American Indians. He served on the National Board of Directors of the American Diabetes Association and on the Board of Regents of the National Library of Medicine. Kelly West was a gentleman, a fine tennis player, and a loyal friend. As a fourth-year medical student, he suffered a ruptured cerebral aneurysm, and a recurrence of this ended his short but productive life.

The Health Sciences Center faculty lost another member on August 15 when Milton J. Serwer, M.D., died. A clinical professor and former acting chair of the Department of Gynecology and Obstetrics, he had served the University as both a salaried and volunteer faculty member for many years. Many young doctors were indebted to him for their superior training in Obstetrics.

DEAN LYNN RESIGNS

In November Dean Thomas Lynn announced that he would resign his position on January 1, at which time he would join the Baptist Hospital administration *[RM, 16199]*. Since July 1974 Tom Lynn had served as dean under four provosts: Donald Brown (briefly); William Thurman (four years), Don Halverstadt (eight months); and Clayton Rich (six months). Dean Lynn recalled that even though he worked well enough with Clayton Rich:

my exit as dean was interesting. I had come to the conclusion in 1979 that the Medical School's next step should be to intensify its research activity. I didn't think I was up to accomplishing that. I thought, however, that I would like to stay in Oklahoma City. So I visited Frank McGregor, medical vice president at Baptist Hospital, and asked if he knew of anything in Oklahoma City appropriate for a former dean. He said no. Shortly after that, he died. I then received a call from Jay Henry, the Baptist administrator, asking if I would be interested in the position. I went to see Clayton and said, 'Clayton, I have this offer. If you would like for me to stay at the University, I'll do that. If you see an opportunity to replace me with somebody that you feel might more effectively develop research, that's OK too.' He called me later and said, 'Why don't you go ahead and take the job?' That's how it happened.[5]

Tom Lynn's years with Provost Thurman were characterized by institutional growth, a fiscal roller coaster resulting from changing federal reimbursement patterns, a legislature and body of State Regents who were seldom supportive, and extensive faculty-administration dissension. During the latter years of his deanship, for the first time there was the prospect of long-term fiscal stability, primarily because of the generous funding of the teaching hospitals by the Department of Human Services (formerly DISRS and the Department of Public Welfare), and the intense interest and support shown by its director, Lloyd Rader, who assured sufficient funds for support of research and clinical faculty, as well as supporting staff. Development of a nationally prominent medical center was at last a realistic possibility as long as this commitment continued. Dean Lynn was a thoughtful, soft-spoken leader with an institutional rather than a parochial viewpoint. His "don't rock the boat" administrative style was well suited to the atmosphere and political realities of the campus at the time. Lynn's own assessment was that his relations with the faculty were always good. "My attitude was that the faculty was almost always right, even though it might not appear to be so. Furthermore, a contented faculty with a good sense of its own worth leads to a much better environment and school. I relied heavily upon the faculty and the Faculty Board."[6] During his tenure at Baptist Hospital, Dr. Lynn was to develop various "Centers of Excellence" which that institution had long desired but had never been able to achieve— e.g., outstanding clinicians in the fields of Oncology, Pediatrics, and Neonatal Medicine. His recruitment efforts brought reality to the aspirations of Baptist Hospital for prominence in the above specialized areas.

G. Rainey Williams, the Schilling Professor of Surgery, was named interim dean of the College of Medicine effective January 1, 1981. A selection committee for a new dean was to be chaired by Solomon Papper, chair of Medicine, with Gordon Deckert, Charles Esmon, Nancy Hall, Donald Halverstadt, Owen Rennert, Lowell Stone, Kenneth Whittington, and Maude Miller as members *[Oklahoma Daily, 11–14–80]*.

The College of Health, which had been created during the fiscal crisis of 1972, was divided once more into a College of Public Health and a College of Allied Health Professions in November. At the same time, the College of Medicine's Professional Practice Plan was amended to include part-time faculty, as well as members of the Tulsa branch faculty.

ACADEMIC ISSUES

The relationship of College of Medicine faculty to the other colleges on the Oklahoma City campus and what, if any, responsibility they had to these colleges, remained unresolved in December 1980. In a report of a Faculty Board committee on cross–listing of courses, it was brought to the attention of Dean Lynn that "The College of Allied Health Professions has seen fit to begin teaching most of the basic science courses with its own faculty, diluting the overall goals of the University of Oklahoma Health Sciences Center and creating intractable problems for the present and future. We do not agree with this approach . . . and advise that all Departments in the College of Medicine withdraw totally from undergraduate teaching" in the College of Health. The Academic Program Council of the Health Sciences Center Faculty Senate believed that the hidden issue in the controversy was "control," and that the provost should seek advice from all units on the campus rather than accept the College of Medicine view.[7] As with most heated academic issues at this time, resolution of conflicting attitudes was postponed rather than finalized.

In a December action, the College of Medicine discontinued its agreement with the Universidad Autonoma de Guadalajara and announced that the college would no longer provide a portion of Guadalajara's clinical education at the University of Oklahoma. As with most such agreements between "offshore" medical schools and LCME-approved institutions, quality control and accreditation of students was almost impossible, and with the decrease in Oklahoma residents in such schools, the incentive for the affiliation no longer existed.

1981

National Board of Medical Examiners, Again!

Nineteen eighty-one may have been a new year, but many of the issues at the Health Sciences Center were the same as in years past when, in mid-January 1981, the Faculty Board conducted a long discussion regarding the "non-requirement" that students "take, but not be required to pass, the NBME Part I examination in order to move from the second to the third year of medical school" *[FBM, 1–20–81]*. This, it may be recalled, was the ultimate resolution (or nonresolution) of the external examination standard disagreement implicit in the degree-granting controversy, which so impinged upon faculty time and effort in 1978 under the reign of Provost William Thurman. After a prolonged discussion, Dr. Edward Tomsovic moved that the requirement be dropped. Dr. Joseph Lee seconded, and the vote was 8–8. A second motion made by Dr. Merrill, and seconded by Dr. Deckert, that both taking and passing the examination be a requirement was defeated. The re-introduced motion—that the requirement be dropped—then passed by a vote of 11–6. Henceforth, neither the taking nor the passing of this external evaluation would be required of students at Oklahoma. The recommendation was forwarded to the administration for transmission to the State Regents *[FBM, 1–20–81]*.

Meanwhile, at the January Board of Regents' meeting, President Banowsky outlined his goals for the near future, including full support of the State Regents' request for $62 million in new money for higher education, with $13.9 million earmarked for the University of Oklahoma. Also, planning was to be initiated for both the Pharmacy building on the Oklahoma City campus and the new Music building on the Norman campus, as well as construction of the Gymnastics building. In other good news, it was revealed that the very successful Associates Donor Program of President Banowsky now had 1,500 members, and the goal for 1981 was an additional 500 persons.

February saw tax-exempt financing finalized for a Laboratory Animal Holding Facility at the Oklahoma City Zoo in order that land owned by the University adjacent to the planned Remington Park Raceway could be utilized by the Racing Commission. The University agreed to a sublease agreement for twenty-four annual renewal options. The animal facility would not be built until 1986, and then not at the Zoo but adjacent to the Colleges of Nursing and Pharmacy, in close proximity to the veterinary faculty in the Pathology Department of the College of Medicine. A review of salary levels at the College of Medicine, conducted in March, revealed that generous raises were possible for sixty-four members of the faculty. This included the professor of Medicine, Dr. Solomon Papper, who saw an increase from $78,154 to $96,000 for the year, while the professor of Surgery and acting dean of the College was raised from $44,694 to $89,694 *[RM, 16327]*. In a final March action, Dee Replogle Jr. was elected president of the Board of Regents for a period of one year.

Campus Fiscal Crisis

In the spring of 1981, primarily because of the loss of federal "formula" funding, the Schools of Allied Health and Public Health were forced to close degree programs in Cardiorespiratory Science and Clinical Dietetics. When members of the faculty of the departments concerned spoke before the Board of Regents, Provost Rich said, "The Health Sciences Center is facing significant cutbacks in federal funding. The two departments being recommended for elimination have been very heavily funded from federal funds in the last few years" *[Oklahoma Daily, 4–7–81]*. This statement was challenged by faculty of the programs involved. Dean Philip Smith of the College of Health said that the Division of Allied Health received no capitation money, and that for the past five or six years had been phasing out other forms of federal financial support. President Banowsky emphasized that as federal funding decreased, the state would have to provide greater financial support than it had been providing the past few years.

Another blow to the Health Sciences Center was the cancellation in March of $4.7 million in contracts for faculty services in the hospitals by the Human Services Commission. This action, in essence, wiped out reimbursement of the University for faculty time spent in hospital activities, as well as threatened salaries for house staff, residents, and interns. Great consternation resulted among faculty and administration, but the order was later modified to lessen the severity of the blow to College and hospital operations. President Banowsky said to the regents: "Unless the people who make the funding decisions in this State take the leadership, this will only be the beginning. . . . No unit in the state system will be more negatively impacted than the Health Sciences Center under the $62 million plan [of the legislature for new higher education funds]. At less than that level, the condition will be worse than severe" *[RM, 16331]*.

Former Provost William Thurman, president of the Oklahoma Medical Research Foundation, also deplored the program's discontinuation, stating that "hospitals throughout the state will have to undertake expensive recruitment activities over the nation" *[Oklahoma Daily, 4–6–81]*. It is of interest to note that at their May meeting, the State Regents for Higher Education approved the discontinuation of the Cardiorespiratory Science Program but voted to continue the program in Clinical Dietetics! These actions clearly illustrated the effectiveness of lobbying at the state level by the well-organized dietitians.

In April, several prominent faculty members received tenure: Stephen K. Young (Pathology, Dentistry), Martha J. Ferretti (Physical Therapy), Dale H.Altmiller (Pathology), Geoffrey P. Altshuler (Pediatric Pathology), Walter H. C. Burgdorf (Dermatology), F. Daniel Duffy (Medicine, Tulsa), and Piers Blacket (Pediatrics).

The requirements of the College of Medicine for promotion and graduation were approved by the regents in early summer, with deletion of the requirement to take and pass Part I of the National Board of Medical Examiners examination *[RM, 16372]*. While this was occurring in Norman, a disagreeable encounter on the Tulsa campus regarding tenure for a member of the Family Practice faculty was resolved by administrators granting him tenure in exchange for a written promise to resign within one year. Even the most cynical of observers found this an unusual solution! *[RM, 16431]*. Also in June, two more prominent faculty members retired and were made professors emeritus: B. Conner Johnson, professor of Biochemistry and Molecular Biology; and Jay T. Shurley, professor of Psychiatry and Behavioral Sciences.

A sad note for the Health Sciences Center was sounded when Regents Professor Emeritus and former Dean and Director Mark R. Everett died on August 17, 1981. A memorial tribute at the Westminster Presbyterian Church in Oklahoma City drew hundreds of former students and colleagues, who paid tribute to his life's work.

In September 1981 inclusion of a health maintenance organization option was included, by federal requirement, in all health benefit plans of the University of Oklahoma. As a result, participation of "Pru-Care" in the University health plan was approved by the regents *[RM, 16596]*.

October saw Christian Norman Ramsey Jr., M.D., appointed professor and chair of Family Practice, with tenure. This appointment heralded a new beginning for that department and a temporary end to the ceaseless bickering that had marked it for the past several years.

Internationally known immunologist-researcher Robert A. Good, former president of the Sloan-Kettering Institute for Cancer Research in New York City, joined the faculty of the Oklahoma Medical Research Foundation to direct the cancer research program in November. He would also join the faculty of the College of Medicine and work at Children's Hospital in the newly developing Bone Marrow Transplant Program. Regents also approved in November a large tuition increase for University students, effective the following year. President Banowsky said that students should pay at least 25 percent of the cost of their higher education *[DO, 11–12–81]*. A final November action by the regents saw David L. Walters, associate provost of the Health Sciences Center and later governor, named an "executive officer" of the University.

On November 18 a new addition to the Dermatology building was dedicated by President Banowsky. The new library in the building was dedicated to Richard Fleischaker, a prominent Oklahoma City oilman and supporter of medical education in Oklahoma, as well as friend and consistent donor to the Department of Dermatology.

The year ended with a focus on two of Oklahoma's most prominent figures in education, Lloyd Rader and E.T. Dunlap. In November, Dunlap retired as chancellor of higher education. At his retirement dinner, almost every note of praise was tempered with comments about his tendency to be long-winded. He was praised by Governor George Nigh, Senator David Boren, and President William Banowsky, none of whom had been enthusiastic about Dunlap's educational priorities, which included, in the words of one speaker, the "development of 41 institutions throughout the state [which] have campuses or facilities that bear his name." Dunlap reacted to some of the speakers' remark by saying, "Hell, I don't pretend to compare to Lloyd Rader or Bill Banowsky" *[DO, 11–21–81]*. His hand-picked successor was Joe Leone, who served for only a few years before being replaced by Dr. Hans Britsch, whose dynamic leadership would bring new ideas and prestige to the office of chancellor of the State Regents for Higher Education.

Lloyd Rader: Decline Before the Fall

The *Daily Oklahoman* in December predicted a battle over legislative oversight and control of Oklahoma's mammoth Department of Human Services. Lloyd Rader, the long-term director, had maintained an "iron-fisted," one-man control of the department's billion-dollar budget. He had once uttered the incendiary statement that half of the state's legislators could be defeated in the following year's elections if they insisted on legislative control of his department. A handful of lawmakers, led by house speaker Dan Draper, maintained that neither elected officials nor the legislature "really know what is going on at the department or have any real input into its policy" *[DO, 12–27–81]*.

In spite of Lloyd Rader's grand plans for his department and the Health Sciences Center, it would be only a matter of time until control of the department would be wrested from him by the legislature. Paul Scott Malone, in the *Daily Oklahoman* on February 21 said of the director, "His relationship with [Senator Robert] Kerr, and other influential Oklahomans, is what has made Rader one of the most powerful and controversial public servants ever to hold a post in state government." But recent allegations by the Gannett News Service about child abuse in the department's juvenile institutions had sent the winds of change blowing through the agency. Continued Malone: "Lloyd Rader is an imposing man. . . . Even in old age with his slumping right shoulder (the result of a collapsed lung) and his wizened countenance, he is charismatic—almost frightfully so, as he trains a spectacled eye on you to catch your response to what he is saying. He is called 'boss' by his cadre of close and fiercely loyal assistants, and 'sir' by most others" *[DO, 2–21–81]*.

Frequently, Rader and his department "took the monkey off our backs," said state Senator E. Melvin Porter recalling that Rader assumed control and funding of many social service programs the state could not otherwise have paid for *[DO, 2–2–81]*. But the current controversy about the juvenile institutions, the diminishing revenue resulting from removal of the once-earmarked two-percent state sales tax, and the increasing demands for funds to support other state activities would bring an end to this fiefdom and the onset of legislative oversight.

One area in which Lloyd Rader's spending helped the Health Sciences Center was faculty salaries. In spite of the continuing financial difficulties for the University and the Health Sciences Center in 1981, base salaries for faculty continued to climb slowly with each passing year. Several faculty salary ranges appear in the table below. In general, the most recent appointments were salaried at a considerably higher level than comparable or better known faculty of long tenure; and Tulsa salaries were, in general, conspicuously higher than those in Oklahoma City. Generally speaking, M.D.s with higher earning potential (e.g., Surgery) were salaried at lower rates than those with lower earning potential (e.g., Pediatrics), while Ph.D.s were salaried at lower levels than M.D.s.

1982

Nineteen eighty-two began auspiciously for pharmacists around the state when in January the regents let a contract for construction of a new College of Pharmacy building in the amount of $7.75 million. The long-delayed facility would at last take its place among the other colleges with free-standing

TABLE 3.   SALARY RANGES AT THE UNIVERSITY OF OKLAHOMA HEALTH SCIENCES
CENTER, 1981

Department	Assistant Professor	Associate Professor	Professor	Department Chair
Basic Sciences	$27–32,000	$30–38,000	$35–45,000	$35–56,000
Clinical Departments	$30–66,000	$50–65,000	$50–90,000	$44–110,000
Tulsa Clinical	$30–68,000	$50–80,000	$60–94,000	$60–95,000
Deans				$89,500
Department Managers				$25–30,000

buildings. Also in January the Faculty Board approved a new code of conduct for medical students, and the dean's office initiated a new orientation program for entering medical students. This introduction to medicine, which often included the student's family members, proved to be an important and welcome addition to the curriculum of entering freshmen *[FBM, 1–26–82]*.

Dean Charles B. McCall

On February 1 Dr. Charles B. McCall assumed the post of dean of the University of Oklahoma College of Medicine. He had previously served as chief of staff at the Oklahoma City Veterans Administration Hospital since 1980, and prior to that as dean of the Oral Roberts School of Medicine in Tulsa *[DO, 2–2–82]*. McCall was given the additional title of executive dean, College of Medicine, to recognize his primacy over the dean at the Tulsa branch, which had been a priority requirement specified by the Liaison Committee on Medical Education which accredits all medical schools. The Committee had been critical of the assignment of the Health Sciences Center provost as Executive Dean, a move which they interpreted (correctly) as a device to assure Tulsa that its dean was not subordinate to the Oklahoma City dean *[RM, 17259–60]*.

Meantime, at the Faculty Board meeting on January 20, Provost Clayton Rich announced that in the future, budget allocations would be determined by overall policy, with allocations related to priorities and program needs as seen by the provost's office. With the tight financial situation at the Center, preservation of core programs would be the central thrust *[FBM, 1–20–81]*.

At their February meeting, the Faculty Board voted that any faculty member with an unmodified title must submit all research grant requests through the office of the dean. This reflected the still-unresolved status of the Oklahoma Medical Research Foundation affiliation agreement *[FBM, 2–17–81]*. Similarly, the Board's Executive Committee adopted as policy a rule that all section heads in College of Medicine departments must have unmodified titles, and be subject to all the rules and regulations of the full-time faculty.[8] Also in February, Dr. Donald Halverstadt, whose current title was "clinical professor of Urology and special assistant to the president for hospital affairs," was given the additional title of vice chair, Department of Urology, effective January 1.

Family Medicine

A superficial, uncritical review of the Department of Family Medicine was accepted by the University Board of Regents at their January meeting—a review that had been requested by the regents some months earlier. The following month, several changes were made in restructuring the Family Practice program in anticipation of the arrival of Chair-designate Christian Ramsey. Dr. Ramsey had become the leading choice for the position following an impromptu trip to Iowa City by Provost Rich, Dr. Rainey Williams, and Dr. Richard Timothy Coussons to consult with the national head of the Family Medicine organization. The latter recommended Dr. Ramsey as the "only candidate" for the position.

In February, the Departments of Family Practice and Community Medicine, separate since 1979, were again combined into a single department, and the Physician's Associate Program was removed from the office of the dean, College of Medicine, and placed within the newly created Department of Family Medicine. The regents also approved inclusion of a new Family Medicine building, budgeted at a cost of $8.3 million, in the Health Sciences Center Capital Improvement Program as "New-Construction Priority One" *[RM, 16889]*. In final February actions, regents renewed leases for space for the Enid Family Medicine Clinic and the Shawnee Family Practice Clinic.

At the annual meeting of the University of Oklahoma Board of Regents in March, retiring regent Dee Replogle was cited for his seven years of dedicated service in improving the quality of the University as an academic institution. Special mention was made of his long-standing interest in and concern for the future of the Health Sciences Center *[RM, 16876; 17087]*. Replogle had been an outspoken advocate for more adequate funding for the University, and he frequently tangled with both the chancellor of the State Regents and with penurious legislative leaders. He had proven to be a strong advocate for the Health Sciences Center. Also in March, the appointment of Dr. Mark Allen Everett and Dean Philip Smith as Regents Professors was confirmed effective July 1, 1982.

Personnel changes were the order of the day at the April 8 regents' meeting. Associate Provost for Health Sciences David L. Walters resigned effective May 14. John Byrne, administrator of Children's Medical Center in Tulsa, was named administrator of Oklahoma Children's Memorial Hospital, which was then a 402-bed acute care facility. Dr. Bertram Sears, professor of Anesthesiology, was given the additional title of interim head of his department following the departure of Dr. Stanley Deutsch for an appointment at another institution. The new permanent head of Anesthesiology, Dr. Lennart Fagraeus, was appointed the following September at a salary of $80,000. Simultaneously, Emeritus Dean Philip E. Smith was reappointed as interim dean, College of Allied Health. And on December 9 Provost Clayton Rich was given the additional title of "Vice president for Health Sciences," indicating his "line," rather than solely "academic," authority over the campus *[RM, 17325]*.

Medi-Flight and the Neonatal Unit

In early 1982 the use of helicopters stationed at Oklahoma Children's Memorial Hospital was well established under the rubric of "Medi-Flight," which was begun about 1980 as an adjunct to the neonatal intensive care program for the purpose of transporting critical care infants to the hospital. The unit quickly became a vehicle for transporting many seriously ill patients to Oklahoma City from the surrounding communities. By 1982 two helicopters were based on the roof of Children's Garrison Tower. It was not long before other Oklahoma City hospitals took note of the dramatic publicity value of the effort (which often overshadowed the medical value or even the necessity of the service), and soon adult patients were transported to a variety of other area hospitals, with no connection to the medical center. The Medi-Flight program was frequently not reimbursed by these receiving hospitals, in spite of efforts of the director of the Department of Human Services, Lloyd Rader, and the teaching hospitals' chiefs of staff (Drs. Halverstadt, Everett, and Thurman) to make transport availability dependent upon a prior agreement to reimburse the agency at the reasonable rate of a $150 lift-off fee and $4 per air mile. The program was very expensive to maintain because of the approximately fifty-five assigned personnel (pilots, nurses, technicians), in addition to the two helicopters and ancillary equipment and maintenance *[DO, 4–25–82]*. For decades the program was to be a very costly one, responsible for annual budget deficits to the hospitals in the region of one to two million dollars.

Medi-Flight was not the only service garnering positive publicity for the Health Sciences Center at this time. The Neonatal Intensive Care Unit was one of the unique and especially visible programs at the Children's Hospital. The unit was designed for the care of premature babies who could not survive outside of a very structured and protective environment. By 1982, the forty-bed unit was served by eighty-five nurses and directed by Dr. Mary Anne McCaffree, who said that 88 percent of the surviving infants of the unit developed normally, while twelve percent had residual brain damage *[DO, 11–14–82]*. In addition to its unique, life-saving value to Oklahomans, it was a focus of attention for the media and the public, with many exciting accounts of survival in the face of overwhelming odds for tiny, helpless infants.

Lloyd Rader Resigns

In May, state newspapers carried rumors that Lloyd E. Rader, longtime director of the Department of Human Services, would resign within the next ninety days *[OKC Times, 5–10–82]*. These reports were stimulated by a series of state and federal investigations regarding alleged child abuse in state institutions for delinquents. Although Rader had said, "I have no thought of resigning; . . . my health is better than it has been in years," on July 14, the seventy-six-year-old director announced that he would step down on December 31. The Daily Oklahoman reported that he had been discouraged recently by financial problems besetting the agency, due in part to reductions in federal funds for social programs, and by criticism from legislators and the media *[DO, 7–14–82]*. Neal McCaleb, Republican representative from Edmond, speculated that the announcement "diffuses [Governor George] Nigh's political problems," and if he is re-elected, Rader might not step down *[DO, 7–14–82]*. Nigh said nothing about being sorry to see the embattled director leave, an action many considered disloyal and reprehensibly "political." That same day, in the *Oklahoma City Times*, reporter Jim Young reflected upon Rader's years of service to the people of Oklahoma: "Legends don't die; changing times erode away the mystical facade and exposes them as mortals with human frailties. And society goes looking for a new legend. . . . Rader was smart because he got in on the ground floor of the revolution in Washington that saw the federal government move deeper and deeper into the social welfare field. Rader helped write much of this legislation and it was tailored to fit Oklahoma's needs and revenues. Rader had much input into the Kerr-Mills Law, later Medicaid. . . . He also knew that you could do anything if you keep the politicians happy" *[OKC Times, 7–14–82]*.

In another article in the *Daily Oklahoman*, Randy Ellis commented that: "The legislature would transfer their troubled programs to DHS and Rader would let his administrative abilities take over. Not only would he pump state funds into the programs, but he always seemed to have an uncanny ability to use state funds to attract matching federal funds. The infusion of new capital into the programs usually filled them with new life and the legislators came off looking like a group of wise men. . . . Stretching of the sales tax finally snapped in 1980 when Rader agreed to take over rebuilding and operation of University Hospital" *[DO, 7–14–82]*.

Cash flow problems developed when Lloyd Rader, in his zeal to transform the University's hospitals, completed extensive construction projects in three years, rather than the six his budget makers informed him it would take. By 1981 there was a move in the legislature to bring the Department of Human Services under legislative budgetary control—i.e., the state sales tax was to be controlled by the legislature, not by the director. At the end of Rader's reign, the Department of Human Services was operating thirty programs, including nineteen institutions for children, the majority of which had been transferred to the department at the prompting of the legislature in order to eliminate the need for legislative appropriations.

Throughout the summer, there was speculation regarding the replacement for Lloyd Rader as director of Human Services. On July 14 the *Daily Oklahoman* indicated that those under consideration included Michael Fogarty, DHS deputy director (and later to become director of the Oklahoma Health Care Authority); former state Senator George Miller (who became director a decade later); Dr. William Thurman; and Dr. Donald B. Halverstadt *[DO, 7–14–82]*. On July 17 the *Tulsa World* reported that Lloyd Rader had recommended that Dr. Donald Halverstadt succeed him. However, on July 22 Governor Nigh reacted negatively to that suggestion, indicating, "They [the Human Services Commission] can hire whoever they please, but I think the person should come from outside the department." On October 1 former Republican Governor Henry Bellmon officially became associate director of the agency, to prepare himself to take over as director on December 21 when Lloyd Rader would retire. Bellmon, appointed by the Human Services Commission at the recommendation of Governor Nigh, recruited Robert Fulton, former chief counsel of the U.S. Senate Budget Committee, to work with him. Within six months, Fulton would become director. When he retired in December, Lloyd Rader had served eight different governors as director and, usually, benign czar of the state's largest and wealthiest agency. In the minds of many observers, Lloyd Rader had no peer as an administrator, politician, and individual who wanted to help children and the less fortunate citizens of his state.

Penn Square Bank Failure

The University experienced significant financial problems in 1982 because of the Penn Square Bank failure. This small banking facility in a shopping mall in Oklahoma City had grown to enormous fiscal proportions through "up-streaming" millions of dollars in loans, chiefly to oil operators, on the predicted basis of $40 a barrel or more for oil. When the price of oil dropped to $15, the bank's loans became untenable, and the collapse of Oklahoma's banking, as well as its building and loan industry, began. The loans originated by Penn Square Bank led to insolvency of major banks in Illinois and Washington, necessitating a federal treasury rescue of billions of dollars. A direct impact on the University was that the University of Oklahoma Foundation lost $573,000 in the August collapse, "just about wiping out our surplus," according to Foundation treasurer Ron Winkler. One week previously, foundation director Ron Burton had said that Foundation losses were "not a matter of public information . . . it's not important." He also said, "There is nothing to be gained" by making information concerning possible losses available to contributors [*DO, 8–19–82*]. The adverse consequences of the collapse of oil prices and state banks would harmfully affect the state budget and the University's operations for years to come.

Dr. Merrill Resigns

In June 1982 James A. Merrill resigned as chair of the Department of Gynecology and Obstetrics, a post he had held for twenty-one years. The regents accepted his resignation effective July 1. Dr. Merrill was a long-time advocate of women's rights, especially their right to determine their own reproductive role. Regarding the social changes he had witnessed among women following the 1960s, Merrill said, "There was a total change in social attitude with regard to reproduction, with the trend toward the concept that women would not be required to reproduce." Today's women "have the right, and indeed the unique opportunity, to decide if and when they will have children. The idea that women were masters of their own bodies was a most revolutionary concept" *[DO, 6–27–82]*. By June of the following year, the obstetrical service at Oklahoma Memorial Hospital was delivering more than 380 babies a month and turning away expectant mothers because of overcrowding. At the same time, St. Anthony Hospital was asking the Health Planning Commission to close its Obstetrical Unit.

Resignation and Return of President Banowsky

On July 22 William Banowsky announced that he was resigning from the presidency of the University of Oklahoma in order to become president of the Los Angeles Area Chamber of Commerce. Provost J. R. Morris was named interim president, and Vice President Gerald Turner was named interim provost *[RM, 17086–87]*. In the *Clinton Daily News* on July 25, the publisher, Mr. Charles Engleman, also president of the University of Oklahoma Board of Regents, stated that Banowsky "is unparalleled in the ability to plan and build houses, but it is yet to be proven that he has the vision to live in them." *The Daily Oklahoman* quoted more of Engleman's comments regarding the departing president:

He loves that spotlight and that exposure, for it enables him to accomplish great things for the causes he espouses. That's why so many people believe that when he became bored with his routine job as a public university president, he decided to use this new job as a stepping stone to becoming president of a large corporation, or more likely use it as a base for running for high political office. What motivates and inspires Banowsky is not always easy to discover. He deserves a lot of credit for a 102 percent increase in state appropriations for the university. . . . Much of the faculty opposed his selection as president, but now they are in his corner and why wouldn't they be? There has been a 45 percent increase in faculty and staff salaries, moving them from the bottom to the top among the Big Eight conference schools. So Bill, as you fly away to your beloved freeways and smog, I salute you, wish happiness for you, and hope to continue our friendship *[DO, 8–8–82]*.

On August 5 at a special meeting, the regents named a search committee and outlined the process for selection of a new president. Several weeks later, on August 24, almost 2,000 well-wishers turned out to bid farewell to Banowsky, who said that he was leaving "for his own personal vitality" *[DO, 8–25–82]*.

Early the next month, Dr. J. R. Morris served as interim president at the regents' meeting, although two days later, on September 11, a special meeting of the board was held to reinstate Banowsky, who reappeared at the November meeting as president *[RM, 17294]*. His return was greeted warmly in an editorial in the *Daily Oklahoman*, but not everybody was pleased with the reinstatement. Over 300 students, faculty, and Norman residents—doubtless some of the same people who bid such a fond farewell three months earlier!—signed a petition questioning the manner and process whereby Banowsky was reappointed without a search process. During his "resurrection" appearance with the regents, Banowsky stated that the projects he had undertaken might suffer during his new term, as Oklahoma was "entering a much more difficult economic climate due to declining state revenues" *[DO, 11–02–82]*.

A bit of Oklahoma medical history went up in smoke when, on September 5, the historic Rolater Hospital building at 325 N. E. 3rd Street, built in 1911, burned to the ground. From 1917 until 1921, the structure had served as the Medical Center's University Hospital *[DO, 9–6–82]*.

Children's Medical Research

An idea which had germinated for more than a year in the mind of the Department of Pathology's Dr. Geoffrey Altshuler became a reality in December 1982. Dr. Altshuler had envisioned an organization dedicated to sponsoring research and research scientists working to cure diseases of children in Oklahoma City. He shared his vision with Mrs. Jean Gummerson, and Children's Medical Research was born at a winter dinner at the Altshuler's. Persuaded by Mrs. Gummerson, Mr. James P. Linn agreed to become president of the new organization. The original incorporators of Children's Medical Research were Dr. Altshuler, Joan Gilmore, James Linn, Jean Gumerson, Ed deCordova, and Dannie Bea Hightower. The nascent group would become a major source of funding for facilities, equipment, and endowed positions for faculty at the Children's Hospital over the years. Additionally, an annual dinner was established to honor outstanding contributors to the hospital and for work with children. On November 1, 1983, the first dinner was held at which four

Oklahomans were recognized by Children's Medical Research for their contributions to the health and welfare of children in Oklahoma. They were Mrs. Mark R. Everett, a founder of the volunteer groups at the University hospitals, Dr. George Garrison, and Dr. Gerald Rogers for their medical care of children, and Mr. Lloyd Rader for his long dedication to the welfare of children and transformation of Children's Hospital under the Department of Human Services *[DO, 10–31–83]*.

1983

At the January 1983 University of Oklahoma Board of Regents meeting, Dr. M. DeWayne Andrews relinquished his position as assistant dean of graduate medical education in order to return to clinical medicine. Later, he would accept a position at the University of Tennessee as vice-chair of Medicine and chief of Medicine at the Regional Medical Center. He would return to Oklahoma in 1987 when Dr. Pat McKee persuaded him to revitalize the section of General Internal Medicine at the Health Sciences Center, and again accept a position in the dean's office as director of graduate medical education *[RM, 17362]*.

At the same January regents' meeting, upon recommendation of Dr. Mark Allen Everett, who was serving as interim chair of Pathology, the "Lloyd E. Rader Professorship in Pathology" was established, initially with practice funds from that department. Ironically, declining state revenues associated with the Oklahoma "oil bust" forced Rader's former Human Services Department to terminate 239 positions at the Health Sciences Center hospitals that month *[DO, 1–12–83]*. Also in January, L. Vernon Scott, Ph.D., retired from his position of head of the Department of Microbiology and Immunology.

The title of the Division of Oral Surgery in the Department of General Surgery, was changed to the Division of Oral and Maxillofacial Surgery in January 1983. Similar department name changes throughout the country reflected the extension of the scope of many surgical disciplines, while also assuring turf battles among the individuals and departments involved. Head and neck surgery became a particularly disputed area between practitioners of general surgery, otorhinolaryngology, plastic surgery, and oral surgery.

In February the *Daily Oklahoman* published an article titled "Doctors on State Payroll Get Top Pay," revealing that Donald B. Halverstadt, executive chief of staff at the Oklahoma Teaching Hospitals, was being paid $102,297 per year. At similar salary levels were Dr. John Barson, president of the

College of Osteopathic Medicine; Dr. J. Gail Neely, professor of Otorhino-laryngology; and Dr. Clayton Rich, provost of the Health Sciences Center. The governor was said to earn $48,000, while Department of Human Services director Henry Bellmon was paid $72,000 per year *[DO, 2–06–83]*.

In March, Gordon Deckert, professor and head of Psychiatry and Behavioral Sciences, was named a David Ross Boyd Professor, while John R. Sokatch, Ph.D., professor of Microbiology and Immunology, was named to a George Lynn Cross Research Professorship. Also in March, Dean Philip E. Smith was named Regents Professor Emeritus and Professor Emeritus of Clinical Laboratory Sciences, and Dr. Norman Levine, head of the Plastic Surgery division in the Department of Surgery, was promoted to full professor.

Governor George Nigh won his fight with the state senate over the replacement of Henry Bellmon as director of the Department of Human Services with his selection of Mr. Robert Fulton, former chief counsel of the U.S. Senate Budget Committee. Fulton was given the position in April on a 5–3 vote of the Human Services Commission, although the Oklahoma State Senate had favored the appointment of former Senator George Miller, who would himself later become the director.

Dr. Tom Lynn, former dean of the College of Medicine and current vice president of Baptist Hospital, announced formation of the "Oklahoma Heart Center" at that hospital in May. This emphasized the trend to competing medical centers for tertiary care set up by area hospitals, with former trainees and faculty of the University of Oklahoma heading the programs. Over the decades, the University and Children's Hospitals' exclusive claim to specialized procedures would be steadily eroded, leading to decreased Health Sciences Center revenues and increased town-gown frictions *[DO, 5–20–83]*. On a less contentious note, in May Mr. Stanton L. Young announced plans to establish a $10,000 Master Teacher Award as an annual prize at the College of Medicine. This generous gesture would recognize outstanding teachers in the College each year *[RM, 17492]*.

At their June 16 meeting, the University of Oklahoma Board of Regents devoted considerable time to an appeal from the attorney of Dr. Arnold Greensher, a former member of the Tulsa medical faculty, whose rancorous letter had contested the imposition of Professional Practice Plan policies on part-time faculty and demanded a financial settlement. The issue was reminiscent of the Donald Halverstadt case some years previously, wherein the physician, a part-timer also, failed to deposit professional revenue into the Practice Plan. Dr. Greensher's petition was denied unanimously by the regents *[RM, 17558]*.

In July amidst much hullabaloo, the Board of Regents approved a preliminary contract with "University Center Associates" to develop a 200-room hotel, conference center, and commercial/retail facility on the Health Sciences Center campus. Like earlier proposals for student housing, nothing other than hot air would rise from this venture.

By September 1983 the $100,000 faculty salary barrier was broken when the Department of Pediatrics announced that Dr. Robert A. Good's income exceeded that sum. On the campus construction front, several significant projects were completed in September, including the College of Pharmacy building, another $2 million addition to the Steam and Chilled Water Plant, and renovation of the College of Health building (the old Medical School). Also in September, Dr. Donald Halverstadt announced his resignation as executive chief of staff of the Oklahoma Teaching Hospitals. In a concluding, if routine action, the regents again approved the annual contract with Oklahoma Health Sciences Facilities, Inc. for rental of some 58,000 square feet of office space on N. E. 14th and 15th Streets, as well as space for the Family Medicine Clinic at 400 N. E. 50th.

Disparate actions dominated the November Board of Regents meeting: Dr. Halverstadt's title as special assistant to the president for hospital affairs was terminated, senior Microbiology Professors Lawrence Vernon Scott and Robert A. Patnode retired, R. Timothy Coussons was named acting head of Medicine, and a "financial emergency" and "program discontinuation" policy was formally adopted *[RM, 17766]*. In a concluding action, the College of Pharmacy building was dedicated on November 19.

At the end of 1983, politics again reared its many-tentacled head in Tulsa, as a contract was approved whereby the Department of Human Services would provide $500,000 in expanded outpatient facility care to low-income patients. The administration and monitoring of the program was not to be the Tulsa College of Medicine branch, but the Tulsa Medical Education Foundation, a consortium of Tulsa hospitals. This Foundation was a longtime player in the Tulsa political arena, as well as a prime champion of the original proposal for a medical school in Tulsa.

Campus on Life Support

Nineteen eighty-three ended with the worst financial crisis in Oklahoma higher education in a decade—a culmination of persistently unenthusiastic legislative support, decreased federal funding, and, especially, the consequences of the oil collapse and nationwide bank failures which had particularly adverse effects on Oklahoma. President Banowsky announced that financial shortfalls since the 1983 fiscal year began had made the current operating picture "far worse than we have imagined. We are being forced to cut even deeper" *[RM, 17753–61]*. Hiring freezes, forced furloughs, and support reductions were the order of the day. The Center's budget was cut by more than $3 million! Searches for deans of the Colleges of Education, Nursing, Pharmacy, and Public Health were canceled, and the planned computerization of the campus was postponed. Vacant full-time, part-time, and adjunct faculty positions were canceled. Equipment purchases were placed on hold. The first University-wide furloughs were ordered for December 29 and January 3, and at the Health Sciences Center on December 23 and January 3 *[DO, 12–15–83]*. A survey of University faculty revealed that fully 32 percent were actively seeking other positions. President Banowsky said:

If something is not done to avoid the disaster looming for the next fiscal year, no state in the nation will have been required to make the deep draconian reductions currently facing institutions of higher learning in Oklahoma. A watershed division is now occurring in the sun belt states of our nation. Texas, Colorado, Arizona, Georgia, North Carolina, and Florida are forging forward with unprecedented speed. Other states . . . in the same geographic region are being left behind. The future of Oklahoma is now being determined. Once it occurs, this division will be fixed for decades to come. Oklahoma is now at the crossroads. We will either pay the price to take our place among the leaders, or be marooned in mediocrity *[RM, 17760]*.

Truly, Armageddon had arrived for the Universities and for the Health Sciences Center.

1984

The financial crisis precipitated by the 1981 "Penn Square oil bust" again dominated University actions during early 1984. As the year began, there were virtually no construction projects underway at the Health Sciences Center, or even in the planning stages, other than additions to the Steam and Chilled Water Plant. An article in the *Daily Oklahoman* on January 29 titled "Teaching Hospitals in Danger of Slipping Into Mediocrity," captured the mood of the day perfectly. State pay freezes had prevented salary increases for nurses for more than three years. Dr. Mark Allen Everett, the chief of staff of University Hospital, stated that although entry-level pay for nurses at University and Children's Hospitals compared favorably with other area facilities, "the inability to offer pay raises has turned the teaching hospitals into a training ground for other hospitals in the area. The legislature wants to know why we haven't opened the 56 new medical-surgical beds on the fifth floor [of Everett Tower] in order to increase revenue. We tried to hire nurses in October for that, but as of this date, we have only 13. That's 61 nurses short of the number needed to operate the unit properly" *[DO, 1–29–81]*.

In addition, "fixed-rate" or "problem-based" reimbursements by Medicare, Medicaid, and Blue Cross, rather than the previous "reasonable cost" basis, further threatened the fiscal stability of the hospitals. Dr. Everett said that what was primarily needed for these institutions was a flexible personnel policy and a top-notch administrator. Although neither the legislature nor the Department of Human Services ever permitted the hospitals to develop personnel policies not dominated by ancient, bureaucratic state rules—incompatible with modern hospital management—in the spring of 1984, a one-year consultant management contract for the hospitals was signed with George Kaludis Associates, Inc. of Nashville, Tennessee. The firm sent William F. Towle, an experienced administrator of troubled hospitals, to serve as a full-time chief executive.

Much of the January 1984 meeting of the University of Oklahoma Board of Regents was devoted to modifying the plan for faculty and staff furloughs in response to various objections from the Norman campus faculty. The principal objection was that the regents specified that classes should not be canceled in order to implement furloughs, and some faculty objected that: "This gives the appearance of subordinating other important responsibilities, particularly research and creative activity" *[RM, 17789]*.

In March, Dr. Mark Allen Everett relinquished the title of interim head, Department of Pathology, and was replaced by Jess Hensley, M.D., formerly head of Pathology at Baptist Hospital. At the same time, Nancy K. Hall, Ph.D., was granted tenure in Pathology.

As part of the Center's campus-wide consolidation policy devised to conserve funds, the baccalaureate degree in Speech-Language Pathology and Audiology was transferred from the College of Arts and Sciences in Norman to the Department of Communication Disorders in Oklahoma City, and merged with the Master's and Ph.D. programs. This represented one aspect of an attempted solution to the ongoing struggle over speech and hearing activities between the Department of Otorhinolaryngology in the College of Medicine and the Communications Disorders Department in the College of Allied Health, a solution which favored the College of Allied Health and its dean. Also, regents modified the College of Medicine's Professional Practice Plan to emphasize that the dean of the College was responsible to the provost for direction of the plan and had ultimate authority over expenditures. This was done to end the contention of some faculty members on the Practice Plan Executive Committee that it was the Executive Committee (which represented the practicing faculty) and not the dean and his administration who held ultimate authority over the plan and who reported to the president and regents on Practice Plan matters.

In March 1984 Stanton L. Young, chair of the Board of Trustees of the Presbyterian Foundation, presented the Health Sciences Center's first "Master Teacher Award," consisting of a significant cash gift, at a formal annual banquet honoring the individual named. The award is funded in perpetuity from a generous endowment to the Center by Stanton Young. Selection was made by the dean from a list of nominees provided by the Faculty Board, the Student Council, and the Alpha Omega Alpha (AOA) Honorary Medical Society. (This nation-wide society honors the top 20 percent of medical students and parallels the undergraduate Phi Beta Kappa award.) The first recipient of Master Teacher Award was James Schmidt, M.D., from the Department of Medicine. Schmidt, throughout his faculty career, devoted himself assiduously to the superior education of medical students and served as a scholarly and concerned role model to the student-clerks on his service.

On April 18 Medical Reporter Jim Killackey wrote in the *Daily Oklahoman* that because of the precarious level of state funding, the two major Oklahoma universities were experiencing an exodus of key faculty members and that "campus morale was at an all-time low." Said Killackey: "Cognizant of Oklahoma's money woes, other universities across the country are aggressively raiding the state's professorial ranks." Norman Provost J. R. Morris said, "Faculty morale is low; it's perceived that there's no light at the end of the tunnel" *[DO, 4–18–84]*. State appropriations for higher education had been cut by $28 million during the preceding year. Although during 1981 and 1982 University faculty had received an average 12 percent annual pay raise, no pay raises were granted in either 1983–84 or 1984–85. Average faculty salaries were $29,747 at the University of Oklahoma, $28,422 at Oklahoma State University, and $47,000 at the Health Sciences Center. Chancellor of Higher Education Joe Leone had recommended an average of $33,200 at the two main campuses. He said that "because the majority of other states no longer are experiencing any budget crisis, they have funds to recruit our faculty to leave Oklahoma" *[DO, 4–18, 84]*. Unfortunately, Leone's effectiveness as the leader of higher education, especially vis-a-vis the legislature, was compromised by charges of financial irregularity in his office.

At the College of Medicine in April, Dr. David Kaplan, head of the Adolescent Service in Children's Hospital and the stimulus for including the hospital in the National Children's Miracle Network Telethon, left for a position at the University of Colorado Medical Center. That same month, Edward K. Gaylord II was named chair for the 1985 Telethon by Children's Medical Research.

At the May general faculty meeting of the College of Medicine, Dr. Mark A. Everett, chair of the Faculty Board, discussed the impact of budget cuts on the mission of the College and on the implementation of recent changes in curriculum and standards adopted by the faculty. He emphasized that a reduction in class size might be needed to avoid major cutbacks in function; and that any retrenchment must be looked at in the context of higher education throughout the entire state, not just on the Oklahoma City campus. Furthermore, said Everett, "all cuts should be programmatic, and not across the board, to avoid irreparable damage to the educational mission of the College. Also, faculty members who bring grants and contracts to the campus must be nurtured with selective raises, in spite of the reduced budget. Earnings of the practicing faculty must be maximized to expand departmental revenues, and the need for a close association of the provost and dean with the executive chief of staff of the Oklahoma Teaching Hospitals is critical" *[FBM, May, 1984]*.

On another topic, Everett added that funds must be found to support the introduction of a six-week elective in Family Practice, pending reexamination of the entire third-year curriculum.

In June 1984 physician-faculty salaries ranged from $50–80,000, with the exception of the chair of Medicine, Dr. Solomon Papper, who received $107,000, and Dr. Robert A. Good, Pediatrics, who received $110,000. Also in June, John Byrne, administrator of Oklahoma Children's Memorial Hospital, resigned following an unfavorable assessment by the interim chief executive officer at the teaching hospitals, Owen M. Rennert, M.D. Robert Fulton, the director of the Department of Human Services, indicated that a replacement for Byrne would await the appointment of a permanent chief executive for the Health Sciences Center.

Dr. Timothy Coussons was named acting head of the Department of Medicine in July, due to the illness and retirement of Dr. Papper, who died on August 19. Dr. Coussons would hold this position until Patrick McKee arrived in 1985. Also in July, Dr. John Fishburne, head of the Obstetrics and Gynecology department at the Oklahoma Memorial Hospital, announced that the department had been "delivering twice as many babies as the Obstetrics department is designed to accommodate." Of these deliveries, 60–100 babies each month were from "low income" mothers *[DO, 7–9–84]*. These numbers threatened the fiscal stability of the Obstetrics units both in the hospital and in the clinics.

In August Children's Hospital announced plans to build a center for a magnetic resonance imaging (MRI) system at a cost of $4.5 million. The only other operating MRI unit in the state was at the City of Faith hospital in Tulsa. Plans for installing MRIs were being made by St. Francis Hospital, in Tulsa, and by a group of Oklahoma City physicians who planned to open a free-standing facility. Also in August an article by medical reporter Jim Killackey in the *Daily Oklahoman* discussed the expansion of University Hospital's Medi-Flight (helicopter) mission beyond its original task of transporting neonatal infants with problems to include adult patients, many of whom were destined for hospitals other than the University Hospitals *[DO, 8–6–84]*. This expansion of service, without guarantee of payment for such service, further contributed to the Hospital's budget deficit.

In September, three new deans were named at the Health Sciences Center: Victor Yanchic was appointed dean of the College of Pharmacy, Lorraine Singer became dean of the School of Nursing, and Charles Cameron was named dean of the College of Public Health. Nancy Hall, Ph.D., an associate professor of Pathology and adjunct associate professor of Dermatology, was named assistant dean for admissions of the College of Medicine. John Robert Sokatch, Ph.D., who was the George Lynn Cross Research Professor of Microbiology and Immunology, was named professor and chair of the Department of Biochemistry and Molecular Biology, replacing Albert M. Chandler, the interim head. Dr. David Hunter, clinical assistant professor of Otorhinolaryngology, was given the additional title of adjunct clinical assistant professor of Dermatology, beginning a long association as the director of surgical training for residents in that specialty.

October saw the continuing exodus of Health Sciences Center faculty, as Dr. Walter Burgdorf, associate professor of Dermatology, resigned to become professor and chair of Dermatology at the University of New Mexico School of Medicine, while Dr. DeWayne Andrews resigned as associate professor of Medicine to become vice chair of Medicine at the University of Tennessee Medical Center, effective November 14. In late October, Children's Medical Research held its annual banquet, honoring Dr. Harris Riley (professor of

Pediatrics) and Dr. G. Rainey Williams (professor of Surgery), as well as Robert H. Anthony (civic leader and chair of the C. R. Anthony company) *[DO, 10–28–84]*.

Changes in the Teaching Hospitals

During 1984, a major change in administration of University Hospital was announced by the regents. The University Hospital returned to an elected chief of staff model with the selection of Dr. Robert McCaffree. The institution had been run for five years by Dr. Mark Allen Everett as chief of staff, with Dr. Jay Cannon as medical director, Dr. Russell Postier as director of admissions, and Donald L. Brown as administrator. These officers had been appointed by and reported to Lloyd Rader, director of the Department of Human Services, through Donald Halverstadt, M.D., the appointed executive chief of staff of all the teaching hospitals. Don Brown, who was later to become chief executive officer and president of the Children's Hospital in Washington, D.C., was relieved of his title of associate dean for administration, College of Medicine, on May 10, 1984. In other personnel changes, Jay Cannon, associate professor of Surgery, would leave the University in April to head the surgical service at the Oklahoma City Clinic, while Russell Postier would later be named chair of the Department of Surgery. Owen Rennert, the interim chief executive officer of the teaching hospitals, was replaced by administrator Antonio A. Padilla, who was also named associate to the provost for hospital affairs in November. Dr. Rennert had served with dedication and distinction since the resignation of Dr. Halverstadt the previous November.

Meanwhile, in the state legislature, the usual impractical schemes for solving the budgetary crisis statewide and at the Health Sciences Center specifically were floated. A proposal for "selling the Oklahoma Children's Memorial Hospital for between $80–100 million" was presented by Representative David Craighead, chair of the House Education Committee *[DO, 10–6–84]*. Craighead was "blasted by the director of the Oklahoma Public Employees Association, Pat Hall, who responded, 'Instead of talking about selling hospitals, let's talk about school district consolidation and closure of some of the 27 fully supported higher-education facilities'" *[DO,10–11–84]*.

The 1984 problems with the teaching hospitals would continue unabated into 1985. The *Daily Oklahoman* carried another front-page story on the continuing financial crisis in January. The new chief executive of the teaching hospitals, Tony Padilla, announced a "forced transfer policy" which would eliminate 225 "non-essential" jobs *[DO, 1–21–85]*. This was in addition to a hiring freeze imposed by Department of Human Services director Robert Fulton. There was continued talk among legislators of "selling the teaching hospitals." Fulton said, "I don't think it makes any more sense than to sell Owen Stadium [the football facility in Norman] or the turnpikes" *[DO, 1–22–85]*. He said that the state subsidy to the hospitals had been cut from $60 million to $45 million per year. The usual "turnpike rivalry" ensued, with Tulsa hospitals and legislators claiming that the state facilities at the Health Sciences Center relieved Oklahoma City's other hospitals from the burden of indigent care, but did not relieve hospitals elsewhere in the state of this burden. Welfare Commission Chair Reginald Barnes (Tulsa) said, "Tulsa hospitals argue that they, too, are teaching hospitals and receive no state subsidy" *[DO, 1–23–85]*. The furor ended when Governor Nigh recommended a one-year delay in considering any major restructuring of the governance of the state-owned hospitals. "This will give the new leadership of the hospitals time to effect additional improvements prior to implementing any major restructuring of the hospitals governance" *[DO, 1–25–85]*. Personnel levels at the hospitals were reduced by 675 persons between December 1982 and December 1984. Padilla said that the hospitals "hired too many employees during the oil boom years." One high-ranking employee said, "Morale is the lowest it's ever been here. Mr. Padilla is nothing more than a hatchet man" *[DO, 3–16–85]*. None of the 3,500 hospital employees had received a raise in three years.

At the Faculty Board meeting of November 27, 1984, three task forces delivered reports. Dr. Joseph Kopta, chair of Orthopedic Surgery, headed a committee considering whether an ambulatory care building should be constructed. The committee concluded that "No" was the appropriate response, because it felt that physician-controlled clinics in University Hospital were sufficient. The committee also considered whether the Site of Practice policy should be modified. Their conclusion was that it depended on whether the teaching hospitals could and would become more responsive to private patient needs. Dr. Christian Ramsey, chair of Family Medicine, headed a committee which examined the desirability of developing a faculty-hospital HMO-PPO and concluded that such an organization was probably worthwhile. Finally, a "committee" consisting of Dr. Jack Sokatch, chair of Biochemistry, studied the desirability of allocating all state "E&G" funds (monies appropriated by the legislature for educational and general purposes), exclusively on the basis of teaching and research loads. The committee concluded that there was merit in the concept, but that extensive selling of the idea would have to take place if there were any hope of implementing it.

Longtime faculty members mourned in November 1984 when Dr. Joseph A. Brandt, sixth president of the University of Oklahoma, died. When he left Oklahoma for the University of Chicago in 1943, Dr. Brandt wrote in an open letter to the governor and the legislature, of his "dismay and distress at the failure of the political leadership to support higher education" *[RM, 18166–67]*. Dr. Brandt would doubtless have been more dismayed to learn that this "failure" would characterize the entire history of the institution he so loved. Joe Brandt, who graduated from the University of Oklahoma in 1921, had been a Rhodes scholar and, subsequently, a reporter for the *Tulsa Tribune*. He was named director of the University of Oklahoma Press in 1928, and then became director of the Princeton University Press. After three years' service there, he was selected as president at Oklahoma. Under his leadership, the University of Oklahoma Foundation was established. The "OU Foundation" would, over the years, accumulate more than $200 million in gifts from alumni and friends of the University. This income constituted a significant percentage of the discretionary funds available for construction, faculty positions, and special projects.

In December, Drs. George and John Bozalis, father and son, the latter currently serving as president of the University of Oklahoma College of Medicine Alumni Association, established the "Evening of Excellence" dinner. They wanted to "get the whole state behind medical research like it's behind Sooner and Cowboy football" *[DO, 12–17–84]*. The first annual recognition award dinner would be held January 23, 1985. Oklahoma's Admiral William Crowe, former chair of the Joint Chiefs of Staff of the United States, was the first speaker, and Dr. Don H. O'Donoghue and Dean A. McGee, President of Kerr-McGee Oil Company, were the first honorees. The occasion was organized by Mrs. G. Rainey (Martha) Williams and Mrs. Pat (Carol) Wilkinson.

The year ended with the resignation, for the second time, of President William Banowsky on December 16 at a special meeting of the Board of Regents. The effective date was to be February 1, 1985. Banowsky told the *Daily Oklahoman* that he had three "chapters" in his professional career: "Chapter one was being a minister, chapter two was being an educator, and I'm now looking forward to being a broadcaster" *[DO, 12–16–84]*. He was to join Gaylord Broadcasting Company, a wholly owned subsidiary of the Oklahoma Publishing Company, which operated television and radio stations, movie and TV production companies, and "Opryland, USA" in Nashville, Tennessee. Said Banowsky: "A school like OU will have its ups and downs . . . a great institution has to endure the lean years as well as the good years. But the financial situation for Oklahoma higher education is very unfortunate" *[DO 12–19–84]*.

1985

At the January 1985 meeting of the University of Oklahoma Board of Regents, Dr. Martin Jischke, dean of the College of Engineering and the interim-president-designate, was in attendance. His appointment had been enthusiastically welcomed by the university faculty, since Dr. Jischke had previously served as president of the faculty senate. A search committee for the permanent president was named at a special meeting on January 26 with Judge Thomas R. Brett named as chair. English professor George Economou, a member of the committee, expressed concern that the criteria for the position of president should stress an academic administrative background and an advanced degree. His recommendation was in reaction to rumors that there was pressure to name a state politician as president, a common occurrence in Oklahoma higher education that continues to this day.

On February 14 Robert D. Foreman, associate professor of Physiology and Biophysics, was named acting chair of that department. At the same meeting, the regents passed a resolution supporting Governor George Nigh's suggestion that the current discussions regarding a possible transfer of the Oklahoma Teaching Hospitals be deferred for at least one year. In another matter, the regents voted to sue a former member of the Tulsa faculty in Anesthesiology for failure to deposit patient care receipts into the Professional Practice Plan. This recurring problem had contributed to the departure of several faculty members, including, as noted earlier, Dr. Donald Halverstadt.

In April the Shawnee Family Medicine training site was closed because of the withdrawal of local practitioners from teaching positions, and a resolution of the Pottawatomie Medical Society requesting that the program be terminated. This request reflected the continued anxiety on the part of many state practitioners of the imagined potential loss of patients and revenue to Health Sciences Center faculty physicians.

During the spring and early summer of 1985, there was a disagreement between the administration and staff of the Oklahoma Memorial Hospital and Robert Fulton, Department of Human Services director, over the admission of prisoner-patients to the hospital. Since the late 1970s, there had been discordance caused by the mandate to make the adult hospital attractive to paying patients and the legislative requirement that the hospital admit Oklahoma

Department of Corrections patients virtually on demand, with no prospect of reimbursement. Chiefs of staff at University Hospital had struggled with this financial and public relations problem since the mid-1970s. Prisoners in irons surrounded by guards who visited the clinics and occupied the wards, discouraged use of the hospital by paying patients. This situation was responsible for the loss of a contract for the annual physical examinations of the executives of the Kerr-McGee Corporation, dooming the hospital's effort to attract a stable and profitable private patient base. Typical of what lay in store for individuals unfortunate enough to share rooms with Department of Corrections prisoners is illustrated in the following account by a patient with a flair for the dramatic:

> I had been admitted late Thursday afternoon for heart studies, which were to be conducted early the following morning. I was surprised— 'shocked' might be a better word—when they wheeled me into a room where one of the two beds was occupied by a very seedy looking character with long, stringy, dirty-blond hair, a four-day stubble that failed to conceal several scars, and tatoos of daggers and naked women on his arms. His stomach was swathed in bandages. Two uniformed deputies, guns strapped to their waists, leaned on each side of the door, looking at me piteously (I thought) as I rolled into the room. During the evening, I naturally had occasion to glance in the direction of my roommate, who not only failed to return my salutations but glared at me in a baleful manner. At one point I overheard a hospital employee querying the guards about the prisoner; I was not comforted to learn that 'somebody tried to gut him in the laundry room at Big Mac' [the state prison at McAlester]. He was hooked up to all these noisy machines that made chugging and gurgling sounds all night, but I think what really kept me awake was the knowledge that, though he was doped and in pain, he was in no way restrained. If I didn't have heart trouble when I got there, I sure had it by the time I left![9]

Dr. Everett had appointed Dr. Russell Postier as the sole physician with authority to admit Department of Corrections patients. No other admission route was permitted. Many service chiefs actively discouraged Department of Corrections admissions by requiring that all such patients be screened and treated at the hospital facility at Griffin Memorial Hospital in Norman—which was staffed by University Hospital residents and faculty—prior to consideration of admission to University. Traditionally, nearly all medical and general surgical patients were treated at Griffin. The biggest problem occurred with attempted referrals of Corrections patients for plastic surgical and orthopedic procedures which were primarily elective and/or cosmetic in nature, and which could not be carried out at Griffin Memorial. The situation led to public complaints and letters to politicians and the media by Dr. John Tillinghast of the Department of Corrections about "unfair" and "insensitive" treatment of the prisoners in his care.

Dr. Joseph Kopta, chair of Orthopedic Surgery, described the Tillinghast brouhaha in these words: "Dr. Tillinghast was a former missionary who had a religious zeal for the idea that prisoners had a 'right' to care equal to that given private paying patients. He and I got into a fight about this right away. I told him that prisoners had no right to the same care as private paying patients; they were entitled only to the same *quality* of care. This was the issue that led Mr. Rader to tear down the 'C' wing [of University Hospital]. He didn't want a prison hospital on the Health Sciences Center campus."[10]

Following the agitation by Dr. Tillinghast, DHS Director Robert Fulton sent a memorandum to Tony Padilla, executive chief of staff at Oklahoma Memorial Hospital, stating, "Frankly, I am getting weary of reports that faculty members and residents at OMH are subverting the state law. . . . If we receive any more reports of refusals by faculty and residents to treat people referred by the Corrections Department, I will cut off DHS funding for whatever people are involved."[11] Dr. Mark Everett, who was also chair of the Faculty Board, replied: "The most favorable interpretation one can put on this letter is that it reflects an almost complete lack of understanding of the facts involved."[12]

Dr. Kopta was outraged by the letter from Fulton to Dr. Everett, and he wrote,

It is patently inaccurate to accuse us of 'subverting state law.' We have not refused to see inmates, and when appropriate have either administered care, or recommended treatment to the Corrections Department physicians. The reports of refusals to which you refer are in reference to *elective* surgical treatment. Because an inmate has a condition which may be amenable to surgical treatment and desires to avail himself of that treatment does not make it a medical necessity. Your blanket acceptance of Dr. Tillinghast's assessment of these conditions belies the fairness and administrative temperance you are reputed to have. (We) do not object to hospitalizing inmates at OMH, but our paying patients do. . . . They object to occupying rooms adjoining prisoners and guards, or being with shackled and prison-garbed patients in the waiting areas. . . . Therefore, when an inmate has a condition which may be appropriately treated by methods that do not require hospitalization, we are disposed to select that form of treatment.[13]

As usual, the furor quickly died down, but the pattern of pressure from the Department of Corrections and resistance by hospital staff continued regarding admission of prisoners with elective surgical and cosmetic problems to the in-patient units. The plan of several legislators some years earlier to create a prison hospital in the "C" wing of the old University Hospital had been thwarted by Lloyd Rader when he demolished the facility overnight, on a weekend, as hospital personnel wheeled patients away from crumbling wards and faculty members peered in shock from their windows as a wrecking ball pounded the walls of the very building in which they were housed! Bill Sylvester, manager of construction projects for Mr. Rader and DHS, later explained that he and his assistants had posted notices on every office door detailing the action Rader was taking. "I personally informed some of them," Sylvester said. "They just looked at me like I was crazy or pulling their leg." He paused in fond recall of the day's activities. "They changed their minds when that big old metal ball came crashing through the walls!"[14] Dr. Joseph Kopta, who was in the building when the ball began its destruction, said, "Rader was something else! I didn't believe things could happen that fast in a bureaucracy!"[15]

Meanwhile, business continued as usual at the University. In April the Board of Regents voted to sell thirteen pieces of property on N.E. 14th and 15th Streets in Oklahoma City because the houses on the property were no longer needed for office space following completion of the College of Pharmacy building. This was the beginning of the end for "Health Sciences Facilities, Inc.," the corporation headed by Dr. Wilson Steen, which had for so long purchased nearby houses and provided temporary space for departments of the College of Medicine and other institutions whose facilities had been displaced during ongoing construction on the campus. In November 1985 Marilyn Pryor Real Estate was selected to sell the properties after establishing a "minimum price" for each of them. Later, in June of 1986, the regents would reduce the minimum price on ten pieces of property because of "the downward trend in the Oklahoma City real estate market as well as the deteriorated condition of the houses, all of which had been vacant for over three years" *[RM, 19070–71].*

Patrick McKee

During the autumn of 1986, Dr. Timothy Coussons, who had served as acting head of the Department of Medicine, was succeeded by a new permanent chair, Patrick Allen McKee. Dr. McKee was a University of Oklahoma College of Medicine graduate who had trained at Duke University and at the National Institutes of Health during the period 1962–1967. He returned to Oklahoma as chief resident in Medicine in 1967 and stayed until 1969 as a fellow under Dr. Robert Bird. The following year, he returned to Duke University where he served as director of the clinical division of the Department of Medicine until 1985. Dr. McKee had been recruited by College of Medicine Dean Charles McCall, who did not divulge that he was leaving his position, although others in the Department of Medicine, including Dr. Timothy Coussons, were privy to this knowledge. Dr. McKee recalled: "When I caught on to what was going on, I had already resigned at Duke, and I was disassembling my laboratory to come out here. I thought, what am I doing. . . . I'm coming out to a place and being recruited by a dean; and you need the dean's support. I'm going to walk in the front door and there's going to be no dean there. By the time I got there [September 5], Rainey [Williams] was the acting dean."[16]

Among numerous accomplishments, Patrick McKee would play a major role in the development of the Warren-St. Francis Research Institute in Oklahoma City, the establishment of the School of Math and Science on the Health Sciences Center campus, and creation of the Center for Molecular Medicine.

The Warren-St. Francis Research Institute

An early result of the enthusiasm and personal contacts of the new chair in Medicine was an affiliation agreement with the William and Natalie Warren Medical Institute of Tulsa. This agreement created a branch of the Institute on the Oklahoma City campus and was a landmark for the Health Sciences Center and the University. For the first time, the Warren Foundation, long a benefactor of medical research and education in Tulsa, would provide money for activities on the Oklahoma City Health Sciences Center campus. The Institute committed itself to fund investigators in the Department of Medicine, under the direction of Dr. McKee, on a continuing basis. At the regents' meeting of November 13 and 14, Dr. McKee reviewed the research programs to be supported by the Institute, as well as other activities of the Warren Foundation/St. Francis Hospital unit on the Health Sciences Center campus. McKee was commended by the regents for his role in effecting this affiliation. The new Medicine chair believed that this important affiliation was probably responsible for his being named to the founding board of the Oklahoma Center for Applied Science and Technology, and to the board of the new Oklahoma School of Math and Science adjacent to the campus.

At the January 1987 regents' meeting, the W. K. Warren Foundation of Tulsa, with matching funds from the Department of Medicine Practice Plan, the Oklahoma State Medical Association, and Dr. C. Alton Brown, provided funds for the establishment of two endowed professorships—the William K. Warren Professorship in Diabetes Studies, and the Natalie O. Warren Professorship in Medicine. Over the next ten years, the affiliation would be responsible for supporting numerous distinguished investigators who were very productive in research. This key association of Dr. McKee with the Warren Foundation was later regarded with ambivalence by senior University officials, specifically Provost Jay Stein and Dean Donald Kassebaum, who would have preferred that Foundation officials relate and report directly to themselves. One of the casualties of their attitude was the mishandling of the search for a chair in Psychiatry (discussed later).

Direct Warren Foundation support to Health Sciences Center programs amounted to more than $3 million per year for the next ten years. (There was some modification of Warren Foundation policy after the teaching hospitals were placed under the auspices of Columbia/HCA in 1997.) According to Dr. McKee, it was important to separate the Warren funds from any appearance of a contribution to the Health Sciences Center budget—especially after the affiliation of the hospitals with Columbia/HCA. McKee felt that if Warren funds were seen as a contribution to the Center, the deans and provosts would want to control them. "Deans and provosts have been a revolving door lately, and each one comes with a different agenda. If you are going to preserve consistency, it must be an affiliation where you still retain a couple of strings. But don't get involved with the College of Medicine's business."[17]

By the spring of 1985, Dr. Charles McCall had served as dean of the College of Medicine for more than three years. Throughout 1984 he had been plagued with ill health, including a coronary occlusion and bypass surgery. In April he announced his pending retirement. Following a series of interviews by provost Rich with several senior faculty members, G. Rainey Williams, head of the Department of Surgery, was named interim executive dean of the College of Medicine effective July 1 for one year.

The Stanton L. Young Master Teacher Award for 1985 was given in early summer to Dr. John Holliman, assistant professor of Pathology. Throughout his residency in Pathology, and as a faculty member following his appointment by Dr. Everett several years earlier, Dr. Holliman had consistently injected wit and warmth into his lectures on the etiology and pathogenesis of disease to sophomore medical students. At the same regents' meeting, the interim head of Microbiology and Immunology, Joseph Ferretti, was made permanent head of that department. Some ten years later, Dr. Ferretti would succeed to the office of provost of the Health Sciences Center.

At the Oklahoma Children's Memorial Hospital, the Bone-Marrow Transplant Unit, which had received much favorable publicity over its two years of operation, was closed due to loss of the two physicians responsible for the unit, Dr. Robert Good and Dr. Nina Kapoor. Meanwhile, a bone marrow transplant unit was in the experimental stage at both the University and at Presbyterian hospitals under the direction of Dr. Robert Epstein. In addition, twenty-four patients undergoing radiation therapy and chemotherapy for leukemia at Children's had been treated for almost two years, with good results in eighteen of the cases.

Controversy again roiled the briefly placid waters of the Health Sciences Center in May when decisions to withhold "vigorous care" from certain patients with spina bifida, based upon their "quality of life" potential, led to a public outcry and threats of a lawsuit by the American Civil Liberties Union. Dr. Joseph Kopta, chair of Orthopedics, described the controversy this way: " The issue was, should hopeless medical problems, such as patients with no hope of ever acquiring functioning ability mentally and physically, have endless community resources expended upon them? We're talking about patients with no expectation of improvement in their quality of life. The spina bifida group decided "No," and felt that nature should be allowed to take its course. The policy of withholding expensive care when there was no expectation of improvement was quickly abandoned, however, and no court cases resulted at the Health Sciences Center."[18]

The uproar in the local and even national media brought much unwanted attention to the Center. The charges of "discrimination" and "human experimentation" were essentially a protest by a political action-pressure group, the "National Legal Center for the Medically Dependent and Disabled, Inc." Their allegations, however, would cloud the professional lives of the physicians involved for months and even years *[DO, 5–9–85; 5–19–85; 5–24–85]*.

The Presbyterian Foundation

The biggest news in July was the sale of Oklahoma City's Presbyterian Hospital to the Hospital Corporation of America of Nashville, Tennessee, for $125 million. This firm also owned other Oklahoma hospitals, including Edmond Memorial and the Wagoner Community. Proceeds of the sale would be used to pay existing indebtedness in the amount of $40 million, while the remainder, between $50–60 million, would be placed in a new, nonprofit "Presbyterian Foundation." This foundation, in the words of the chair of the Presbyterian Hospital Board, Mr. Stanton Young, would be "dedicated to the support of medical education, research and clinical pastoral education" *[JR, 7–25–85]*. This event heralded the beginning of a significant, long-term contribution of the new foundation to excellence in medicine and medical research on the Health Sciences Center campus.

In August, the 1985–86 state educational budget was approved. It provided, for the first time in four years, an increase, rather than a decrease or a standstill budget, for higher education in Oklahoma. More than $6 million of the increase was reserved for the Health Sciences Center campus. According to Interim President Martin Jischke, who discussed the increase at the midsummer regents' meeting, this brought the level of funding of the Health Sciences Center to "about 60 percent of the national average for comprehensive medical centers. A total of about $65 million would be needed to close these funding gaps" *[RM, 18523]*.

The Board of Regents welcomed new University of Oklahoma President Frank E. Horton in September. The forty-six-year-old Horton, with a Geography degree from Northwestern University, came to Oklahoma after serving as chancellor of the University of Wisconsin at Milwaukee. Initially met with much faculty good will and the first growing budget in several years, Horton rode a wave of approval and success for a time. However, his tenure was characterized by the least cooperative and/or constructive Board of Regents in memory. After three years of rancor and attacks from two of the board members who wished to micromanage the institution rather than set policy, he left the University to serve as president of the University of Toledo in Ohio, where he found a more helpful and congenial board.

In October the University again voted to bring suit against a former Tulsa College of Medicine full-time faculty member because he had failed to deposit clinical income from care of personal patients into the Faculty Practice Plan. Such a lawsuit was evidence that, after years of income control by University administrators, there was still resistance to the concept that income earned by faculty while doing private practice was to be treated as "state money."

The Kemp/Sarrat Imbroglio

Throughout the mid-1980s, there was considerable acrimony and dissension among the members of the University of Oklahoma Board of Regents, with Regents Thomas Elwood Kemp and Charles F. Sarratt frequently championing a "hands on" management role for members of the board. For example, there was a very uncomfortable atmosphere at a retreat with the new president, Frank Horton, in December 1985. At this meeting, Kemp and Sarratt challenged the executive authority of the president and advocated active administrative decision-making by the regents. At one point, Mr. Sarratt requested an inventory of everything the University owned, including its people! At the regents' request, a guest professor from Wisconsin, Dr. Joseph Kauffman, reviewed the responsibilities and duties of university governing boards such as the regents, including the appropriate times for delegation of authority to the president. He urged that the regents attempt to "create an effective environment for effective leadership." Regent Sarratt worried about the administration "keeping secrets from the board." Both Kemp and Sarratt expressed concern over University faculty members meeting with state legislators. Regent Sarah Hogan defended the faculty, stating that they were "trying to be helpful in a difficult time, and . . . legislators need to be educated about education" *[RM, 18742–66]*.

This was not the first time—nor would it be the last—that members of the Board of Regents tried to exert control over matters better left to the administration. In November 1985 a "pressing jurisdictional matter" relating to the relationship between the University of Oklahoma Foundation (OUF) and the University was discussed by the regents at the request of Kemp and Sarratt. (The relationship was similar to the one originally proposed for the Oklahoma Medical Research Foundation and the College of Medicine. However, while the regents remained the sole beneficiary of the OUF, the College of Medicine quickly became tangential to the mission of the Oklahoma Medical Research Foundation.) The regents, spurred by Kemp and Sarratt, desired to make it clear that they had the "right" to inspect all books and records of the OUF at any time *[RM, Exhibit D, 3–21–85]*. In June 1986 Regents Kemp and Sarratt were defeated 5–3 in an attempt to affirm that "any regent can serve on any search committee and out of deference, the senior regent on the committee should be chair of the committee" *[RM, 19141]*. Search committees for Medicine, Law, and Arts and Sciences, as well as for the Norman campus provost position, gave reports of their efforts to find suitable candidates to fill these positions. Regent Kemp indicated that he might want to attend all such committee meetings. He also suggested that the president should not make the final selection but should forward the names of several candidates to the regents. Kemp was later condemned by a resolution of the University of Oklahoma Faculty Senate, in November1986, on a vote of 37–5, which stated that Kemp's "words and actions impugn the integrity of the administration, faculty and staff," and that further, some of his actions and statements "falsely accuse and insult administrators, staff and faculty" *[DO, 11–12–86]*. The resolution was presented by History Professor Gary Cohen. Faculty Senate chair Penny Hopkins told the regents that Kemp "made the irresponsible implication that the faculty and staff at OU were criminally culpable. To have the faculty's devotion to the institution answered by disdainful and pejorative accusations is shameful" *[DO, 11–12–86]*.

Regents Kemp and Sarratt did not dominate all phases of activity at the November 1995 meeting, though newspaper accounts indicate that little else occurred. A progress report by the search committee for the new dean of Medicine, chaired by Dr. Timothy Coussons, was delivered. In the words of Dr. Coussons, "the search was slow going" *[RM, 1869]*. Also at the November meeting, Provost Clayton Rich discussed the College of Medicine budget for 1985–86. This budget gives a clear picture of exactly how important physician income was to the Center and why administrators fought so hard to control it.

TABLE 4.   COLLEGE OF MEDICINE BUDGET 1985–86

Type of Funds	Amount	Percentage of Total
1. Clinical Funds:		
Physician Practice Plan	$23,612,275	37
Teaching Hospital Contract	$8,382,000	13
"Dean's" Fund (PPP)	$1,571,049	2
SUBTOTAL	$33,565,324	53
2. Other Funds:		
From State: College Budget	$15,060,425	24
From State: Campus Support	$8,100,330	13
Grants, Gifts, Contracts	$7,113,319	11
SUBTOTAL	$30,274,174	47

Provost Rich pointed out that well over half of the operational budget came from clinical income and that the fiscal problems of the teaching hospitals had led to a recommendation from hospital administrators to the Department of Human Services that support for the College of Medicine, especially the house-staff budget, be reduced. A joint University-Hospital task force was formed to study and make recommendations regarding this proposal, which was so threatening to the College of Medicine budget. Fortunately, no drastic reductions followed.

State of Oklahoma Preferred Provider Organization

In 1982 development of a statewide health plan for employees was undertaken by the legislature and the Health Sciences Center administration. It was to be a "preferred provider organization" (PPO) utilizing the Health Sciences Center faculty and hospitals to provide care. During the approximately three years in which the plan operated fully, it became a principal source of income for the clinical faculty and the College of Medicine. Later, agitation from physicians statewide to be included in the plan would cause Health Sciences Center administrators, led by Dean Edward N. Brandt, to recommend "opening up" the PPO to physicians and hospitals throughout the state. A prominent faculty member remembered this action as "tragic—the most unfortunate thing to ever happen to this institution." He added, "I pled with Brandt to just go out there [to the legislature] and say you want 30 percent of the contract—to maintain an underpinning for this Health Sciences Center. But he just gave it away because it had become a lightening rod with private physicians." As a result there was an enormous decrease in revenue to the faculty practice.

At the November 26 Faculty Board meeting, Dr. Everett articulated the Executive Committee opinion that "any alteration of the budget should reflect 'where we want to be' rather than any across-the-board cut." Additionally, Dr. Everett asked Provost Rich to review and clarify the recently distributed policy on sick leave, as the Executive Committee "believes that the wording has resulted in unreasonable sick leave benefits being provided." Added Everett, "the policy should make a clear distinction between leave for disability, and leave for sickness. In a period when fiscal prudence is called for, this policy portends a hemorrhaging of funds which we cannot afford as a University" *[FBM, 11–26–85]*. Despite recognizing the destructive effects of this policy on institutional budgets, no University provost or vice president ever recommended repeal, even though they acknowledged the enormous adverse fiscal impact on department and University personnel costs. An additional adverse effect was that in many instances the resulting escalation of personnel costs rendered departmental services uncompetitive in bids for managed care contracts. Due to timidity on the part of the administration, the error of this policy was never corrected and it remained in force as late as 1998.

The year's final Board of Regents meeting on December 12 was brief and relatively uneventful. Dr. Jess Hensley, at his own request, was relieved of his title as head of the Department of Pathology, and a new chair, Dr. Richard Leech, was appointed.

Welcome Progress

In spite of continued fiscal problems for the University, 1985 was an improvement over the previous two years for the College of Medicine and the Health Sciences Center. The Presbyterian Foundation had been established, and several outstanding investigators made important clinical contributions: Dr. Dwight Reynolds implanted the world's smallest heart pacemaker; a team headed by Dr. Donald B. Halverstadt made a new bladder for a fifteen-year-old; Dr. Robert Epstein initiated the Bone Marrow Transplant Unit for treatment of adult leukemia and other cancers; and University of Oklahoma scientists were among the first to use interleukin 2 in renal carcinoma [*DO, 10–6–85; 12–6–85*]. Even the financially starved program for perinatal care of indigent women was growing, assuring healthier babies [*DO, 12–20–85*].

Looking back at this period in the history of the Health Sciences Center, Dr. Patrick McKee recalled that when he arrived at Oklahoma, "clinical practices were pretty sluggish in the Department of Medicine, the clinic was very mediocre in design, and amenities were severely lacking. I said we needed to juice up the clinical activity . . . get some recognition in the community for excellence in clinical care."[19] He believed that marketing was best done through excellent clinical care and word of mouth from satisfied patients, rather than by "billboards and pamphlets." The clinical staff and its executive committee, largely at the instigation of Dr. McKee, designated four "centers of excellence" to be given special support and attention by the teaching hospitals: the transplant program; critical care for newborns; geriatric medicine; and a trauma center [*DO, 12–20–85*]. In June of 1986, a joint agreement with the teaching hospitals was approved for construction of a Bone Marrow Transplant Unit in Oklahoma Memorial Hospital. The teaching hospitals were to provide funds for renovation of the space, while practice funds from the

Department of Medicine would be used to move the four laminar flow patient isolation units from Children's Hospital to the new site. The Department of Medicine invested some $300,000 in clinical income establishing the Bone Marrow Unit. In another step forward, Dr. McKee induced the clinical departments to invest collectively more than $500,000 to create a "VIP" ward on the tenth floor of Oklahoma Memorial Hospital. According to McKee: "There was a domino effect, because you saw, over the '85–'88 period, floor nine, then eight, and then other clinical units refurbished and upgraded. There was an air of excitement. There were a lot of differing opinions, and examination of the issues in a non-contentious way, rather than confrontation. Things were really happening then."[20]

1986

Nineteen eighty-six opened with amendments to the University of Oklahoma policy on endowed chairs and professorships providing that "interest income" would be the first source of funds for these positions. Interest on such endowments would become a major source of funding for distinguished investigator-faculty chairs in the future. Later, in April, Mr. Edward L. Gaylord provided an endowment of $1 million to establish the Gaylord Chair in Ophthalmology at the Dean A. McGee Eye Institute. It was a signal event that the University would provide matching funds for a chair for a faculty member located in a private institution such as the Eye Institute. Also in January, an external audit report showed that the "unrestricted fund balance" at the Health Sciences Center was now $19.47 million—a balance that was exclusively the result of bringing practice-generated funds into the university system! Of interest is the fact that at this same January meeting, the regents adopted a definition of "auxiliary enterprise funds" (i.e., Practice funds) which stated that such enterprises are expected to be self-supporting, but "while it apparently is not prohibited by law, the auxiliary enterprises and service units should not be called upon to provide support for the Educational and General activities of the institution" *[RM, "Attachment 1," January 20, 1986]*. This latter admonition was never heeded in the College of Medicine; on the contrary, practice funds rapidly became a significant—and in many instances the major—source for the operational budgets of many departments in the College.

Salaries in the fiscal year 1985–86 were at $50–65,000 for assistant professors in the Department of Medicine, while full professors in Psychiatry and Behavioral Sciences were at $35–40,000. Regents expressed concern that incorporation of Practice Plan funds into the base salary (rather than restricting Practice dollars to income supplements) would mandate an increased University commitment for fringe benefits. They asked for a month's advance notice in the future when auxiliary (Practice) funds were to be employed to fund base salaries. Rather than increasing the demand on appropriated college funds, Practice funds for base salaries quickly began to supplant university funding. Furthermore, funds coming from the teaching hospitals or the Department of Human Services as reimbursement for "teaching and supervisory services" were still traced to the individual receiving the funds. Later, like practice funds, hospital transfers would be merged unrecognizably into the general budget of the College. An example of such funding was the salary of Dr. Jenq Chang in Dermatology, who was paid from the Children's Hospital "Sharing-clearing B Account" and from Practice Plan funds, rather than from the general educational budget, in spite of the fact that he was a tenure-track faculty member.

The Stanton L. Young Master Teacher award for 1986 went to Nancy K. Hall, Ph.D., another faculty member from the Department of Pathology. Since her arrival on campus, Hall showed exceptional concern for the welfare of students, both in her direction of the class in etiology and pathogenesis of disease, as well as outside the classroom. Dr. Hall had come to the Department of Pathology from Stanford University as a research faculty member, but quickly found that her chief interest was as an educator and mentor of students.

The Department of Human Services as a reliable source of funding came into question in January 1986 when the Public Welfare Commission approved sweeping cuts in medical and emergency services to the poor, in an effort to "spread the pain" of a nine-percent budget reduction *[DO 1–29–86]*. Cutting the Department's "Medically Needy" program meant the loss of health care for an estimated 13,500 persons. Commission Chair David Walters said, "This action will push some hospitals over the brink" *[DO, 3–04–86]*. The Oklahoma Teaching Hospitals would suffer a $12 million cutback in funds. The College of Medicine was notified that there would be, in addition, a $1 million reduction in the master reimbursement contract which paid for faculty services in the hospitals. One cost-cutting measure—privatizing the hospitals' food service activities (supported by a teaching hospitals task force and the chiefs of staff)—was opposed by the Oklahoma Public Employees Association, as well as by Senator E. Melvin Porter of Oklahoma City, who feared a loss of the jobs of 200–300 food service workers, most of whom were his constituents. Privatization of food service was never implemented, even though at the time the direct cost of food service operations was almost $6 million per year *[DO, 2–16–86; DO, 2–25–86]*.

In another lobbying effort by the Department of Human Services, an intense "human interest series" in the *Daily Oklahoman* succeeded in arousing the public sufficiently to oppose successfully the end of the Medically Needy program *[DO, 5–04–86]*. On May 22, the Legislature notified the Department of Human Services that the Medically Needy and the Vendor Drug Programs would be saved, and that a reduction in welfare checks would be avoided. The solution of Governor George Nigh and the legislature to this fiscal crisis was to tap the state pension reserve fund. (Because the pension funds for state employees—primarily teachers, but other classes of employees as well—were already seriously underfunded, the severe crisis predicted for early in the twenty-first century by opponents of such a solution would become a reality in the mid-1990s.)

On March 13 an Evening of Excellence dinner was held in Oklahoma City at which Dr. George Garrison, beloved pediatrician and longtime secretary of the Faculty Board, and Stanton L. Young, president of the Presbyterian Foundation, were honored. Gifts of $1 million from Dorothy Miller and a similar amount from Edward L. Gaylord were announced. The Gaylord gift, as noted earlier, was to endow a chair in Ophthalmology, and the Miller gift was to be shared by the School of Geology and the Department of Surgery *[DO, 3–14–86]*. Dr. G. Rainey Williams announced that the Evening of Excellence raised more than $100,000 for the Health Sciences Center's research efforts.

Despite an era of coping with fiscal austerity and a constant struggle to maintain program excellence at the Health Sciences Center, a negative note was sounded in March with the announcement by Mental Health Commissioner Frank James of his intention to create a 20-bed detention unit and 20-bed detoxification unit on the Oklahoma City campus and close the Acute Medical and Surgical Unit of Griffin Memorial Hospital in Norman, which had cared for most Department of Correction in-patients. Closure of this facility would increase the presence of prison inmate patients in the struggling teaching hospitals, that had been trying to alter their "indigent" image. Realizing that this was hardly a move to alleviate the problem, Dr. G. Rainey Williams suggested that the "best solution would be for the governor to say 'No' to Commissioner James' request" *[FBM, 3–18–86]*. Unlike many ill conceived plans before it, this one was not implemented. (However, a similar unit would later be opened in the defunct O'Donohuge Rehabilitation Hospital in the mid-1990s, without closing the facility at the Norman mental hospital.)

Cogeneration: A Cautionary Tale

In 1984, a proposal surfaced at a University of Oklahoma Board of Regents meeting to contract with "Smith Cogeneration" of Oklahoma City to build a steam plant south of the Health Sciences Center which would obviate the need for the University's Steam and Chilled Water plant. The cogeneration plant would provide electricity, created as a by-product of steam produced by burned garbage, for heating and cooling the campus. The Oklahoma Gas and Electric Company (OG&E) would be mandated to purchase the electicity at an artificially high price *[RM, 18180]*. The Corporation Commission on March 1, 1986, had ordered OG&E to buy electricity from a 300 megawatt cogeneration plant to be built in LaFlore County. Opinion was divided over whether the revenue from sales would primarily benefit the University or the cogeneration developers. The *Daily Oklahoman* stated in an editorial: "Cogeneration without regard to projected power demand makes no economic sense. It would be a burden instead of a blessing for consumers. In this category are cogeneration proposals at the OU Health Sciences Center. . . . OG&E can buy kilowatts for peak demand at relatively low cost from other utilities in the region . . . but if . . . it is forced to buy kilowatts it doesn't need, those extra costs will be passed on eventually to consumers. The grandiose cogeneration claims ignore the old axiom that there is no such thing as a free lunch" *[DO 5–13–86]*.

Several months later, at their meeting of October 16, the regents approved seeking competitive bids from proposed "venture participants" for construction of the project. In November, the regents named Smith Cogeneration Management, Inc. of Oklahoma City as the "venture participant" to proceed with development of the project, despite alleged irregularities in bidding *[DO, 11–20–86 and 11–21–86]*. The project foundered several months later when OG&E was successful in warding off the mandate to buy the proposed electricity.

Another Fiscal Crisis

The February 1986 Board of Regents meeting was devoted to a discussion of the grim prospects for adequate operational funds for the 1986–87 fiscal year, with dire predictions regarding state revenues. University President Horton said, "The events and pronouncements of the past several days regarding the status of State revenue projects, and the probable impact on State support for higher education, and more specifically, the University of Oklahoma, will have a devastating impact. . . . I indicated that we would most likely request each state-supported budget unit to identify 13–17% in budget reductions" *[RM, 18849–59]*.

On the Oklahoma City campus, not only was there an adverse impact from a decrease in state-appropriated funds, but the teaching hospitals likewise were experiencing budgetary reductions, which in turn required a reduction in the contract with the College of Medicine from $8.3 million to $7.1 million. The negative image of the hospitals due to reduced funding and the rancor of employees who might be declared "redundant" was aggravated by reports of favoritism and improper personal conduct by the head of the hospitals, Tony Padilla, who had come to the Center in 1984 at a much-criticized annual salary of $93,000. As executive director of the hospitals, he had been given the titles of "associate to the provost" and "adjunct professor of health administration."

Affirmative Action

The Title VI Affirmative Action Compliance Program was a University of Oklahoma document submitted to the Oklahoma State Regents for Higher Education in compliance with the court-ordered "Extended Revised State Plan for Desegregation of the Oklahoma State System for Higher Education." It was approved by the regents in 1976 and implemented in 1977. Compliance was to be reviewed at five-year intervals, initially in 1982, which report was accepted by the reviewing agencies in 1983. The annual update of the Affirmative Action plan for the Health Sciences Center campus was presented, and goals for increasing representation of minorities in all job categories, as well as in the faculty, "were established only for the College of Pharmacy and the Tulsa Medical College, because the apparent deficiencies revealed in other colleges were so small" *[RM, 18872]*. However, the professional schools at the Health Sciences Center had "consistently been the target of intense scrutiny" from the U.S. Department of Education's Office for Civil Rights.

As of 1986, 12 of the 148 incoming medical students were Blacks (a term later to be replaced by the phrase "of African-American descent"), constituting 8.17 percent of the current class, which exceeded the goal of 6.8 percent and established "what appears to be a new record" *[RM, 19052]*. The College was praised for faculty efforts to increase Black faculty representation as well. At this same time, a State Regents' report suggested that College of Medicine enrollment should be decreased by at least 8 percent because of an anticipated oversupply of physicians by 1995. Currently, there were 188 places in the freshman class at the University of Oklahoma and 80 at the osteopathic school. Because of both a shrinking applicant pool and financial constraints due to low state appropriations as well as decreased federal subsidies, the University of Oklahoma had left 28 of its first–year positions for the fall of 1986 unfilled. Adding to the problem was the fact that federal government funds for the operating budget of the College of Medicine, had dropped from 44 percent to less than 25 percent.

Family Medicine Project

The status of the "University Center/Family Medicine Project" was reviewed by provost Clayton Rich at mid-year of 1986. In 1982 the State Regents had allocated $850,000 for this building project, with additional state-appropriated funds to be allocated upon approval of a detailed plan. At that time, the total cost for the project, consisting of a Family Medicine facility, the aerobics center, and the student center, was estimated at approximately $12.1 million. Initial plans had been approved by the regents in 1984 requiring an anticipated $3 million funding from the governor as well as support from the Department of Human Services with an additional $3 million. The fiscal crisis in state government now made both sources of revenue unlikely, and the project seemed as distant as in past years. Other options for funding were explored by the regents: revenue bonds and private financing. The University attorney determined that bond funding for this project was not feasible. Only "investment financing" of the project now seemed attainable. At the October regents' meeting, a feasibility study for a free-standing Family Medicine construction project was approved. Other solutions considered by the regents included: remodeling the Pauline Meyer Building owned by the Department of Human Services; remodeling the South Pavilion; constructing an outpatient building by or with the teaching hospitals; and partnering with the Oklahoma Health Center. The regents authorized exploring all these alternatives.

Dean Donald Kassebaum

In June 1986 after a search of nearly one year, Dr. Donald G. Kassebaum was appointed University of Oklahoma Health Sciences Center executive dean, with the additional title of dean, College of Medicine, at $99,500 per year, effective August 1. President Horton said that, "Dr. Kassebaum has shown great skill as an academic leader and clinical administrator at the University of Oregon and his experience will benefit the University of Oklahoma and our College of Medicine" *[RM, 19060; DO, 6–14–86]*. Kassebaum, who had been director of the Oregon Teaching Hospitals for ten years, followed by the position of director of Health Policy Studies, was selected by Provost Clayton Rich. In the words of another University provost, Kassebaum was selected because he persuaded Rich that "he could get more done in Washington than any other single human being." It was, continued the former provost, "typical Clayton Rich concern for appointment of a person to do a specific job rather than to be a dean. When Kassebaum was here—and he traveled all the time, you know—people said he was a lot like former president Hollomon. He wines you and dines you, he rents big cars . . . then he gets hung up on the most minute details."

Another long-time faculty member stated that: "Kassebaum's style contributed to the disagreements between the basic science departments and the clinical departments and among the various colleges. In addition, Kassebaum was a master of the 'retreat' philosophy. That's what they told me in Oregon: if you want to have a lot of retreats, hire him as dean. . . ."

Dean Kassebaum certainly did not fulfill President Horton's hopes that his past experience would greatly benefit the College of Medicine. He did have admirers, however. Another prominent faculty leader said:

My impression of Kassebaum was that he was a very smart man. He had a lot of experience and knew people who respected him. But he had mannerisms, and a way of interacting with people, that always made you feel that he had to be kind of 'one-up' on you. He had to play the superior card to show you that he was the big Dean. He could be pompous, but in retrospect, the man was very smart. He would entertain differing opinions. He not only tolerated them, but respected them. He almost looked forward to a contentious interaction. And he would change his mind. It was not fruitless to discuss things with him. He may have been the smartest dean we've had here since the 1970s.

Meanwhile, on the Health Sciences Center campus, Dr. Thomas Acers, head of Ophthalmology and director of the Dean A. McGee Eye Institute, presented a report in July on the growth of that institution after ten years' existence. According to Dr. Acers, there were eight full-time physicians with clinical academic appointments and four full-time University of Oklahoma faculty physicians. Also in July, Dr. Steven J. Gentling was appointed as the new Veterans Administration Hospital administrator, just in time to be consumed by another in a sequence of hospital crises, this one the threatened closure of the Open-heart Surgery Unit. Closure was averted when the national veterans office announced that, following reexamination of the issue, the unit would not be eliminated. It had received negative national publicity due to what was perceived as an abnormally high percentage of patient deaths compared to other such units [*DO, 10–11–86*].

In the summer of 1985, the office of the provost had initiated a current-status analysis of the Health Sciences Center. The document, which was summarized by Provost Rich to the regents in April 1986, emphasized the growth of the Center from 1971–1981, noting the development of seven colleges, an increase in faculty numbers from 271 to 667, completion of eighty percent of the "programmed" buildings on campus, and comparable expansion of the teaching hospitals. The provost continued:

> The intense expansion which characterized this period outstripped resources, but an almost new and extensively redirected academic health center emerged as a result. . . . The exceptional facilities, excellent leadership, . . . and increased state funding on two occasions during this period (1982–1985), were important factors in bringing about improvement and an increased local and national reputation for the center. However, this recent period has been plagued by economic reverses; because first, basic federal capitation support for health professional colleges was discontinued and, secondly, since 1983, the serious downturn in the State's economy had a very adverse effect on financing of the center. As a result, much of the effort in the past several years has been aimed at minimizing the negative impacts of budgets which have fallen well below the average amounts for health sciences centers nationally, and well below the amounts established by the State Regents, as well. The gross overdependence of the Health Sciences Center on Practice Plan revenue and Teaching Hospital contracts not only threatens to distort the College of Medicine's operations, but it creates a serious financial exposure. . . . After years with minimal to no pay increases, compensation of faculty and staff is slipping well below national averages. Equipment is becoming obsolete. The level of State support remains far below the average nationally. . . . Oklahoma funds medical education at 49 percent of the national median, i.e. $20,000/student rather than $42,000/student. . . . The result of these

cutbacks [has been] faculty flight, deteriorating equipment, and poor morale *[RM, 19277]*.

In spite of the provost's dire warning, the University's budget request to the State Regents for the Health Sciences Center was reduced from $22 million to $10 million. Provost Rich had always believed that the emphasis should be upon increasing external dollars for research funding, and he pointed out that research funding had tripled to $15 million in the years since he became provost in 1980 *[DO, 4–06–86]*. Unfortunately, other forces mitigated against a really significant role for research dollars in the College's budget—i.e., the decrease in research funding at the national level (National Institutes of Health) and the inability to recruit significant numbers of top quality research faculty because of the penurious funding of Oklahoma higher education by the legislature. Fortunately, a white knight would come to the rescue, if only temporarily. The young Presbyterian Health Foundation would award the Center $3.3 million in grants in September for research and medical education *[DO, 9–7–86; 9–26–86]*.

The Animal Facility and the Zoological Society

In 1981 University regents had arranged for tax-exempt financing of a Laboratory Holding Facility. Such a facility had not been built earlier because of disagreements among affected individuals and organizations concerned about its location. There was a small Department of Pathology animal facility on University land adjacent to the Oklahoma City Zoo. Many University faculty members wanted the facility to be located on the Health Sciences Center campus. Following announcement of a plan to build the Remington Park Race Track, it became apparent that the University land near the zoo would be needed for the track. In September 1985, regents struck an agreement with the Oklahoma City Zoological Society to lease 24–35 acres of land for the track, in exchnage for funds to build a $900,000 animan research unit on land on the health sciences campus owned by the Department of Human Services. That Department's director, Lloyd Rader, leased the land to the regents for 75 years at a nominal rent. Remington Park was thus able to use the university land near the zoo in exchange for funding the new facility on Lottie Avenue near the College of Nursing, as well as providing funds for student scholarships. The result was a modern, one-story animal facility with indoor runs, in close proximity to the interested colleges.

The mid-1980s witnessed a period of active faculty involvement in governance of the Health Sciences Center, chiefly through a series of faculty task forces initiated by the chair and Executive Committee of the Faculty Board and culminating in numerous reports and recommendations, especially relating to College of Medicine standards for admission, promotion, and graduation; HMO-PPOs; Site of Practice; bylaws; research; feasibility of an M.D./Ph.D. program; and the utilization of faculty Practice Plan revenues.

The report of the Task Force on Enhancement of Research, formulated by Drs. Sokatch, Ferretti, Kopta, McKee, and Tang, was presented to the Faculty Board on July 29. It pointed out the rise in extramural support from $7.8 million in 1981 to $12.5 million in 1986. This growth, while commendable, aggravated the need for laboratory space on campus. The first recommendation of the task force was that assignment of all laboratory space be made by the dean, not by departments, and that it be made on the basis of funded research grants held by faculty. Second, it was suggested that planning should begin immediately for the construction of a new research building.

A committee headed by Dr. Patrick McKee recommended that the College of Medicine initiate an M.D./Ph.D. graduate program, and also initiate a program in biotechnology and molecular biology. The important roles of the Presbyterian Foundation, the Warren Foundation, and the Evening of Excellence for their support of research was recognized, as was the need for the College to increase private giving for research.

The seven active endowed chairs at the University of Oklahoma were reviewed by the Faculty Board in September, including four in the College of Medicine: the Eason Chair in Oncology, the Gaylord Chair in Ophthalmology, the Rader Chair in Pathology, and the Schilling Chair in Surgery. All but the Gaylord Chair were fully funded, and that would be funded with $350,000 in 1987 and $300,000 in 1988 *[FBM, Exhibit B, 10–86]*.

October saw J. R. Morris named a Regents' Professor. His citation noted that he exemplified the required criteria for the honor: "Outstanding service to the University, to the academic community, or to an academic or professional discipline through extraordinary achievement in academic administration or professional service" *[RM, 19003]*. In another October action, regents approved the transfer of $400,000 in Department of Psychiatry practice funds to the University of Oklahoma Foundation to establish an endowment, the earnings from which would "support the salary of an established educator/ clinician on an annual basis" *[RM, 19064]*.

Lloyd Rader Dies

In November Lloyd E. Rader was awarded the "Distinguished Service Citation" by the University of Oklahoma Board of Regents for his "dedication to public service, devotion to the welfare of man, and abiding concern for children" *[RM,19343]*. Then, early in December, the "Father of welfare in Oklahoma" died. Beginning with Johnston Murray in 1951, Rader had served eight governors, the last being George Nigh, a governor whom many accused of using Rader when he needed him but abandoning him when the political waters grew hot. Rader retired in 1982, living modestly, as he had throughout his life, in a small home in a downtown Oklahoma City condominium.

Many doctors at the Health Sciences Center viewed Lloyd Rader as an autocrat who operated a "my way or the highway" regime, holding the most powerful University administrators in contempt if they did not follow his dictates. Others, however, saw a far more reasonable administrator. Dr. Joseph Kopta, chair of Orthopedics, described a heated encounter with the white-thatched Rader: "On one occasion Mr. Rader decreed that 'No OCMH patient will ever receive a bill.' The Health Sciences Center faculty argued that private patients with insurance should be billed just as they are at every other hospital. Don Halverstadt called a meeting to mollify the faculty, at which Drs. Kopta and Moran challenged the order. Rader shot back, 'You are on the master reimbursement contract, which is in lieu of balance billing!' After much give and take, Rader agreed to allow insurance billing as long as no 'dun' letters were sent to patients who received treatment at Children's."[21]

Dr. Kopta also recalls that Lloyd Rader's word was his bond: "[Mark Everett] had arranged a meeting between Mr. Rader and me shortly after I became chairman of Orthopedics. The scheduled one hour meeting turned into an all-day session. Vera [Rader's secretary] brought in lunch. Each time we would discuss some improvement Rader favored, he would call in Lyle Coit [the director's liaison with the hospitals] and tell him to 'Write this down, Lyle. Do it for the doctor.' Later, when a power play developed in Neurology to take some of our space, I said, 'Lyle, you remember that Mr. Rader said this space was mine? You were there when he gave it to me.' We didn't lose an inch of it."[22]

The 80-year-old director of the Department of Human Services had been a devoted public servant who tenaciously pursued his goal of better health for the poor, a safety net for the needy, and outstanding facilities for children and adults at the University of Oklahoma teaching hospitals. With Senator Kerr, he had been the force behind the Kerr-Mills Bill which founded Medicare. Former Dean Tom Lynn credits Rader with "basically saving the University's two hospitals, although his management style was problematic."[23] A selfless, ruthless, and driven man, he was the dominant figure in Oklahoma politics, health, medical education, and welfare for decades. While some of his political enemies excoriated him for working so relentlessly for his vision of Oklahoma, others lauded him as the state's single greatest man. Regardless of their feelings or affiliations, however, everybody addressed him with the moniker by which he will always be remembered: "Mr. Rader."

1987

The new year opened with persistent media focus on the state of higher education in Oklahoma, with special interest paid to the University of Oklahoma and its teaching hospitals. Favorite media targets in no particular order were: the chancellor of higher education, Joe Leone; a proposed reorganization of the higher educational system, including elimination of some smaller schools; questionable activities of the director of the Oklahoma Teaching Hospitals, Tony Padilla; the management style and decision making of the director of the Department of Human Services, Robert Fulton; and accusations by Regent Kemp of a conflict of interest by the president of the University of Oklahoma, Frank Horton, vis-a-vis the University of Oklahoma Foundation.

The year began with a presentation to the Board of Regents by the new dean of the College of Medicine, Dr. Donald Kassebaum, of a summary of medical education in the United States. According to Kassebaum, there were 127 medical schools in the United States, graduating almost 17,000 physicians annually. As the number of schools grew, the number of applicants to them decreased, nationally by 23 percent and in Oklahoma by 21 percent. The Admissions Board had reduced the size of the entering class to 146 from the authorized 176. However, the University of Oklahoma remained in the upper 20 percent of medical schools in class size. Salaries of faculty were at approximately the 35th percentile nationally, although those of clinical faculty were supplemented somewhat by a disproportionate reliance upon income from private practice, with state appropriations and external research funding being well below the national average *[RM, 19404–406]*. Following Dean Kassebaum's January report, Regent Kemp objected to any policy which would limit College of Medicine enrollment. His objection was duly noted by the Board.

Professor Lorraine Singer was named to another term as dean of the College of Nursing in January 1987. She had been instrumental in obtaining the Parry Grant for Geriatric Nursing, the single largest grant to a College of Nursing in the United States at that time. Dean of Nursing since 1983, her term was extended to June 30, 1988.

February witnessed the death of Dr. Kurt Weiss, the beloved, longtime professor of Physiology. A former vice president of the Hebrew Christian Alliance of America, he had recently been chair of the board of Oklahoma's "Feed the Children" program. Joining the faculty in 1961, Dr. Weiss, a concentration camp survivor of World War II, had rapidly involved himself in the cultural and intellectual life of Oklahoma City, and was greatly loved by his students and colleagues.

On March 13 Dr. Jerry B. Vannatta, director of medical student education for the Presbyterian Hospital, associate professor of medicine, and later dean of the College of Medicine and associate provost of the Health Sciences Center, was named the fourth recipient of the Stanton L. Young Master Teacher Award.

The death of another revered faculty member occurred in April: Edgar W. Young Jr., professor of Medicine and associate dean of the College of Medicine. A 1947 medical graduate of the University of Oklahoma, he had worked for the Upjohn Pharmaceutical Company in Michigan, practiced family medicine in El Reno for fifteen years, and had served as chief executive officer of the Oklahoma State Board of Medical Examiners. Beloved of both faculty and students, the annual Alumni Association "Physician of the Year" award, which Young received in 1986, was named in his memory *[DO, 4–14–87]*. Also in April, regents changed the name of the "University of Oklahoma Tulsa Medical College Clinics" to "The University of Oklahoma Tulsa Medical Center," an action noted with approval by much of the state's media.

Fate of The Teaching Hospitals

The University of Oklahoma hospitals had a brief flurry of favorable publicity in 1987 as the long-awaited Bone Marrow Transplant Unit opened at Oklahoma Memorial Hospital on January 20. This good news was rapidly succeeded by a refocusing of media attention on the fiscal problems of the Center and its hospitals, as Governor Bellmon named a seven-member task force to study possible changes in their management. Members of the task force were familiar names in the state: William Talley, Ph.D., Oklahoma City, chair; William Bell, Tulsa; Dr. Ed Calhoon, Beaver; Mrs. Nancy Davies, Enid; Dr. Donald B. Halverstadt, Oklahoma City; Mr. Sam Noble, Ardmore; and Mr. W. K. Warren, Tulsa. The governor pointed out that if the state sales tax were applied to hospital bills, and the revenue used to pay for indigent medical care in the state, it would be possible to reduce the annual subsidy to the teaching hospitals from $35 million to $5 million. He directed the committee to consider four courses of action: (1) privatization, (2) leaving the hospitals under the umbrella of the Department of Human Services, (3) creation of a nonprofit corporation, and (4) creation of a public authority *[DO, 1–28–87; Dallas Morning News, 1–28–87; JR, 1–28–87]*. In March the task force recommended that the hospitals be placed under a governing authority similar to the Oklahoma Turnpike Authority, stating that the institutions "must have the ability to issue bonds, receive state appropriations to satisfy operating losses, and have employees eligible for the state retirement system" *[DO, 3–10–87]*. The governor indicated that he would not request consideration of these recommendations by the legislature until its 1988 session. A house-senate appropriations subcommittee took the plan under advisement in June. On June 26 state Senator Bernest Cain bluntly informed Governor Bellmon that legislation to create a separate governing board for the three hospitals was "dead for this session" *[DO, 6–16–87]*.

The University of Oklahoma Foundation and "Regential Oversight"

At the April 1987 Board of Regents meeting, Regent Elwood Kemp questioned the expenditure of funds by the University of Oklahoma Foundation on behalf of the president of the University, citing a conflict of interest with his role as a voting member of the board of trustees of that Foundation. After a heated and prolonged discussion, a study of the issue by accountants was requested. In May, Kemp's agitation regarding Foundation funds continued unabated. He "questioned whether it is improper that the president of the University receive money from the Foundation inasmuch as he is an ex-officio voting member of the board of trustees." The regents voted 4–3 against considering the issue, because "it is a decision to be made by the Board of Trustees of the University of Oklahoma Foundation as to whether or not the payments they make are in conformity with their Articles of Incorporation" *[RM, 19756]*.

Headlines about President Horton and the Foundation appeared in both Oklahoma City and Tulsa newspapers in May and June. "OU President Paid Illegally" bannered the *Daily Oklahoman* on May 15 as a result of the release of a letter by Regent Kemp to Chair John Imel in which he said, "I have studied the relationship between the foundation and regents with intensity because of my belief that there has been mismanagement and dereliction of duties." The article noted that Regents "Kemp and Sarratt have repeatedly indicated their displeasure with Horton's performance as OU president" *[DO 5–15–87]*. Regents president John M. Imel responded, "What we have before this Board of Regents is an irresponsible allegation." He quoted the accounting firm of McAfee and Taft in their conclusion that "neither the foundation's articles of incorporation nor any Oklahoma law prevent the president's office from receiving funds from the foundation" *[DO, 6–12–87]*. Regent Kemp replied that "it was not fair to assault me like this," that all he wanted "was a legal opinion. I never made an irresponsible charge. . . ." *[RM, 19806–809]*. Kemp failed to attend meetings again until October 10. In that month, a University of Oklahoma Foundation audit revealed that the total assets of the Foundation were $92.5 million, up 17.2 percent from one year previously *[JR, 10–02–87]*.

Meanwhile, more than just the extensive publicity over Kemp's allegations engendered newspaper interest in college-related foundations. Questionable financial activities at a number of other state educational entities had aroused the curiosity of reporters and led to at least one grand jury investigation. Among the major "scandals" were: (1) the daughter-in-law, and also the wife, of former Southeastern State University President Leon Hibbs received low interest loans from the foundation of that college; (2) former Higher Education Chancellor Joe Leone received $1,250 per month and use of a car for serving as president of a State Regents foundation; (3) the president of Northern Oklahoma College in Tonkawa and several former Oklahoma higher education officials had been hired as "consultants" by their school's respective foundations; and (4) an Oklahoma County grand jury was formed to examine the embezzlement of funds at Rose State College in Oklahoma City. Chancellor Joe Leone—E. T. Dunlap's hand-picked successor—resigned after disclosure of payments from Rose State, the Regents Foundation, and other "fiscal irregularities" *[DO, 4–23–87]*. Leone was ultimately indicted by the jury on a felony charge of filing fraudulent travel claims. Vice chancellor Dan Hobbs, a twenty-six-year employee with no hint of scandal and a "hard working, behind the scenes architect of higher education reform," was unanimously chosen as interim chancellor *[DO, 4–24–87]*. Representative James Hamilton introduced a bill in the legislature to assure fiscal oversight and "reduce widespread abuse of the purposes of some (university) foundations, through exorbitant and extravagant spending in some questionable areas. These foundations can no longer take the position that they are separate and private, since their public purpose is to support an entity of state government" *[DO, 4–17–87; 5–29–87]*. In June, House Speaker Jim Barker said such legislation "may discourage people from donating to higher education and the measure, Senate Bill 26, will not come up for a vote." He appointed a committee to study the matter *[DO 6–3–87]*.

Regent Kemp also questioned the lack of "regential" oversight of "Agency Special Accounts" at the University of Oklahoma, such as the athletic department, the bookstore, food services, and the Professional Practice Plan. Several of these accounts were reviewed, and the policy reaffirmed that "agency funds consist of amounts held by an institution as custodian or fiscal agent for others such as student and professional organizations. As is typically the case, the University provides no more than a bank function for these groups" *[RM, 19420]*. At this time, of the $47 million in "Agency Special Accounts," $37 million was in the Professional Practice Plan of the College of Medicine. The status of such special accounts on the Health Sciences Center campus is shown in the following table.

TABLE 5.   AGENCY SPECIAL ACCOUNTS FOR PROFESSIONAL PRACTICE PLANS

Entity	$	Entity	$	Entity	$
Dean	1.67	Anesthesiology	2.1	Dermatology	0.45
OB/GYN	3.4	Medicine	3.4	ORL	0.82
Pediatrics	3.1	Family Medicine	0.64	Psychiatry	1.6
Radiology	4.2	Animal Research	0.03	Neurology	0.39
Orthopedics	1.0	Ophthalmology	0.80	Anatomy	0.05
Biochemistry	.034	Microbiology	.085	Pharmacology	.064
Physiology	0.12	Surgery	4.83	Urology	0.62
Pathology	0.76	Dean (T)	0.41	Family Medicine (T)	0.96
Medicine (T)	0.86	Surgery (T)	0.48	OB/GYN (T)	1.6
Pediatrics (T)	0.38	Psychiatry (T)	0.20	OB Cl (T)	0.69
College of Dentistry	1.8	College of Nursing	0.52	College of Public Health	0.6
College of Allied Health	0.22				

($) = Annual volume in millions of dollars.
(T) = Tulsa Medical Branch

At their April 1987 meeting, the Board of Regents approved a plan designed to "improve" (again) their control over agency accounts, which had been submitted by the Practice Plan Executive and Advisory Committees, through implementation of a centralized data base system for billing, collection, and management of funds. This would replace the current patient accounting systems operated by each individual clinical department.

On June 11 the old issue of requiring medical students to pass Parts I and II of the National Board of Medical Examiners examination was revisited. The regents unanimously approved a Faculty Board resolution requiring students to pass Part I at the end of second year of Medical School, and part II prior to graduation. The readopted policy would be initiated with the entering class of autumn 1988. There was no opposition to the requirement, which also provided that promotion and graduation decisions would be made on the basis of "composite evaluation of the cumulative grade point average, performance on the review course, and performance in the NBME examination (Part I or Part II)" *[RM, 19780]*.

In early July there was campuswide consternation and a flurry of negative commentary over Governor Henry Bellmon's veto of HB 110, which provided funds for the Physician Manpower Training Commission. This program supported most of the Health Sciences Center's training programs and provided residency stipends in Family Medicine, Pediatrics, and General Internal Medicine, as well as a percentage of those in Obstetrics and Gynecology. Following an outpouring of protest from the residents and departments concerned, the program was reprieved.

Psychiatry Chair Search

Later in July, an administrative nightmare developed over the impending appointment of Dr. Michael Janike as chair of the Department of Psychiatry, that resulted in his withdrawing his candidacy after he had accepted the position and had purchased a home in Oklahoma City. Janike, whose appointment the department faculty considered a *fait accompli*, apparently came to believe that Dean Kassebaum was still negotiating with another candidate, which constituted a breach of integrity, and he withdrew his candidacy. Another candidate, Dr. C. Robert Cloninger, also withdrew after a second visit to the Center *[FBM, 5–26–87, 7–28–87]*. Dean Kassebaum apparently felt that "helping" the Warren Foundation participate in the evaluation of candidates would serve to increase administrative rapport with Foundation officials and, along the way, hopefully provide access to their large reserves of money. Warren Foundation officers had already interviewed both Dr. Janike and Dr. Joseph Westermeyer of Minnesota. After Janike had been offered the position, Kassebaum decided that the Foundation, which was committing about $1 million per year to the chair of Psychiatry to spend as he saw fit, wanted to hire Dr. Westermeyer, not Dr. Janike, so the Janike offer was withdrawn. Dr. Janike, not surprisingly, was furious. On July 20 Joseph Westermeyer, formerly of the University of Minnesota Hospital and Clinics, was named professor and chair of Psychiatry and Behavioral Sciences, at a salary of $90,000 plus a guaranteed Practice Plan supplement of $85,000 per year—a total annual package of $175,000. He assumed the position formerly held by Dr. Gordon H. Deckert (who served until September 1986), and by Dr. LeRoy Gathman, who occupied the chair until he died on July 7, 1987. Dr. Ronald Krug had served as interim chair during Dr. Gathman's illness. Later, the new provost, Dr. Jay Stein, would ask for Westermeyer's resignation when fiscal mismanagement within the Department of Psychiatry, including the Warren Foundation funds, was alleged. The "big mess in Psychiatry," as the situation was known around campus, harmed the image of that department at Oklahoma for a number of years.

During the summer of 1987, the Health Sciences Center's hospitals were again in the news. There was public and private concern about the managerial style of the administrator, Antonio Padilla, and there were alleged personal activities which were unrelated to his duties as head of the hospitals. The *Daily Oklahoman* described Padilla's majority ownership in a company that offered referral services for doctors, nursing homes, and other health providers, an activity which had attracted criticism by the governor as well as by state lawmakers *[DO, 6–17–87]*. On June 19 Department of Human Services Director Robert Fulton wrote, "I hereby accept your resignation as proffered by your letter of June 19, 1987. Your resignation will become effective August 31, 1987" *[DO, 6–20–87]*. Bobby G. Thompson was named the interim chief executive officer of the Oklahoma Teaching Hospitals in July. Then, in August 1988, Andrew Lasser, the newly appointed administrator of the Oklahoma Children's Memorial Hospital, was named chief executive officer of the entire Oklahoma Medical Center. He would serve with distinction in this position through the transition of the hospitals to an independent hospital authority in 1992–1993. In late 1993, because of differences with Provost Jay Stein, who served on the governing authority, Lasser resigned. Dr. Richard Timothy Coussons then succeeded him as interim and then permanent chief executive officer until amalgamation of the hospitals with Columbia Presbyterian in 1994.

At the July regents' meeting, the Family Medicine/University Center Project was reviewed. A report from Peat Marwick Mitchell concluded that the previous investment model of this project was not feasible. A study committee recommended that the project be reconfigured "to include 38,000 square feet of academic space, 54,000 square feet of clinical space, 46,000 square feet of aerobic center, and 13,000 feet of student center." The cost was estimated at $25 million, of which $17 million would come from a bond issue. The 1986 and 1987 legislatures had authorized a bond issue for these purposes. The regents approved the proposal and requested that the State Regents authorize funds for a feasibility study and schematic plans. Placing the issue squarely on the front burner was the fact that, as of July 1987, the University was paying $48,000 per year for leasing the Family Medicine Clinic in Enid, $52,000 for the North Family Medicine Clinic in Oklahoma City, and $165,000 to the Oklahoma Medical Research Foundation for space in the Rogers Building. Little more than a month later, at the September meeting, Regent Sarratt questioned the statement that some $240,000 of the regents' $850,000 Family Medicine project had been expended on "schematic plans and the Peat Marwick study." Regent Noble responded that "none of the $850,000 allocated by the State Regents for this project has been expended" *[RM, 19899]*.

Dr. Patrick McKee announced in August 1987 that the new Oklahoma Health Research Act provided $1 million for research, which would be distributed in thirty-seven grants, seventeen of which would go to the University of Oklahoma Health Sciences Center and six to the Oklahoma Medical Research Foundation. He also announced that the governor was providing money to study the feasibility of a state School of Math and Science to be located at an unspecified site. Oklahoma City was one of six cities vying for this proposed school, to be located in the Health Sciences Center area. Dr. McKee also discussed his first efforts to establish a Center for Molecular Biology on the Health Sciences Center campus. As an initial step, he proposed to the Oklahoma City Chamber of Commerce that a chair in Molecular Biology be developed. A thirteen-member committee was to identify the funds needed for the project *[JR, 8–7–87]*.

Also during the summer of 1987, a State Regents study titled "Oklahoma's Secret Crisis" became the focus of attention of a newly constituted committee under the leadership of Interim Chancellor Dan Hobbs. The study was originally released in December 1986 but had been ignored during the crumbling chancellorship of Joe Leone and other state higher education scandals, including those engulfing Rose State College and Southeastern State University in Durant. Particularly notable in the study was a recommendation by the committee that

"State funding for college programs needs to be changed so that budgets are based more on quality and less on enrollment" *[DO, 9–20–87]*. The committee also advised that a massive consolidation of college governing boards and mergers of schools and programs was needed. The report stressed that the four-year state colleges should have tougher entrance requirements and stricter measurements of academic progress.

Later in August, Governor Bellmon caused a stir by announcing that the Oklahoma College of Osteopathic Medicine and Surgery should be merged with the Tulsa Medical College. "It seems a little ridiculous to me to have two state-supported schools in Tulsa" *[DO, 8–6–87]*. Earlier in April, Bellmon and a member of the Tulsa Board of Health had been reported in favor of closing the University of Tulsa Medical College to save money. These reasonable and frequent conclusions were, as usual, never implemented. Under the title "Proposals to Close State Colleges Dead," the *Daily Oklahoman* reported that senate leader Roger Randle said the governor's proposal to close either the Tulsa Medical College or the Oklahoma College of Osteopathic Medicine and Surgery "is dead." In the words of Randle, "The two proposals are clearly unsound economically. They would deprive Tulsa of the very few state-supported programs it enjoys as compared to Oklahoma City. The Senate will not allow this to happen. With all due respect to Governor Bellmon, I want him to know that the Senate will simply say no" *[DO, 4–30–87]*. As always, constructive suggestions were ignored by parochial politicians, who chose not to face hard realities—and voter dissatisfaction—when sacrifices might be required among their constituencies.

In September Gary L. Smith, vice provost for administration and finance, was promoted to vice president of administrative affairs, Health Sciences Center. Also in September, Oscar Parsons, long-term George Lynn Cross research professor of Psychiatry, and an authority on alcoholism and brain dysfunction, received the Distinguished Contribution of Science Award of the American Psychological Association *[DO, 9–25 87]*. Late September saw Dr. William E. Brown named regents professor, and later regents professor emeritus and dean of Dentistry emeritus, effective December 31, 1987, while Dr. Webb M. Thompson, Jr., the pediatric cardiologist, retired effective the same date. Thompson had been recruited in 1963 to open the Pediatric Cardiology Unit at Children's Hospital. He served conscientiously for over twenty-five years, and after retirement, he continued to attend clinics weekly. Dr. Thompson's loyalty and friendliness to students and staff were legendary. He died suddenly in 1999.

On November 24 the Faculty Board discussed the report, "Strategic Planning Consensus: Preparation for the 90s," which had been developed from a faculty retreat held on November 14. This report dealt primarily with the Center's financial needs and how to increase revenue from its hospitals (suggested solution: increase the number of private patients) and from private practice of the faculty (suggested solutions: create a state network; add faculty to increase PPO service possibilities; increase contributions of departments to the Dean's Fund; use the Dean's Fund for "venture capital," not for basic departmental support; develop quality assurance; and market services better) *[FBM, 12–24–87]*.

At the fall general faculty meeting, a revision of the bylaws of the College of Medicine was presented. These revisions had been proposed by a Faculty Board committee one year previously, amended by the Faculty Board, and discussed at the spring general faculty meeting, where other suggestions were made. It was then edited by Dr. Everett and Dr. Knisley prior to presentation to the general faculty. At the request of Dean Kassebaum, consideration of its findings was tabled "pending a report from the dean." The only substantive change made by him, prior to final adoption by the faculty on May 24, 1988, was the limitation on the term of office of the Faculty Board chair. This would assure that no faculty member would ever again achieve the prominence as a leader equal to that of the dean.

In December a new dean of the College of Dentistry was named to replace founding dean, William E. Brown. He was Russell J. Stratton, a University of Oklahoma professor since 1977. He assumed leadership of a college that had received opposition from practicing dentists throughout the year and who had supported an earlier closure recommendation by Governor Bellmon. In a survey of Oklahoma dentists, about one-half of those practicing in the state had supported closing the College *[DO, 2–17–87]*.

Searches for qualified individuals to fill empty chairs at the Health Sciences Center continued into December. Search committee heads groused about the impossibility of luring good candidates to Oklahoma in light of the relatively low salaries being proffered. The Departments of Psychiatry and Pathology reported that they were stalled in their efforts. A consultant visit to Pathology by Dr. William Hartman, former head at Vanderbilt University and future executive secretary of the American Board of Pathology, was termed "disappointing in its superficiality" by Dean Kassebaum,[24] although Dr. Hartman's report was well received by members of the faculty *[FBM, 12–87]*.

1988

The recurring issue of utilization of the National Board of Medical Examiners Parts I and II examinations as criteria for promotion and graduation was again revisited in January 1988. This time, the State Regents' staff expressed "concern about the imposition of a nationally standardized examination on decisions about promotion and graduation, especially as these relate to underrepresented minority students" *[RM, 20089]*. As a result, the policy adopted by the University of Oklahoma Board of Regents in June 1987 was rescinded by unanimous action of the board upon recommendation of Provost Rich. Although students would be required to take the two examinations, the results would be used only "to alert the student of poor . . . preparation in time for corrective action." Many senior faculty at the Health Sciences Center accused the regents and provost of "copping out" to ease pressure from students, parents, and politicians who received complaints about the exams. One influential faculty member went so far as to observe that, "This continuing controversy over absolute national standards for competency and the action taken on this date by our provost reflects the persistent influence of 60s permissiveness in the higher educational establishment, much to the detriment of professional standards" *[FBM, 1–88]*.

Also in January, the regents established a Professional Practice Plan committee composed of regents, faculty, administrators, and an attorney to recommend a reorganization which would clearly assign management of the plan to the dean of the College of Medicine rather than to a faculty committee. This action ended direct communications between the Practice Plan Executive Committee and the regents, clearly defining the chain of authority through the Health Sciences Center administration.

The Oklahoma Center for the Advancement of Science and Technology

The January 26 Faculty Board meeting focused on the new Oklahoma Center for the Advancement of Science and Technology's "Centers of Excellence" program. This program was created by the 1987 legislature for the purpose of instituting applied science and technology programs that would foster cooperation between business and the educational community to develop Oklahoma's economic potential. Three potential "Centers of Excellence" were proposed for the Health Sciences Center campus: (1) "Addiction," headed by Dr. Oscar Parsons from the Department of Psychiatry; (2) "Reproductive Biology," headed by the Department of Obstetrics and Gynecology, in conjunction with Oklahoma State University; and (3) "Cardiovascular Biology," headed by Dr. Robert D. Foreman, chair of Physiology. Patrick McKee, chair of Medicine and vice chair of the Faculty Board, would play a seminal role in bringing such centers to the Oklahoma City campus.

In May Oklahoma launched the "Centers of Excellence" program with an $18.89 million budget and guidelines stressing cooperation between higher education, various branches of state government, and private industry *[JR, 5–24–89]*. Together with committed private investments, the funds for the centers totaled $33 million *[Tulsa World, 5–26–89]*. Three centers were initially selected, two of which involved the Health Sciences Center: (1) the Molecular Medicine Research Center (based at the Center); (2) a Laser Development and Applications Center (a joint project between the Dean McGee Eye Institute and Oklahoma State University); and (3) a Center for Integrated Design and Manufacturing. The first private company to locate on the Health Sciences Center campus was Houston-based CytoDiagnostics, Inc. The company employed technology developed by Dr. George Hemstreet and licensed from the University of Oklahoma. The company later became UROCORP and occupied two large buildings on the Oklahoma Health Center campus between Lincoln Boulevard and the Centennial Expressway *[DO, 6–22–89]*.

On January 18 the Tulsa Chamber of Commerce issued a report by its medical education task force which emphasized the "in kind" financial contribution made by area physicians and hospitals working at and with the Tulsa Medical College, and which "subsidized the TMC operated clinics ($1.1 million in fiscal year 1988)." The report did not mention that a primary purpose of the clinics was provision of care by salaried faculty and house staff to uninsured indigents, thus relieving practicing physicians of the burden of uncompensated care. The greatest benefit of a Tulsa College of Medicine branch to the private hospitals was that it permitted them to continue their residency programs, assuring both future specialists for the area as well as an immediate profit from the services rendered by these physicians. The report noted that "it is virtually impossible to get accreditation for postgraduate education without medical school sponsorship." The report suggested that basic science education (currently available only at the osteopathic college) should be provided "to students of both TMC and OCMS, as well as graduate and undergraduate students." The report assumed that a free-standing medical program, with the first two years of College of Medicine being a joint effort with the Osteopathic program, would be approved by accrediting agencies. In the longer term, the report envisioned that the University Center in Tulsa would become a free-standing university with both the Osteopathic and Medical training programs becoming colleges in a large new state university. This dream was not to be realized, since the LCME consistently refused to consider the Tulsa program as anything other than a branch of the University of Oklahoma College of Medicine in Oklahoma City. Furthermore, by 1997, politicians had created "Rogers University," another untenable fantasy of area senators. Ultimately, Oklahoma State University would operate the area's undergraduate programs and, jointly with the University of Oklahoma, provide graduate programs. Health-related education in Tulsa (other than in the Osteopathic degree) would be the purview of the University of Oklahoma.

At their February 1988 meeting, University regents approved an optional Doctor of Pharmacy degree to replace a Ph.D. degree in Clinical Pharmacy. The purpose of this action was not entirely clear, as the difference between the two degrees appeared primarily political rather than scientific, not to mention that up to $427,000 in incremental funding would be required, an element not commented upon by any of the regents.

Very little activity relating to the Health Sciences Center occurred in the spring of 1988. In March, Elwood Kemp, now serving his final year as a regent, was elected chair, following the practice of that Board, while in April, longtime professors Glen S. Bulmer (Microbiology), Webb M. Thompson, Jr. (Pediatrics), and Phyllis Jones (Dermatology) were made professors emeritus. The 1988 Master Teacher Award was given to P. Alex Roberts, Ph.D., director of the program in Neuroanatomy in the Department of Anatomy.

In Oklahoma City, at an Oklahoma Biomedical Research Symposium sponsored by the Presbyterian Foundation and the University and the Oklahoma Medical Research Foundation, Dr. Patrick McKee, the chair, stated, "There is an air of excitement in this state. A new set of hopes and expectations is developing as we talk." He referred to the recently established Oklahoma Center for the Advancement of Science and Technology (OCAST), the Oklahoma High School for Math and Science (situated adjacent to the Health Sciences Center campus as a result of a cliff-hanging 10–9 vote of its board of trustees), and pending state legislation to establish endowed professorships and chairs. The $15 million provided to establish this program, as well as the initial funds for the School of Math and Science, were spared a gubernatorial veto in July when Governor Bellmon, exercising his line-item veto power, killed the omnibus appropriations bill which he characterized as "pure pork barrel," but spared the other initiatives. Included in his veto was $2.5 million for the Family Medicine Center, regarding which the governor stated that the "regents could allocate funds without interference from the legislature" at any time *[DO, 7–8–88]*.

In May annual leases were approved for academic space for the Department of Ophthalmology in the Dean A. McGee Eye Institute, at $116,250 annually, and for commercial space in Tulsa for the Tulsa Family Medicine Clinic, at $68,000 annually. The remainder of the May regents' meeting focused on the minority recruitment program for University faculty. At the Health Sciences Center, 14 percent of new faculty were minority and 34 percent were women. The conclusion by the Board of Regents following receipt of this data was that "our affirmative action programs will continue to enjoy success" *[RM, 20255]*. On the Norman campus, new faculty included 17 percent minority employees and 10 percent females.

At a special meeting held on May 26 to address personnel issues, the regents announced that Donald B. Kassebaum, dean of the College of Medicine, had resigned effective June 30. A search committee to identify a successor was appointed. Dr. Kassebaum, who had also served as a professor of Medicine, was named assistant to the provost for health policy analysis for the period July 1988 to June 1989. At the same time, Dr. Timothy Coussons was named associate dean for clinical affairs and Nancy K. Hall was promoted to associate dean for student affairs and admissions. Dr. G. Rainey Williams, professor of Surgery, was named interim executive dean and interim dean of the College of Medicine.

In May the Department of Human Services changed the names of the Center's hospitals from the Oklahoma Teaching Hospitals and Oklahoma Children's Memorial Hospital to The Oklahoma Medical Center and Children's Hospitals of Oklahoma *[DO, 5–10–88]*. This occurred shortly after a commotion in which the Department of Human Services "borrowed" $4 million from the teaching hospitals in order to pay departmental bills and the subsequent resignation of University Hospital chief executive officer Bobby Thompson, who transferred to St. Anthony Hospital at a great increase in pay *[DO, 4–26–88]*. In other hospital-related news, a monument to the late Lloyd Rader on the Health Sciences Center campus at the corner of Stanton L. Young Boulevard and Everett Drive was dedicated on April 28 by Senator David Boren and Governor Henry Bellmon.

In June University of Oklahoma President Frank Horton submitted his resignation effective August 1. David Swank, dean of the Law School, was named interim president. An editorial in the *Journal Record* stated that Horton resigned because he was: ". . . under pressure from several members of the board of regents. . . . Regents Sarratt and Kemp have been critical publicly, with Sarratt quoted as saying the 'chemistry' of the board was not in Horton's favor. That's vague, and no reason to run off a president who has represented the university and the state so well. . . . Horton's role in helping Oklahoma prepare for a new diversified economy has been almost beyond measure. During Horton's three years here, Oklahoma has come a long way toward developing the basic thinking we need for cooperation between public education and private enterprise" *[JR, 6–4–88].*

A search committee was appointed to find a replacement for President Horton, with instructions that although "an earned doctorate is not a requirement, it is the expectation of the Board of Regents that the next President will have an earned doctorate or its equivalent" *[RM, 20476].* Many faculty members believed, and fretted, that this wording left open the possible selection of former Governor George Nigh to fill this position.

Private Patient Billing

As of June 1988 the IDX Corporation was providing patient billing/accounts receivable systems for seven clinical departments at the Health Sciences Center: Orthopedic Surgery, Psychiatry, Pediatrics, Medicine, Pathology, Obstetrics/Gynecology, and Anesthesiology. The company also provided software for three Family Medicine clinics. Oddly, although the University administration and regents were persistent champions of centralized billing, in July the purchase of a new billing system for the Department of Surgery, independent of the central billing and collecting unit, was approved. This action testified to the skill and influence of the chair of Surgery, G. Rainey Williams, who clearly felt he knew a better way. Then, in September, the regents approved purchase of a free-standing billing system by the Department of Radiological Sciences, while at the same meeting hiring Peat Marwick Main and Company to "advise regarding a standardized patient accounting policy and procedure for its 360 full-time faculty members in twenty-one clinical departments in Oklahoma City and Tulsa" *[RM, 20532].*

The University's first endowed chair in Molecular Biology was funded in October through gifts from several of the largest state foundations—Presbyterian, Noble, Kerr, and Sarkey's—with a significant contribution from OCAST *[DO, 10–12–88].* The regents named the chair for Ed Miller, president of the Presbyterian Foundation, who played such an important role in campus development.

Cogeneration Revisited

In November 1986 the regents had selected Smith Cogeneration Management to develop and operate a 100 megawatt cogeneration facility on the Health Sciences Center campus. In April 1987 the firm applied to the Oklahoma Corporation Commission to set a "fair rate" for selling power to Oklahoma Gas and Electric, since direct negotiations with the utility had been unsuccessful. After extensive discussion, it was apparent that the project was still very much in the planning stage, including the physical location of the facility, and there was doubt it would ever be built. In October regents voted that "The University shall have no ownership in the plant nor in the land upon which the plant is constructed" *[RM, 20358–9]*. The final acts of this drama would be played out before the Oklahoma Corporation Commission in 1991. Oklahoma Gas and Electric opposed construction of plants on the Health Sciences Center campus as well as at Will Rogers Airport on the basis that, if built, these plants would cost ratepayers an extra $75–95 million on the "highly speculative chance that they would break even 22 to 30 years down the road" *[JR, 1–23–91]*. Opposition was also voiced by the Audubon Society of Oklahoma, which advocated that the Commission adhere to a strict conservation policy rather than approve the construction request. It was revealed that Smith Cogeneration would make $3 million on the financing and another $2 million when the plant was activated. The *Journal Record* reported that the Oklahoma Attorney General's office, which often appeared as a consumer advocate in Corporation Commission hearings, was not participating in this proceeding. "Attempts were made to inquire about the lack of participation in these cases but no response was received" *[JR, 2–13–91]*. This statement was a clear hint that impropriety almost certainly dogged the entire enterprise. It would be only a very short time until the fanciful dream of a University-owned, income generating power plant came to an end.

The 1987–88 University of Oklahoma budget was reviewed during the June 1988 regents' meeting, and it was revealed that faculty salaries ranked sixth in the Big Eight Conference, or fourth if benefits were included in the calculations. The average faculty salary at Oklahoma was $36,000, compared to $43,000 at Colorado, $47,000 at the University of Texas at Austin, and, by comparison with another conference of schools, $50,000 at the University of Michigan. Oklahoma still had a long, long way to go before it could hope to browse in the same fiscal pastures with benchmark universities. The "tenuous financial state" at the University of Oklahoma was attested to by the fact that approximately 200 faculty positions had been totally eliminated, chiefly because in fiscal 1985–86 the University sustained a $10 million reduction in state appropriations! This cut "followed a severe budget reduction in 1982–83 and another in 1983–84," according to President Horton *[RM, 20393]*.

A new revision of the College of Medicine Faculty Bylaws, approved by the faculty on May 24, was accepted by the regents at their June meeting. The major substantive change was a limitation of the term of office for the Faculty Board chair to four years. This revision had been inserted at the insistence of Dr. Kassebaum, who regarded the position as too visible and powerful, and hence a potential threat to the authority of the dean. At the same meeting, the regents formally recommended a "stand-alone" facility for Family Medicine be built at a cost of $6.3 million; following this recommendation, they authorized President Horton to request $300,000 from the State Regents for architectural and engineering studies.

In September the search committee for a new dean of the College of Medicine met with regents to discuss candidates for the position. At the same meeting, Dr. Patricia Brown Forni was named dean of the College of Nursing. Gary Smith, the Health Sciences Center vice president for administrative affairs, announced his resignation to become executive vice chancellor of the State Regents. Mark Lemons, Health Sciences Center controller, was named interim vice president for administrative affairs, to report directly to the president "but with coordinated reporting to the Health Sciences Center Provost" *[RM, 20528]*.

Construction and Endowed Chairs

The Health Sciences Center's Master Plan for Capital Improvements on its campus, was released by the Board of Regents in September 1988. It contained several major items: (1) the Family Medicine building ($6.3 million); (2) a biomedical research tower (two phases of $16 million each); (3) a student activity center ($4.4 million); and (4) two parking structures ($7 million). (One of the items on this list—the first phase of the research tower—would not be completed until 1997.) In Tulsa, purchase of the currently leased campus for $5.6 million, a clinic building for $9.9 million, and a $4 million education building were the chief priorities.

On September 18 the University of Oklahoma Board of Regents met with the State Regents to review this campus master plan, as well as the endowed chair and professorship program. The previous legislature had appropriated $15 million for matching funds for endowed chairs and professorships. This program, which was intended to benefit the entire higher education establishment, primarily benefitted the two comprehensive universities and the Health Sciences Center due to the skill of faculty and supporters of these institutions in raising private funds. The smaller four-year schools found the sledding very tough in generating sufficient donations to fund endowed chairs of any description.

As of October 1988 there were eleven fully funded and six partly funded chairs at the University of Oklahoma, including the Eason, Schilling, Parry, Gaylord, and Rader chairs on the Health Sciences Center campus. In December the Department of Medicine provided $500,000 in matching funds for two endowed chairs, with an additional $1.5 million anticipated from the W. I. Warren Medical Institute to fund two additional chairs. The Department of Dermatology established a chair with grants from the Carl Herzog Foundation, gifts from alumni, and a substantial contribution from current faculty, especially Dr. Mark Allen Everett and Dr. Dennis Weigand. These actions would bring to sixteen the number of chairs funded on the campus at year's end.

Also in October, Dr. Charles R. Brown was promoted to associate provost, retaining his title of associate dean for administration, College of Medicine. A month later, Dr. Fred G. Silva II was appointed Lloyd E. Rader professor and chair of the Department of Pathology, while Dr. James Wenzel was named interim chair of Pediatrics.

Edward N. Brandt

Edward N. Brandt Jr. was named executive dean of the College of Medicine in December 1988, at a salary of $125,000 plus $50,000 from the faculty Practice Plan. Dr. Brandt was a native Oklahoman who had graduated from the University of Oklahoma College of Medicine. Formerly assistant dean of the College 1958–70, he served as vice chancellor for health affairs in the University of Texas system at Austin 1977–81, as acting surgeon general of the United States in 1981, and as assistant secretary of health 1981–1984. He then served as president of the University of Maryland at Baltimore 1984–1988. His appointment was greeted with enthusiasm by faculty and administration, all of whom believed that Dr. Brandt, through his national contacts, would usher in a new era of federal largess in research and construction funds for the Health Sciences Center. One administrator, who wished to remain anonymous, later remarked that: "[Clayton] Rich misjudged that; he thought Brandt had contacts across the board. But the 'assistant secretary for health' has absolutely nothing to do with NIH . . . nothing to do with the agencies appropriating funds for buildings and equipment. His contacts were primarily with the CDC. Furthermore, he spent too much time trying to keep himself in the national eye rather than fighting for the institution. Talk about hating facing issues! Ed just *hated* facing issues. I don't think we've been blessed with a good strong dean for quite a while."

Why did Ed Brandt not meet the (admittedly high) expectations of the faculty? One senior faculty member believed that, after so long a period of fiscal constraint and unmet personnel needs at the Health Sciences Center, the expectations were too great for Brandt or anybody else. Others thought that Brandt had, in a sense, already completed his career and merely wanted a respectable title and a "genteel retirement" at Oklahoma. Later, when a new provost was selected to succeed Dr. Rich, many, including Ed Brandt himself, could not believe that he was not selected for the position.

"Closing Tulsa" Laid to Rest

It is clear from the Board of Regents' discussions of September 1988 that Governor Henry Bellmon had a continued interest in medical education in Tulsa and in the University of Oklahoma Dental College. Obviously, said one regent, "the (recent) transfer of the College of Osteopathic Medicine to Oklahoma State University did not settle that issue" for the governor *[RM, 20583]*. Provost Rich indicated that, in his opinion, the real issue to be studied was the incremental cost of the dual Tulsa/Oklahoma City system as opposed to one limited to Oklahoma City. The University Center at Tulsa was also hotly discussed. Deliberation of each of these items would prove to be more political than educational, and debate would continue for decades.

As the year drew to a close, a study committee appointed by Governor Bellmon recommended that the Tulsa Medical Branch be maintained "because it provides needed residency positions, and receives a great amount of support from the city's hospitals." Furthermore, the proposal to combine the Tulsa branch with the Oklahoma College of Osteopathy was inappropriate because, "any attempt to unify the clinic programs into one primary care organization would be extremely difficult" and "the recognized difference in the curriculum for, and practices of, medical and osteopathic doctors," by all medical professionals, supports the continuation of the two schools in Tulsa, rather than a single combined school offering all four years of training *[DO,12–23–88]*. This report officially put to rest the attempt to consolidate or close either or both of these politically inspired schools.

A December budget analysis provided to the regents revealed that for the first time, the College of Medicine's Professional Practice Plan revenue was nearly equal to the entire appropriated budget for the Health Sciences Center campus ($25 million vs. $26 million, for six months).

1989

The new year dawned with Governor Henry Bellmon asking the legislature for $65 million for higher education, including $5.5 million for the Tulsa Medical College, and $1.7 million to convert the O'Donoghue Rehabilitation Center in Oklahoma City into a research facility *[Tulsa Tribune, 1–23–89]*. The latter recommendation was due to the "phenomenal growth in research grants at the Health Sciences Center" *[DO, 2–05–89]*. The Tulsa proposal was for purchase of the 10.5 acre campus currently occupied by the Tulsa branch. At this same time, there was a shortage of intensive care beds and emergency room facilities in the University's teaching hospitals in Oklahoma City, causing ambulances to "divert patients to private hospitals" with increasing frequency *[DO, 1–24–89]*.

Saint Francis Hospital Medical Research Institute
in Oklahoma City—Again

Early in 1989, remodeling of space in the Basic Sciences Education Building for the Saint Francis Hospital Medical Research Institute was completed, at a cost of some $2 million. Funds for this project were provided by the Warren Foundation and the Oklahoma Center for the Advancement of Science and Technology (OCAST). The Research Institute was originally established at the College of Medicine in Oklahoma City in June 1985 with Dr. Patrick McKee as director. Faculty were to be recruited jointly by the Institute and the University, with tenure being given by the University and salaries being reimbursed by the Institute on a renewable annual basis. The relationship between the College of Medicine and the Institute was "based upon a mutual commitment to the highest quality of biomedical research," and highly productive investigative work [RM, 21440]. Other consequences of this relationship were the partial endowment of four chairs by the W. K. Warren Foundation, funded with $1.5 million, and a grant of $2.5 million over five years to help develop research in the Department of Psychiatry. An additional expenditure of $1.2 million on renovations in the area of the Biomedical Science Education Building for the OCAST Molecular Medicine Center of Excellence had been approved the previous September.

The 1989 Master Teacher Award winner was F. Daniel Duffy, M.D., chair of the Department of Medicine in Tulsa, and the most prominent and energetic mentor of students at the Tulsa branch.

In March there was a great tempest in the teapot known as the University of Oklahoma Board of Regents. Regent Chair Kemp opened the proceedings by asking that in the future, board members should "raise their hands" if they wished to speak. Apparently Regent Kemp had forgotten his own well-earned reputation for breaking into the presentations of other regents without a by-your-leave or so much as a request to the president to be heard. Charles Sarratt was then nominated for the position of chair by Regent Sylvia Lewis, who was acting more out of conformance to tradition than of respect for Sarratt; he was the regent with the most longevity who had not served as chair. Sam Noble countered by nominating Ron White for the same position. Chairman Kemp suggested that the second nomination was illegal, inasmuch as it "is a break with tradition." Following a request for an opinion, the legal counsel pronounced Mr. Noble's nomination "legal." Sarrat said, "My viewpoint has conflicted with those members of the University community who believe that the administration and faculty should govern the university" *[RM, 20930].* After much deliberation, Regent White was elected chair on a vote of 4–2–1. Regent Kemp then asked for "Regent White to resign from the Board of Regents of the University of Oklahoma for gross conflict of interest on several different fronts. [Also] I am asking that Regent Noble resign because of the appearance of violation." Kemp called the election a "raw steal of power" *[Tulsa World, 3–16–89].* Kemp and Sarratt had for years voted as a "bloc" in opposition to the other regents, opposing tuition increases and tougher admission standards while criticizing University auditing practices and expenditures by the University of Oklahoma Foundation. Later, Kemp stood up and said he was "leaving." The University of Oklahoma Faculty Senate was so incensed by Kemp's action that it at once issued a public condemnation, calling him "terrible" and "offensive" *[Tulsa World, 4–04–89].*

During the spring of 1989, two physicians were appointed by Governor Henry Bellmon to the State Board of Regents for Higher Education: Ed Calhoon of Beaver in May, and Dr. Donald B. Halverstadt of Oklahoma City in November. The latter was named to complete the unexpired term of Joffa Kerr, who had recently resigned. Halverstadt would serve until 1993. Also in the spring, the name of the Oklahoma Tulsa Medical College was changed by act of the legislature to the University of Oklahoma College of Medicine-Tulsa, to reflect the subordinate relationship of the Tulsa campus to the executive dean in Oklahoma City *[Tulsa Tribune, 5–19–89]*. Regents approved the change in June.

At a special meeting of the University of Oklahoma Board of Regents on May 2, 1989, Dr. Richard L. Van Horn was named president and chief executive officer of the University, to be effective July 15, at an annual salary of $140,000, with a "president's fund" of $50,000 per year.

On May 17 at their regular meeting, regents named Dr. Ralph Lazzara as the Natalie O. Warren Professor of Medicine, and Dr. James R. Gavin as the William K. Warren Professor of Diabetes Studies. At this time, full professors in clinical departments in the College of Medicine were salaried at $70–80,000 per year (a level comparable to that of deans on the Norman campus), and associate professors usually at $50–65,000, unless they were "high earning" practitioners. Also at the May meeting, regents let contracts obligating Professional Practice Plan funds on behalf of the Surgery department at Tulsa for space at Hillcrest Hospital at $42–50,000 per year for five years *[RM, 20971, 20978–21282]*.

Admission Standards

In May, the State Regents set admission standards for the College of Medicine and the College of Osteopathic Medicine at identical levels—i.e., a grade point average (GPA) of at least 3.0 and a Medical College Admissions Test (MCAT) score of at least seven. (At this time, the University of Michigan, for example, was interviewing only students with an MCAT of ten or more.) Up to 15 percent of admissions could be under "alternative criteria" defined by the College *[RM, 21277]*. Because 100 percent of students admitted in 1988 with a GPA below 3.0 and an MCAT below 7.0 were on probation their first year, while only 7.9 percent of those with a GPA above 3.0 and an MCAT above 7.0 were on probation, the faculty and provost approved offering all students admitted under the alternate criteria the option of taking three years to accomplish the first two years of College of Medicine. The obvious solution of requiring "alternative admissions" to meet the 3/7 minimum was deemed politically incorrect by University administrators.

In another example of raw politics at work, the Health Sciences Center vending services were commandeered by the Department of Human Services, which promptly assigned them to its own Division of Visual Services (formerly

"Aid to the Blind"). Previously, vending services in University Hospital had been a function of the Women's Auxiliary. This had been the principal source of income of that organization since it was established in the 1950s by the Council of Jewish Women, Mrs. Mark R. Everett, and Mrs G. Rainey Williams. Women's Auxiliary income was earmarked for hospital improvements, while Visual Services income was spent outside the Center. The original purpose of assigning ancillary food services in state institutions to the Visual Services Division of DHS—providing employment for the visually impaired—was not met by this transfer, as the individuals servicing the vending machines throughout the medical facilities were never noticeably visually impaired.

Central Billing and the State PPO

In September 1989 the Board of Regents renewed a contract with IDX Corporation for billing systems for nine of the Health Sciences Center's clinical departments at a cost of $700,000 per year. The services of this vendor never equaled in speed of collection, or in percent of gross charges collected, the efforts of the several independent department billing and collecting units— i.e., Ophthalmology, Surgery, Otorhinolaryngology, and Dermatology. Central Billing's record at the time was comparable only to that of Family Medicine's, which is to say, rather unsatisfactory. Clinical departments participating in the central system had remained solvent, in spite of the poor collection record of IDX, primarily because of the State of Oklahoma Preferred Provider Organization. State of Oklahoma employees treated by Health Sciences Center faculty provided an income of $10.5 million to the Center in 1988. However, the total cost of medical care to employees on the state health plan escalated because of easy access, overutilization, and high prescription costs. The generous benefits of the plan caused other physicians and hospitals in the state to eye these reimbursements with envy, and on October 9, twenty-four state hospitals sued to end (or enter) the program, stating that they were unfairly excluded and had become victims of an arbitrary and capricious bidding process.

Health Sciences Center departmental revenues decreased further when, in October, the College of Medicine's Professional Practice Plan was once again amended, this time to increase the amount of money in the "Dean's Enrichment Fund" with a flat tax of 3.7 percent on all gross revenues, and a surtax on income of "higher earning faculty"—i.e., 7.5 percent on total income from $100–150,000, 15 percent on income from $150–200,000, and 20 percent on all income over $200,000 *[RM, 21395–7]*. Likewise, a ceiling was imposed, equal to the 90th percentile of levels for comparable faculty nationally. In June 1990 the regents would once again turn their attention to the College of Medicine's Professional Practice Plan, primarily because "reimbursements for patient care are necessary to sustain the operation of the clinical departments and the College, including faculty compensation, and are necessary for the Oklahoma Medical Center." Faculty practice income accounted for approximately half of the funding of the College. For the 1989–90 fiscal year, the Professional Practice Plan generated nearly $60 million, of which $20 million (30 percent) was returned to the faculty as salary supplements. That same year, state appropriations were approximately $57 million for the Health Sciences Center, and grants and contracts generated $27 million *[RM, Schedule I–III, Exhibit A, July 1990]*. The regents concluded that "current policy allows for an excessive degree of decentralization that interferes with the plan's business operation . . . and an executive committee . . . will be responsible for operational decisions rather than the individual departments" *[RM, 21847]*. This policy was the beginning of the end for relative fiscal independence of clinical departments, and signaled a period of significantly decreased collections, increased siphoning of funds into general University operations, and, especially, an expanding bureaucracy in the Practice Plan office. The contract with IDX, as the provider of patient billing and accounts receivable, was extended to include additional clinical departments—e.g., Neurology and Urology. Surgery, Otorhinolaryngology, Ophthalmology, Family Medicine, Radiology, and Dermatology still maintained independent billing and collecting units.

On September 15, 1989, pioneer oilman and civic leader Dean A. McGee died at the age of 85. He had been a longtime and unstinting lay supporter of the development of the Health Sciences Center, which was the "achievement of which he was proudest," according to the *Daily Oklahoman* of September 16. That same week, the *Tulsa World* announced that Evangelist Oral Roberts would close the City of Faith Hospital and shut its College of Medicine in order to eliminate a $25 million dollar debt and save his Oral Roberts University. This marked the denouement of one of the evangelist's grandest visions *[Tulsa World, 9–14–89]*.

A variety of other events took place at the Health Sciences Center in September. Mr. Jerry B. Farley was named vice president for administrative affairs at an annual salary of $93,000, and Associate Dean William H. Knisely retired from the College of Medicine. William Knisley had served as the principal confidante of the dean for many years, as well as occasionally filling the role of acting dean. Previously he had been president of the University of

South Carolina at Charleston. In other September actions, schematic designs for the Family Medicine building were approved, and the regents also purchased nine lots on the south side of N.E. 14th Street west of Phillips Avenue for the purpose of constructing a surface parking lot. (This lot would not be completed until 1998!) Finally, the regents adopted resolutions of appreciation for Governor Henry Bellmon, the Oklahoma Legislature, and the State Regents for Higher Education and its chancellor, Hans Brisch, for instituting Oklahoma's "matching program" for endowed chairs. Under the matching program, the state would provide $250,000 or $500,000 for each similar amount in "private" money pledged to establish a chair or professorship.

At the regular regents' meetings of April 1988, July 1988, and May 1989, plans were developed and approved for a new Oklahoma Museum of Natural History (successor to the Stoval Museum on the Norman campus) to be built on the south campus at Chautauqua and Timberdell. These actions set in motion the process culminating in a splendid $58 million museum to be completed in 1999 and opened in the new millennium.

On the political scene, former State Senator Phil Watson, serving briefly as director of the Department of Human Services, defaulted on a $360,000 loan in October and filed for bankruptcy *[Tulsa Tribune, 10–14–89]*. This was soon followed by his departure from office amidst widespread editorial comment that someone who couldn't manage his personal finances probably couldn't manage Oklahoma's billion-dollar welfare empire either.

Provost Clayton Rich presented the Health Sciences Center Strategic Plan to the Board of Regents in December. This plan, which praised the improvements and facilities built over the previous twenty years, pointed out that the legislative funding base for the Center is "marginal for achieving major stature nationally." Rich called primarily for growth in research activity. His plan envisioned the use of $600,000 per year of "seed" money to recruit fifty new investigators to the campus, all with external funding, by December 1994. "But attaining the national average in state funding is essential, and currently the legislative appropriation is only 50 percent of the national level. The current state operating budget must be doubled." The need for a new research building (which would not be completed until 1998) and "seed money" for other projects were deemed critical by the provost. Regents adopted the plan unanimously *[RM, 21497–21502]*.

On December 20 a division of Dermatopathology was established at the Health Sciences Center. This division was to be "a joint and equal function of the Departments of Dermatology and Pathology" *[RM, 21540]*. And, in a final decade-concluding note on the same date, thirteen Oklahoma City hospitals became smoke-free on midnight, December 31 *[JR, 11–17–89]*. These hospitals would now boast of their new "pure air" standards, but their dispossessed smokers quickly learned to congregate just outside entry doors, often forcing visitors and patients to pass through a reeking, hazy gauntlet on the way inside.

1990

As the new decade opened, the top priorities for capital construction at the Health Sciences Center were: (1) the Family Medicine building (projected cost: $6.3 million); (2) the Biomedical Research Tower, phase I ($25.2 million); (3) purchase of the Tulsa campus ($5.6 million); and (4) a Student Center in Oklahoma City ($5.5 million) *[RM, 21608]*. If this list appears familiar, it was almost a verbatim rehash of the priorities of 1989.

The 1990 Master Teacher Award was bestowed upon M. Alex Jacocks, M.D., a physician in the Department of Surgery. Dr. Jacocks had served as secretary of Alpha Omega Alpha for several years and was an invaluable mentor of students on the general surgery clerkship.

Three new endowed positions were announced for the Health Sciences Center in March: the Frances and Malcolm Robinson Chair in Gastroenterology (a major gift by Dr. Malcom Robinson), the Grayce B. Kerr Centennial Chair in Biochemistry, and a Centennial Professorship of Visual Science. In addition, $425,000 was added as a match for the Lloyd E. Rader Chair in Pathology, originally established by Dr. Mark Allen Everett in 1984 when he served as interim chair of that department. In July gifts were announced establishing the John S. Gammill Chair of Polycystic Kidney Disease (Reserve National Insurance Co.), and the James R. McEldowney Chair of Immunology (James R. McEldowney Trust). In October 1990 the Centennial Professorship of Dermatology Research was established with funds donated by Dr. Everett, Dr. Dennis Weigand, and alumni of the Department of Dermatology. The professorship was later changed to a chair and named for Richard and Adeline Fleischaker, in honor of their generous gift and long-term interest in Dermatology.

Physicians as Independent Contractors

For physicians at the Health Sciences Center reporting income to the Internal Revenue Service, funds received by them as income supplements from private practice activities had always been considered to be "schedule C" income, permitting them to report such funds as income from a profession, and subject to deductions for professional expenses, rather than as a salary from the University. This policy stemmed from the faculty practice document in which the regents stated that when caring for private patients, faculty were not acting as state employees. The IRS raised the issue of "holdover" private practice income, retained in University accounts beyond the end of the fiscal year, which the IRS would consider as taxable to the earning physician in the year earned. At their November meeting, regents reaffirmed the 1973 recognition of physicians as employees of the University when performing academic functions, but as independent contractors when caring for patients. However, they modified the accounting procedures so that "carryover" funds would not be used as physician income supplements, in order to conform to the "constructive receipt doctrine" of the IRS *[RM, 22075–6, 7]*. (Later, the regents would renounce the "private contractor" policy, causing major dislocations in physician tax reporting.)

In June 1990 a policy applicable to full-time Health Sciences Center faculty was adopted which provided that all clinical income was to be deposited in University accounts, and which stated that "this policy applies to the geographic full-time faculty. . . . Part-time faculty are excluded from application of this policy" *[RM, 21873; RM, Exhibit C, June 1990]*. Also, Site of Practice exceptions were approved for two positions in the Department of Gynecology and Obstetrics to be based at the Presbyterian Hospital Obstetrical service. The following month, the Site of Practice policy was further modified to permit institution of a Family Medicine training program at Presbyterian Hospital, with three full-time faculty and twelve residents. Later, in November, an exception was made to provide a faculty surgeon at Presbyterian Hospital. These policy exceptions reflected an increasing educational presence of the University in Presbyterian Hospital, usually stimulated by grants from the Presbyterian Health Foundation.

A lease for 15,000 square feet for the Department of Ophthalmology in the Dean A. McGee Eye Institute at a cost of $116,250 per year was also approved in March. Unlike the Family Medicine leases, which had always been paid from the College of Medicine budget, the Ophthalmology lease was to be paid from departmental practice funds.

In April 1990 Dr. Hervey A. Foerster, clinical professor emeritus of Dermatology, died at age 87. Commander of a U.S. Army station hospital in London during WW II, he returned to Oklahoma City where he practiced dermatology until his death. He served as a clinical professor in the College of Medicine for many years, and after retirement in 1982 he founded the Retired Doctors Club *[DO, 4–18–1990]*.

On June 23, the first James F. Hammarsten Physician of Excellence Award was presented by the Department of Veterans Affairs, Oklahoma City Veterans Administration Hospital Center. The recipient was Dr. Dennis A. Weigand, chief of Dermatology at the hospital, for his dedication to teaching, his professional manner with patients, and his long service on Veterans Administration Hospital committees and boards. The award would be presented annually to the Veterans Administration Hospital physician "who has made significant contributions to patient care, research and education" *[DO, 6–24–90]*. Named for James F. Hammarsten, former chief of medicine at the Veterans Administration Hospital from 1953–1962 and chair of the Department of Medicine, this first award was presented personally by Dr. Hammarsten.

Oklahoma Model for Medical Education for the 21st Century

In August, Dr. Gordon Deckert, the David Ross Boyd Professor of Psychiatry and Behavioral Sciences, was named director of programs for curriculum change, in the office of the dean of the College of Medicine. His chief responsibility was to chair a study, announced in March 1990, of the "process and content of medical education" at the Health Sciences Center, and to recommend a plan for the future. Called the "Oklahoma Model for Medical Education for the 21st Century" (OMME–21), Drs. Gordon Deckert, Mark Allen Everett, Robert Foreman, John Holliman, Patrick McKee, Daniel Duffy, and Philip McHale constituted the steering committee. The group met weekly in intensive sessions for three months, and in October 1991 submitted a report with a number of key recommendations, including: (1) early College of Medicine admission for up to 30 percent of the incoming class; (2) an overall reduction in the length of medical training; (3) a more cost-effective grouping of courses; (4) increased "hands-on" training—"the way medicine will be practiced in the 21st century"; (5) an annual increase of 5 percent in the number of highly qualified applicants to the College of Medicine (high MCATs and grade point averages) in each of the next six years; (6) an increase of 100 percent in the number of graduates entering academic medicine and primary care prior to the year 2000; (7) establishment of a mix of knowledge-based and problem-based learning in all courses; (8) a generic basic-science knowledge-based examination; and (9) a generic clinical sciences knowledge-based examination for all medical students. In addition to these recommendations, the report suggested that by 1996 each student should be required to produce two scholarly works during his/her time in medical school; the basic sciences were to be shortened from two to one and one-half years, and the required clinical rotations were to be reduced to one year by 1993. Finally, the report empha- sized that although "lumping educational material around a particular disci- pline, such as biochemistry, may be an efficient way to teach [medicine], physicians always discover later that they simply cannot practice medicine within that organizational framework."

In October the Faculty Board adopted a series of specific objectives related to recruitment, admissions, curriculum, and student evaluation. These included: (1) increasing the number of qualified resident applicants to the College of Medicine to achieve an applicant/admission ratio of 2.25:1 by the year 2000 (this would be accomplished by 1994); (2) increasing the number of highly qualified matriculating students by a minimum of five percent per year over the next five years, requiring an MCAT score of 10.0 or greater and grade point average greater than three on a four-point scale (this was accomplished in 1993–1994 after a decrease in such students in 1990, 1991, and 1992); (3) increasing, by 1995, the number of students admitted after three years of college to 30 percent of the class (there was no substantial increase in this category through 1995, presumably because the number of highly qualified applicants with the degree increased so markedly during the same time frame); and (4) increasing, by the year 2000, the number of American Indian applicants to the College of Medicine by 100 percent (this was accomplished by 1993, although the number of matricu- lating American Indians increased by only 25 percent, primarily due to the fact that as a group, their MCAT scores were less competitive, and the most highly qualified American Indians frequently received more generous scholar- ship support from other institutions). Thus, the faculty objectives regarding *admissions* were, for the most part, achieved more quickly than had been envisioned; on the other hand, the objectives regarding *evaluation*—a stan- dardized course- and student-evaluation system—were introduced more gradually. The faculty objectives regarding the career choices of graduates were only partly successful—i.e., a 100 percent increase in the number of graduates entering academic medicine was not achieved, but a 100 percent increase in students entering primary care did occur. Thus, three-fourths of the faculty objectives for the College of Medicine admissions procedures and standards were accomplished prior to the envisioned date. Clearly this represented a worthwhile, but modest, outcome for OMMI–21 and all the faculty effort devoted to articulation of these goals. The curricular and educational objectives of OMMI–21 were less completely realized or not at all. Problem-based learning was introduced slowly in all courses; an integrated program for, and examination in, clinical skills for all students was not accomplished; a basic sciences knowledge-based examination (in lieu of the NBME I exam) for minimum competence was not introduced; and a required scholarly research project for each student was not instituted *[FBM, 1–23–95]*.

Oklahoma School of Science and Mathematics

In September the first class of sixty-two students of the newly constructed Oklahoma School of Science and Mathematics arrived on campus. Six cities had vied to have the institution located in their midst, and the final selection came down to either Stillwater or Oklahoma City, on the Health Sciences Center campus. State Senator Bernice Shedrick of Stillwater campaigned doggedly for the school to be located at Oklahoma State University. A consultant from the North Carolina School of Math and Science recommended that the committee select the site on the Health Sciences campus, at Lincoln and N. E. 13th Street, as best for the students. Dr. Patrick McKee worked to secure this prime site from the Oklahoma City School district and Urban Renewal Authority, with the assistance of the local Chamber of Commerce. Ed Miller of the Presbyterian Foundation agreed to donate a large piece of land for the site. During deliberations and balloting by a governor-appointed selection committee to pick the winning site for the prestigious school, hearts pounded and tempers flared. At one point in the proceedings, there was a tie vote between Oklahoma City and Stillwater. The committee chair, Dan Little, had to make the final decision about where it would be located by casting the tie-breaking vote. According to Dr. McKee, "Mr. Little sat and thought. And thought. And thought some more."[25] One observer felt Little had "gone into a fugue state." People began to stretch and disappear on bathroom breaks. Finally, after almost 15 minutes of concentrated deliberation, Little said simply, "Oklahoma City." When queried about his decision later, Little said, "The proximity to great facilities and mentors in the College of Medicine and elsewhere on campus made my decision for me."[26] Students would live on the Norman campus in the Cross Center until a dormitory was finally built in the autumn of 1997.

Governor David Walters

At the general election in November 1990, David Walters, former associate provost and later chair of the Human Services Commission, was elected governor of Oklahoma. His transition team was dubbed "The Gang of Five" in the newspapers, many of which never looked with favor on his term of office. The "gang" included Jack Clarke, Shawnee banker; Larry Brawner, an Oklahoma City attorney who had worked with Walters while he was with the University; businessman Ron Yordi, a longtime political friend who would later become director of the parking enterprise at the Health Sciences Center; and businessmen John Kennedy and Michael Samis. Three of these men, Yordi, Kennedy, and Samis, once held second mortgages on Walters' Oklahoma City home as part of a controversial "loan" during his previous try at the governorship. In spite of his former position as associate provost at the Health Sciences Center, Governor Walters' term was not characterized by consistent support for the Center or its programs. Fond of the editorial "we", Walters pronounced, "We were perceived as the governor on November 7th." He promised Oklahoma voters a "very dynamic, active period of time" *[DO, 12–30–90]*. These words would prove prophetic from a man who eventually would be the object of a grand jury investigation and possible impeachment. During his tenure on the Health Sciences Center campus, Walters played a pivotal role in two major initiatives, i.e. the purchase of the Tulsa campus, and consolidation of colleges and programs during the 1970s. He later recalled that when several program closures were begun, attorney Robert Henry represented the faculty, and successfully forestalled the closure of one of these. It was Walters' first battle with this knowledgeable and effective legislator, attorney, and future federal judge.

At the Health Sciences Center in November, a four-alarm fire destroyed four of the Steam and Chilled Water Plant cooling towers, causing $1.5 million in damage and necessitating rental of temporary cooling equipment for several months *[DO, 11–16–90]*. For more than twenty-four hours, the teaching hospitals were without refrigerated air and were forced to resort to fans. Also in November, the resignation of Edward J. Tomsovic as dean of the University of Oklahoma College of Medicine, Tulsa, was announced by the regents "because of the pressures of the job."

In December actions, regents approved an exclusive contract with the Medical Arts Laboratory of Oklahoma City to provide laboratory services to the Family Medicine clinics. Because a requested bid from the Oklahoma Medical Center (University Hospital) was never submitted, the only other bidder for this contract was Smith-Kline-Beecham. The regents also approved an increase in the projected cost of the Family Medicine Clinic to $7.1 million from the previously approved $6.3 million, as well as raising the expected cost of phases I and II of the Biomedical Research Tower to $39.8 million from $37.9 million. The Family Medicine Clinic was currently the number two building priority of the entire University, with phase II of the Catlet Music Center in Norman listed as number one, built at a cost of $8.72 million. The proposed Health Sciences Center student activities center was estimated to cost $5.5 million.

1991

The new year began with the announcement that Dr. Jesus Medina, professor of Otorhinolaryngology, had received the state's first professorship of Clinical Oncology from the American Cancer Society, one of two such physicians in the country so recognized. This honor provided $40,000 per year for three years. The new year's Evening of Excellence honorees were Dr. Robert G. Tompkins of the Tulsa Hospital Medical Foundation, and prominent Oklahoma businessman Edward C. Joullian. At the festivities, the Presbyterian Health Foundation was lauded for its support of medical research and education. Also in January, Childrens' Medical Research committed itself to funding two more chairs in Pediatric Research. In addition, a Francis Duffy Professorship in Oncology was announced by the Department of Medicine, and a $106,000 gift from the Rumsey family initiated the Virginia Briscoe Rumsey Endowed Professorship in Pulmonary Research.

The IRS and Faculty Practice

On a less salubrious note, the regents, upon recommendation of President Richard van Horn, altered the Professional Practice Plan document so that all practice income currently distributed as "independent contractor" income (1099 income) would in the future be considered to be part of the University "salary" (W-2 income). Thus the role of physicians as independent contractors was terminated, and while they were engaged in professional practice, "all faculty are to be considered employees of the University of Oklahoma" *[RM, 22192]*. The president's recommendations were accompanied by the comment that clinical departments "are given a degree of autonomy that may interfere with the effective conduct of an interdependent group practice." Although considered to be University income through adoption of the new IRS policy, "PPP supplements [were to] be excluded from the University of Oklahoma's 401-k retirement plan" *[RM, 22197]*. These recommendations were unanimously approved by the regents. Thus, the worst of both worlds was thus thrust upon the medical faculty! Regent White, made the dissimulating statement that the changes proposed were "for the benefit of the plans and the participants of the plans." This was, in the minds of many faculty members, an incorrect interpretation. University Vice President Jerry Farley said that he believed the president should have the authority to implement these changes "once the issues are resolved with the faculty members" *[RM, 22198]*. Clearly, many of the faculty thought that the changes were not in the best interests of University faculty members, especially the loss of the ability to report schedule C income, and that the changes should be opposed. Dean Edward Brandt and Provost Clayton Rich agreed that "the issues can be resolved and that additional time to work with faculty concerns should be allowed." Later, in partial response to faculty dissatisfaction, the plan was amended to provide that the "University" would contribute on a limited basis to the retirement plan based upon supplemental income—i.e., 10 percent on supplements between $25–100,000; 15 percent on supplements $100,001–150,000; and none on amounts above $150,000. However, these benefits were to be paid from the supplemental income, and not the University budget! In April Dr. Brandt and Dr. Rich reported that a faculty vote "to confirm changing practice income to salary income passed overwhelmingly." Implementation was to be completed by July 1 *[RM, 22307]*. Thus ended the entrepreneurial era of faculty practice. The era of "physicians as employees" had begun.

The Oklahoma Center for Molecular Medicine

In the winter of 1990–1991, the Oklahoma Center for Molecular Medicine (OCMM), developed conceptually by Dr. Patrick McKee, became reality with a "Center of Excellence" designation and funding from the Oklahoma Center for the Advancement of Science and Technology. Dr. Phil Comp was selected as director. The Center was under the joint aegis of the College of Medicine, the University of Tulsa, the William K. Warren Medical Research Center, and the Oklahoma Medical Research Foundation, with its own students and faculty and a core interdisciplinary curriculum. The operating committee consisted of basic science department heads, the Oklahoma Medical Research Foundation section chiefs, and graduate faculty members responsible for establishment of, and recruitment to, the endowed chairs. Students were to enter the graduate program as unclassified students; take a multidisciplinary, combined course in molecular biology; participate in the "Molecular Biology of Human Disease" course; and rotate through the laboratories of three members of the OCMM faculty. At the end of the second semester, each would declare a major area of basic science interest, enter the laboratory of a graduate faculty member, and begin doctoral research. Much of the third floor of the Basic Sciences Education Building was remodeled for center laboratories with OCAST grants and strong support from the Presbyterian, Warren, and Noble Foundations. Dr. McKee believed that the success of the program lay in wedding the entire effort to the M.D./Ph.D. program: "Nobody at this institution ever understood how powerful such an amalgamation can be, if you have M.D. scientists laced with Ph.D. investigators. Not one dominant over the other, but working together. If you can believe it, at one time we had all three Foundations supporting the program. And we blew it!"[27]

This program, initially funded jointly by the Noble, Warren, and Presbyterian Foundations, was submitted to the National Institutes of Health for continuation funds. Dr. McKee remembered that "we applied to NIH, and we knew that it was going to be unlikely we'd get approval on the first application. We had a site visit from them, and we finished just below the cut mark for funding. We were told we would likely be the next center funded."[28] When a subsequent application was prepared in 1992, Provost Stein and then-Dean Voth opposed the program as "too expensive" for the College, with little prospect for full self-support. Additionally, the graduate dean, Ray Cling, and some of the basic science chairs were not enthusiastic supporters of the M.D./Ph.D. program because they believed that all Ph.D. training should follow the M.D. years, virtually assuring that no medical student would ever select the program. The lack of enthusiasm of the administration lessened the interest of the Foundations in funding it. Additionally, the basic science faculty was unhappy with the "undifferentiated" initial year in Molecular Medicine, fearing that the graduate stipends granted to these interdisciplinary students would reduce graduate slots available to individual departmental programs. Thus, for lack of vision, various territorial jealousies, and unfounded and unspecific fears, the Center for Molecular Medicine atrophied, and the M.D./Ph.D. program died. The Center received $8.7 million in grants over the five years of its existence.

In March 1991 the new Health Sciences Center Library was named for former Dean Robert Montgomery Bird, who died on December 31, 1976. The Robert M. Bird Society, founded by Dr. Patrick McKee and contributed to by many physicians whose lives were touched by Dr. Bird, had raised over

$500,000 for library support. The dedication was presided over by Health Sciences Center officials and Governor David Walters. Dr. Donald Lindberg, director of the National Library of Medicine at the National Institutes of Health, was the featured speaker.

Also in March the regents approved a planned addition to the Dermatology building and associated parking space, to be built with $314,000 in faculty practice funds, money held in trust for Dermatology at the University of Oklahoma Foundation, and recent gifts to the department. In other actions, Governor Walters appointed Dr. C. Victor Williams of Lawton to the University of Oklahoma Board of Regents, replacing Dr. Ronald White. Dr. Williams was to have a very short term, as he died suddenly on May 1, 1992. About the same time, Dr. Fred Silva was appointed to replace Patrick McKee on the OCAST board.

In a final March action, the 1991 Master Teacher Award was given to G. Rainey Williams, M.D., chair of the Department of Surgery, for his skill and leadership in surgery, dedication to mentoring students and residents, and his service as interim dean of the College of Medicine.

April began on a bright note when the Upjohn family of Kalamazoo, Michigan, announced a gift in the amount of $500,000 to fund the Upjohn Chair in the College of Medicine. Dr. L. N. Upjohn had been the first head of what was to become the University of Oklahoma School of Medicine—i.e., the first dean. Also in April, three of Dr. Upjohn's children, E. Gifford Upjohn, Roda Cookson, and Esther Sharp, together with Don Parfet, grand nephew and executive vice president of the Upjohn Company, joined family friend Mrs. Mark Everett and college officials to make a formal presentation of the award *[JR, 5–18–91]*. The following month, Dean Edward Brandt Jr. was named occupant of the chair.

Another chair was announced for Children's Medical Research in May in honor of the late businessman C. R. Anthony, when the Presbyterian Foundation matched a gift of $150,000 from the Anthony Foundation and friends. Then, in September, the Ungerman Trust of Tulsa provided $392,000 and the Presbyterian Health Foundation added $150,000 to endow the Dr. Arnold and Bess Deldich Ungerman Chair in Cross-Cultural Psychiatric Care *[DO, 9–9–91]*.

Presbyterian Health Foundation

In July regents honored the Presbyterian Health Foundation, its chair, Stanton Young, and its president, Jean Gumerson, for their commitment to the University of Oklahoma Health Sciences Center. The Foundation had made grants to further medical education and research in excess of $17 million during its first one-half decade of operation. Established in October of 1985 with $65 million from the sale of Presbyterian Hospital to Hospital Corporation of America, the Foundation gave vital and generous support to medical education, scientific research, clinical pastoral education, community health programs, and technology transfer related to health care. That same month, the Foundation gave $150,000 toward establishment of the James A. Merrill Chair in maternal-fetal medicine in Gynecology and Obstetrics. Faculty and friends donated $350,000 to complete funding of the chair. In August the Foundation gave $275,000 toward two endowed chairs in Psychiatry and Behavioral Sciences, in addition to one in cancer research *[JR, 8–07–91]*.

By 1990 external research funding at the Health Sciences Center had risen to $18.4 million for the fiscal year, up from the $8.6 million in 1986. Federal sources provided another $8.6 million for research. Other sources included state funds (OCAST) of $3.3 million, private foundations $4 million, and industrial sponsors $2.5 million. According to newspaper reports, approximately 62 percent of research proposals by Health Sciences Center faculty were receiving funding of one kind or another *[JR, 4–03–91]*.

The Robert Wood Johnson Foundation awarded $1 million to the Health Sciences Center in August for AIDS prevention and service. In addition, the grant was to be used in a program to improve American Indian health and the minority education program at the Center *[JR, 8–21–91]*.

Largely at the instigation of Dr. Nancy Hall, associate dean of the College of Medicine for admissions and student affairs, a summer academy program was initiated to provide acclimatization to health sciences careers for high school students from all over Oklahoma. In the summer of 1991, some ninety-eight students studied under and worked one-on-one with faculty members in the health sciences. This was the largest of twenty-three summer programs sponsored by the Oklahoma State Regents for Higher Education and was designed to attract students with aptitudes for the health sciences to the campus.

September 1991 witnessed a series of important personnel changes among Health Sciences Center faculty. Dr. Jesus E. Medina, the American Cancer Society Professor of Otorhinolaryngology, was named chair of his department. Dr. Carl R. Bogardus, professor and vice chair of Radiological Sciences, was elected president of the American College of Radiology. Lela Ann Lee, M.D., was appointed to the Carl J. Herzog Chair in Dermatology effective October 1. She would work for six years with Dr. Morris Reichlin, internationally renowned researcher in lupus erythematosus at the Oklahoma Medical Research Foundation. She resigned to return to the University of Colorado following the appointment of a new chair of Dermatology. Meanwhile, Oscar A. Parsons, long-term George Lynn Cross Research Professor of Psychiatry and Behavioral Sciences, retired after a very distinguished career at the Center. William L. Parry, professor and chair of Urology, likewise retired effective October 29, 1991.

In November, regents divided the Family Medicine Clinic building project into two phases: Phase I would be the first floor, with a shelled area; Phase II would be the second floor. It was felt that such a division would allow more expeditious progress toward completing the overall project.

The Health Sciences Center Site of Practice Policy was revisited in December and provision was made to permit "specialized patient care activities" at non-campus sites. Furthermore, "with the approval of the dean, full-time faculty members shall be permitted to act in a professional capacity in specific instances not covered above." These changes would introduce flexibility into the Center's relationship with Presbyterian Hospital, especially, while not alarming the administration of the teaching hospitals *[RM, 22704]*. Also in December, Dr. David W. Parke II was named professor and chair of the Ophthalmology Department.

1992

Nineteen ninety-two dawned as a year of severe financial retrenchment for higher education in Oklahoma, partly due to the failure of the state's economy to recover from the 1990s recession as quickly as the rest of the country, but principally due to the passage of House Bill 1017, which committed the legislature to mandated annual increases in funding for elementary and secondary education. In Oklahoma, as elsewhere in the body politic, "the squeaky wheel gets the grease," and the elementary education forces in the state had petitioned and cried for increased funding so incessantly—to the point, even, of parading statistics that revealed how ineffective some of their own programs were in educating Oklahoma's children—that the legislature finally folded and gave them most of what they wanted. The mandated spending under House Bill 1017 was a colossal shift of responsibility for primary and secondary education in Oklahoma from local property taxes to the state general fund.

With a large slice of the general revenue pie carved out for elementary and secondary education for the foreseeable future, supporters of state colleges and universities knew they were in trouble. Dr. Donald Halverstadt, chair of the Board of Regents for Higher Education said, "This is a perilous time for higher education. It's the most critical time for higher education that we've faced in a couple of decades." Legislative commitment to funding of House Bill 1017, concluded Halverstadt, "indicates that Oklahoma higher education institutions will be fortunate to have a standstill budget for the 1992–1993 academic year" *[DO, 4–25–92]*.

Higher education forces fired the few guns they possessed at this time. "Have you repaired your home since 1968?" asked Chancellor Hans Brisch of the legislators, referring to the last capital bond issue for higher education. Unfortunately, Brisch's was the only effective voice being raised for higher education at this perilous time. Neither of the large state universities could boast a president with the muscle to influence the legislature (a situation that would continue until former governor and senator David Boren arrived in Norman in 1995). Added to the lack of effective voices, there was in the legislature at this time a persistent populist feeling that higher education was "elitist" and that "professors spend too much time on research, grants, committees and consulting, and not enough time in the classroom"—an old diatribe oft delivered by the uninformed *[DO, 4–25–92]*.

On January 30, Dr. Stewart G. Wolf Jr, first full-time chair of the Deparment of Medicine, and John S. Gammill, chair of the board of Reserve National Insurance Company and a University benefactor, were honored at the Evening of Excellence held at the University of Oklahoma College of Medicine banquet. Also in January, Dr. J. Moore Campbell III, clinical professor emeritus, died at the age of 80. A thoracic surgeon practicing in Oklahoma City from 1932 until the mid-1980s, Dr. Campbell was a pioneer in cardiac valve replacement surgery and, when the author was a student in 1947, he was usually followed around the campus by one of his canine experimental patients—often identified by a clicking sound with each heart beat! He also was an accomplished organist who for decades played at College of Medicine graduation ceremonies.

The John W. Records Chair in Obstetrics and Gynecology was initiated with a gift of $150,000 from Mr. and Mrs. George Records of Oklahoma City in February. The regents also announced two new "Laureate Psychiatric Chairs" in Molecular Medicine on February 20.

In March, the cash-strapped Department of Human Services once again "transferred" $8.7 million from the Oklahoma Medical Center to fund other, more "pressing" departmental programs. Such transfers contributed greatly to the chronic inability of the teaching hospitals to replace aging equipment and facilities. At the same time, a $10.7 million supplemental appropriation was approved by the legislature to fund the operational deficit of the hospitals.

The Board of Regents took time from a busy schedule to note, in March, that the eight Oklahoma physicians included in the book, *The Best Doctors in America*, were all at the Health Sciences Center. These were Regents Professor Mark Allen Everett (Dermatology), Professor Dennis A. Weigand (Dermatology), Dr. Bradley K. Farris (Neurology), Dr. Warren Jackman (Cardiovascular Disease), Dr. James Little (Ophthalmology), Professor Jesus Medina (Otorhinolaryngology), and Dr. Betty Pfefferbaum (Psychiatry) *[RM, 22836]*.

Gordon Deckert was named interim chair of Psychiatry effective March 6, 1992. At the same time, numerous faculty based at the Veterans Administration Hospital experienced significant salary reductions, including professor Jan V. Pitha ($20,000 pay cut) and George Hemstreet ($6,000 cut). Only Dr. Robert McCaffrey, Dr. Norman Levine, and Dr. Dwight Reynolds received increases.

Two newly appointed University of Oklahoma Board of Regents members were sworn in at the Board's March meeting. They were University of Oklahoma Law School graduate Ada Lois Sipuel (to fill the unexpired, one-year term of the recently resigned Sylvia Lewis); and Melvin C. Hall, who was appointed to succeed Sarah Hogan. Also in March, regents authorized the purchase and installation of a Health Sciences Center wide fibre optic network, which connected the seventeen agencies on the campus with those in Norman, Tulsa, and the worldwide internet.

J. Andy Sullivan was named chair of the Department of Orthopaedic Surgery in April. Dr. Sullivan, chief of Pediatric Orthopedics, was secretary of the Pediatric Orthopedic Society of North America. In a sad note, Dr. Don H. O'Donoghue, for whom the Rehabilitation Institute on the Health Sciences Center campus had been named, died on April 21, 1992. He was an internationally known orthopedic surgeon and former head of the Department of Orthopedics, as well as the first Faculty Board chair.

Dr. Harold L Brooks was named dean of the University of Oklahoma College of Medicine, Tulsa branch, in May. At the same time, the Oklahoma Medical Research Foundations honored several of its scientific staff: Dr. Paul Kincade, immunobiologist, was named to the William H. and Rita Bell Chair in Biomedical Research; Dr. James H. Morrissey was designated the Fred Jones Distinguished Scientist; and Jordan J. N. Tang was awarded the Edward L. and Thelma Gaylord Prize for Scientific Achievement because of his work on genetic factors in the acquired immunodeficiency syndrome (AIDS).

An announcement in May that a "comprehensive breast institute" would be created at the Oklahoma Memorial Hospital elicited a cry of anguish from the *Tulsa World*: "It is outrageous that the State of Oklahoma continues to expand taxpayer supported health care in Oklahoma City while it virtually ignores Tulsa and the rest of the state" *[Tulsa World, 5–16–92]*. Although an Oklahoma City newspaper indicated in June that ground-breaking for a "5,500 square foot building enclosing the lower level of the South Pavilion" for the breast institute would take place *[JR, 6–6–92]*, the reality proved far less grand. The small former offices of Dr. Donald Halverstadt when he served as chief of staff of the teaching hospitals, and of Dr. Mark Everett when he was chief of staff of University Hospital, would be remodeled into a "breast health" suite—hardly an "outrageous" expansion of taxpayer support in neglect of Tulsa! Many such complaints from Tulsa physicians and the press resulted from the large number of indigent patients throughout the state—patients who were a burden on all hospitals, but especially resented in Tulsa because of the state-supported hospitals in Oklahoma City, which shouldered much of the capitol city burden. In Tulsa, neither the Osteopathic College nor the University of Oklahoma College of Medicine branch owned its own hospital. Because of the huge number of medically uninsured citizens in Oklahoma, there was a push for a health care provider tax on hospitals, nursing homes, and pharmacies to support indigent care. The tax was voted down in November. A typical comment from a Tulsa health leader was, "We are supporting a huge, thirsty medical facility (in Oklahoma City) with virtually no access to it" *[Tulsa World, 8–19–92]*. More important, many informed Oklahomans wondered why the medical care industry should be the principal source of funding for indigent care, rather than a yearly legislative appropriation from the general fund.

On June 10 state Representative Tim Pope, a vocal conservative politician, addressed the regents to protest the presence of Anita Hill—the accuser of U. S. Supreme Court nominee Clarence Thomas—on the University payroll. He especially objected to a movement to create an endowed chair in her name, and to the fact that she had been granted a sabbatical leave of absence, "during which she will be making speeches around the country for which she will be paid large sums of money and also may be endorsing and working for political candidates" *[RM, 22925]*. This was followed by questioning from representative Leonard Sullivan about "why the state is spending more than $1.3 million on paid sabbatical leaves of absence this academic year for fifty-seven faculty members at Oklahoma colleges and universities" *[DO, 8–17–92]*. Anita Hill was one of three University of Oklahoma law professors who received $45,000 for a six-month leave.

Also in June several members of the faculty were promoted to full professor: John B. Harley; Warren M. Jackman, Peter J. Sims (Oklahoma Medical Research Foundation), Gary Thurnau, Robert A. Wild, Lester A. Reinke, Russell Postier, David W. Tuggle, and Dala R. Jarolim. Audits were authorized for the clinical departments of Medicine, Orthopedic Surgery, Surgery, Dermatology, Medicine-Tulsa, and Pediatrics-Tulsa. Additionally, the regents established a policy on naming buildings, facilities, and positions for individuals: "A building may be named for one-half of the private funds required for the project, or for one-half of the estimated cost of construction" *[RM, 22963–7]*. One wonders what Everett Tower or Evans Hall would have been called if money, rather than honorable service, had been the principal determinant of building names.

Provost Rich Retires

Provost Clayton Rich, announcing his retirement at the end of June 1992, bid the University of Oklahoma farewell, saying , "I had fun as provost, but I'm looking forward to doing something different now. Over 29 years in academic administration is enough" *[DO, 6–7–92]*. Clayton Rich had been named provost in 1980 during the Oklahoma oil boom, when educational budgets were awash with money, and everything seemed possible. Thirty-six months later, several years of flat budgets began, and with it, retrenchment and penury throughout the higher education system of Oklahoma, most notably at the Health Sciences Center. Clayton Rich was an effective provost for those times—deliberate, low-key, gentle-speaking, and tending to avoid conflict when possible. The chair of the Department of Medicine described Clayton Rich as:

a very intelligent man. He was somewhat indecisive, but always a gentleman. Some people thought that he avoided difficult decisions; and in spite of his good ideas, he did not know how to build a consensus, or get people to do what he wanted. He would listen to you. He felt that his role was to protect the faculty and keep them out of harm's way. He was more concerned with trying to keep things safe and peaceful, rather than saying, 'Here's my vision; here's what I want to do with the Health Sciences Center.' As a consequence, the legislature and community leaders came to think of him as placid. He recruited deans for each of the seven colleges, and focused on increasing research activity and funding of the campus, especially the College of Medicine. He was particularly proud of the endowed chairs program created by the State Regents. He left saying, 'We would love another oil boom.'

Another long-term faculty member lauded Clayton Rich as a "most effective provost" because he didn't always feel that he "had to do something" to solve issues. Said Dr. Joseph Kopta: "Rich preferred to just talk at committee meetings, serving excellent wines, until the committee died a natural death of inanition. He wanted to avoid controversy and emphasize the joys of good wine. On one occasion he delayed a proposed action to take over the PPP [Professional Practice Plan] from its Advisory Council on the grounds that it was a divisive issue and, as such, should not be implemented. [Provost] Thurman, on the other hand, and [later Provost] Stein, would take a position and never change, regardless of the consequences."[29]

Overall, Clayton Rich was a successful provost for the turbulent times in which he served.

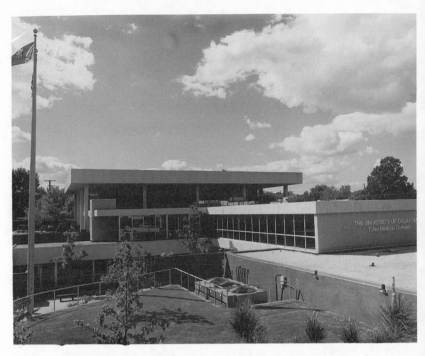

The University of Oklahoma College of Medicine, Tulsa Branch. (OUHSC)

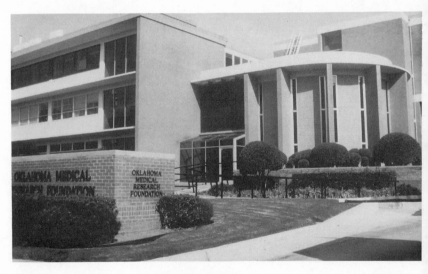

The growing Health Sciences Center's Oklahoma Medical Research Foundation. (OUHSC)

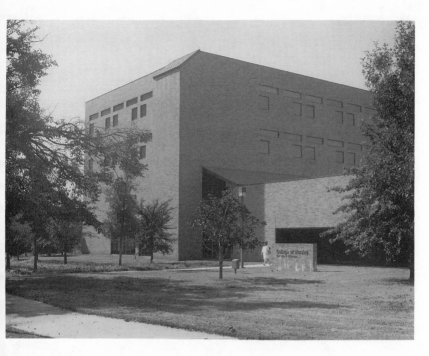

The Health Sciences Center's College of Nursing. (OUHSC)

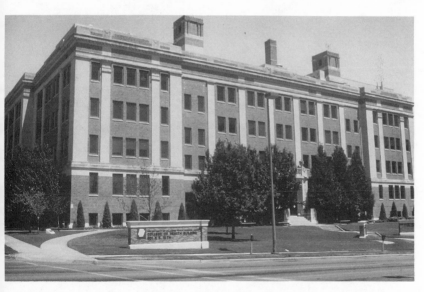

The Health Sciences Center's Colleges of Allied Health and Public Health. (OUHSC)

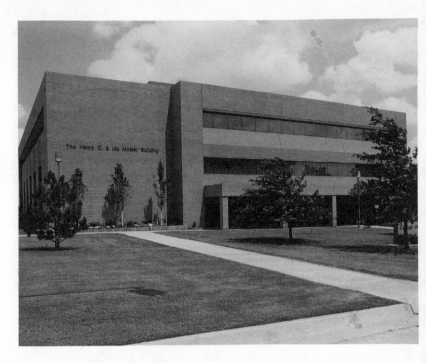

The Health Sciences Center's College of Pharmacy. (OUHSC)

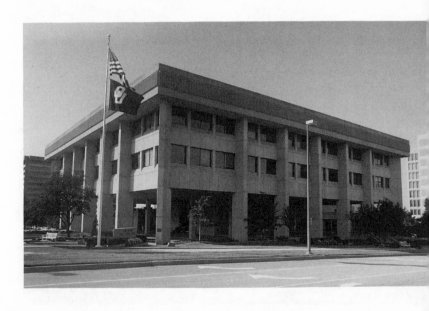

The Health Sciences Center's Robert M. Bird Library. (OUHSC)

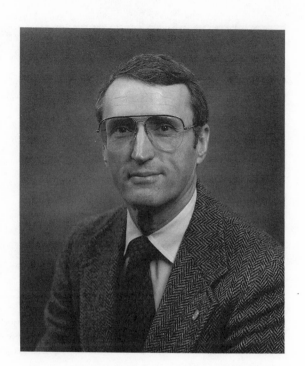

Charles B. McCall, M.D.,
Executive Dean of the
College of Medicine.
(OUHSC)

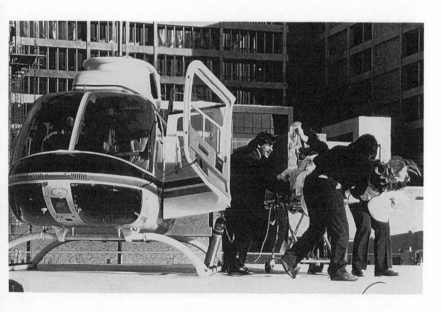

A Medi-Flight helicopter on the landing pad of Children's Memorial Hospital. (DHS)

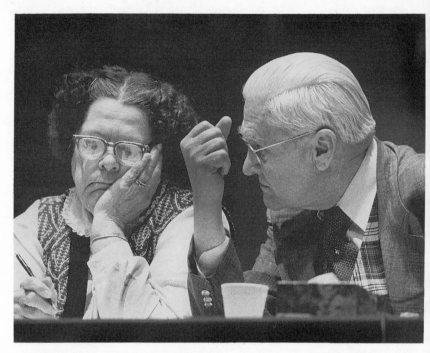

Lloyd Rader (right), Director of the Department of Human Services, with assistant Vera Alder (left), Secretary to the Oklahoma Welfare Commission. (AAE)

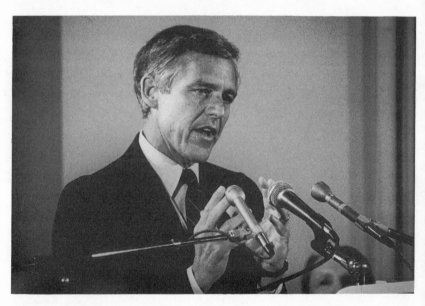

William Banowsky, Ph.D., President of the University of Oklahoma. (OUPA)

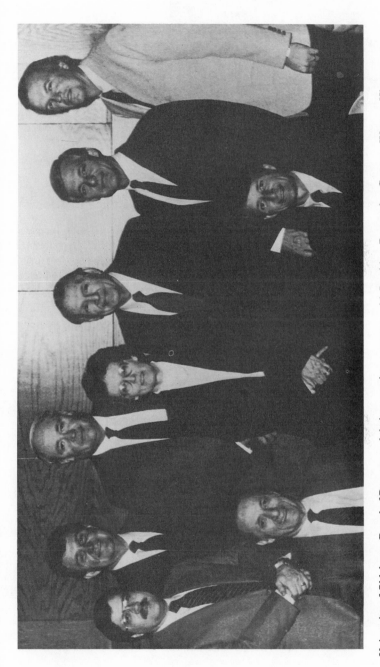

University of Oklahoma Board of Regents and their executive secretary, with President Banowsky. Courtesy Western History Collection University of Oklahoma Libraries. (OUPA)

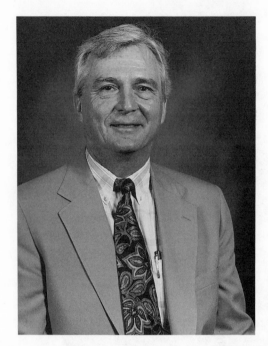

Joseph Kopta, M.D., Professor and Chair of the Department of Orthopedic Surgery and Chair of the Professional Practice Plan. (OUHSC)

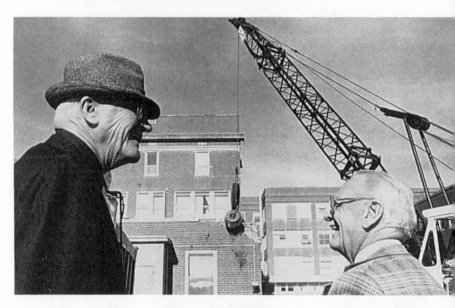

Lloyd Rader and architect Ralph Hudgins with the infamous wrecking ball at the "C" wing of Old Main. (AAE)

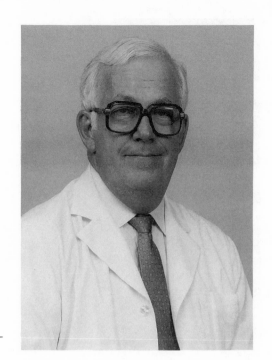

Patrick A. McKee, M.D.,
Professor of Medicine and
Director of the Warren
Institute of Medical Research—
Oklahoma City. (OUHSC)

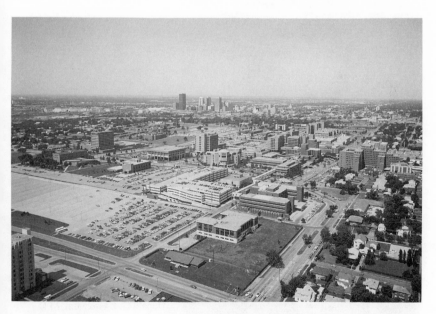

View of the University of Oklahoma Health Sciences Center and downtown Oklahoma
City, 1985. (OUHSC)

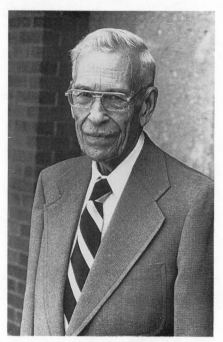

George Garrison, M.D., pioneer
Oklahoma City pediatrician. (OUHSC)

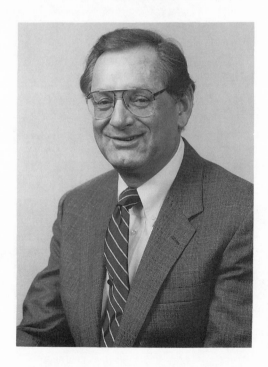

Donald G. Kassebaum, M.D.,
Executive Dean of the College
of Medicine. (OUHSC)

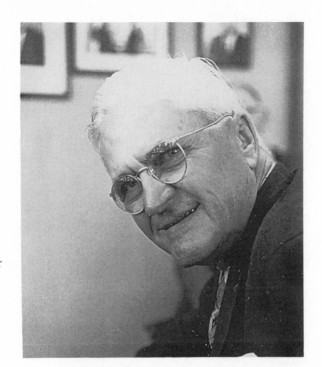

Lloyd Rader, Director of the Department of Human Services, champion of children and the Health Sciences Center. (DHS)

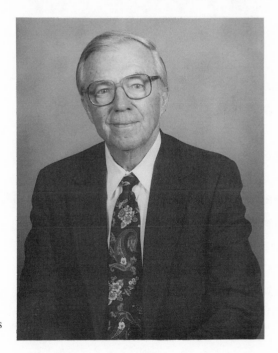

William E. Brown, D.D.S., founding Dean of the College of Dentistry and Interim Provost of the Health Sciences Center. (OUHSC)

303

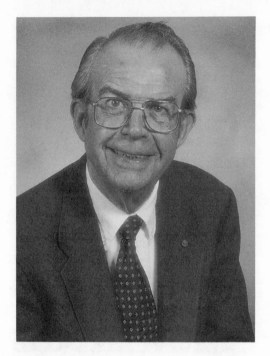

Edward N. Brandt, Jr.,
M.D./Ph.D., Executive Dean of
the College of Medicine.
(OUHSC)

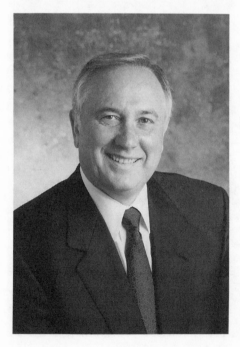

Hans Brisch, Ph.D., Chancellor of
the Oklahoma State Regents for
Higher Education. (OUHSC)

Chapter VI.
The New CEOs: Academe Lost,
1992–1996

THE NEW PROVOST

New Provost Jay Stein made his first appearance at the University of Oklahoma Health Sciences Center on October 14, 1992. The inside story of his appointment is not widely known. Four candidates for the position were being considered by the search committee which was appointed by the University Board of Regents. One obvious candidate had been Dr. Edward N. Brandt, current dean and presumed heir apparent. Of the three external applicants, the individual most favored by the search committee withdrew from consideration during the interview process. Although the *Daily Oklahoman* stated that Jay Stein was appointed after "an exhaustive national search" *[DO 6–11–92]*, many members of the senior faculty, and most of the members of the search committee, believed that it had not been exhaustive enough. A delegation of senior faculty, including the chairs of Medicine, Surgery, and the Faculty Board, visited University President Van Horn and suggested that the three remaining candidates had not sufficiently impressed the committee with their backgrounds and administrative abilities to warrant a hasty appointment. The faculty leaders recommended that he reopen a national search for a truly qualified successor to Clayton Rich. The president made it clear that the issue was not up for discussion, informing them that, "I have made up my mind. I will appoint Dr. Stein."[1] And that is exactly what he did.

In a *Daily Oklahoman* interview in November, Jay Stein stated, "I've crossed the Red River permanently" *[DO, 11–27–92]*. He previously had been chair of Medicine at the University of Texas Medical School in San Antonio. He was reported to have come "with a hefty, unprecedented salary ($338,400 per year) and equally lofty ideas about turning the Health Sciences Center into a nationally recognized hub of medical research and patient care." The *Oklahoman* compared "Stein's proposed salary as provost . . . to the $189,000 made by Dr. Edward N. Brandt Jr., former executive dean of the University of Oklahoma College of Medicine, who was considered the leading candidate for the provost's job until it was unexpectedly awarded to Stein" *[DO, 11–27–92].* The *Tulsa World* pointed out that at the same meeting at which President Van Horn announced that the new provost would have "the highest pay of any state employee," he revealed that "tight money" would force a reduction in the size of the staff at the University *[Tulsa World, 6–11–92].* Van Horn's hiring of the new provost at such an exorbitant salary in the midst of "tight money" was not one of his more astute or endearing acts as president of the University—especially in light of the fact that his selection was opposed by senior faculty at the College of Medicine.

On June 10 Dr. Jay Stein was named by the regents as senior vice president and provost of the Health Sciences Center. His task as administrator was made easier by the passage, on November 3, of a long-awaited $350 million bond issue for higher education capital improvements, which finally assured construction of the Family Medicine building and the new Biomedical Research building. The *Daily Oklahoman* had strongly supported the passage of State Questions 649 and 650, which included $22.4 million for the Health Sciences Center (of which $17.9 million was for Phase I of the Biomedical Research Center) and $4.5 million to complete the Family Medicine building *[DO, 10–26–92].*

Jay Stein as Provost

The hard-driving Jay Stein was a wine connoisseur, golfer, and former cigar smoker who was always "on the go." The thrust of his administration would be reform of the health care delivery system on the campus, and biotechnology partnerships with the business community. Administrators and chairs who did not share his vision became an endangered species *[JR, 11–6–93].* In November Stein shared his vision for a medical research park located between the old Oklahoma Publishing Company (OPUBCO) building in downtown Oklahoma City and the Health Sciences Center campus. He indicated that the Oklahoma Medical Research Foundation, which planned to utilize the old OPUBCO building for research, was one of the ingredients essential for development of a vigorous biotechnology industry in Oklahoma. Other key elements in Stein's plan were the staff and facilities of the University of Oklahoma Health Sciences Center; the state's Oklahoma Center for Science and Technology (OCAST); the Presbyterian Health Foundation; and "available

space,"—i.e., nearby land for construction. "Oklahoma has all the prerequisites," Stein informed the *Journal Record* early in 1993. The new provost was
expert at conveying his idea of what needed to be done to the media as well
as to community leaders. However, his skill with a third large and very necessary element—the political—was somewhat lacking. For reasons that few
understood, Stein did not court the Oklahoma legislature as assiduously, and
with the deference they not only expected, but demanded. Hence, his success
in the political arena was far less than it might have been, and consequently
his great plan never came to fruition.

In July 1992 despite the concern of many on the Health Sciences Center
faculty, the Board of Regents authorized the sale of 16.3 acres of land between
8th and 10th Streets on Lincoln Boulevard to Presbyterian Hospital for construction of a "Healthy Living Center, conference and related facilities." The
instrument created by the regents, which displayed their lack of awareness of
the possible long term consequences of such a sale, was the issuance of a
Request for a Proposal (RFP) for a health, fitness, and rehabilitation center
on University of Oklahoma Health Sciences Center property—to which only
Presbyterian Hospital could provide a complete proposal in August 1992.
Assistant Provost Tom Godkins said, "I don't know what we'll see. We're
hopeful that we will receive proposals and the land will be developed" *[JR,
8–11–92]*. Godkins' remarks suggested that the development was a natural
successor to the previously proposed student fitness center, sports medicine
center, and student union frequently discussed by the regents through the
years. In November the parcel of land on Lincoln Boulevard desired by
Presbyterian Hospital was sold by the regents for $2 million. Unfortunately,
relocation of a parking lot currently located on the property was to cost $900,000,
making the transaction of little immediate, and no permanent, value for the
University, especially since the land included the only remaining frontage on
Lincoln Boulevard. What resulted was an office building—primarily used by
faculty fleeing the requirements of the Professional Practice Plan—a fitness
center, and an outpatient laboratory and surgical facility which, for the most
part, excluded participation of University Hospital and its staff.

Also in July the M. A. Wells Construction Company was awarded a contract
to build a new wing on the Dermatology building at a cost of $354,270. Of
human interest is the fact that M. A. Wells, the current owner of the company,
had been a construction worker on the original building erected in 1969–70.

At the regents meeting of September 9, 1992, the major fund-raising priorities for the next few years at the University of Oklahoma were enumerated.
They were, in no specified order, a new School of Music, a Museum of Natural

History to replace the various buildings in which dinosaur skeletons and other artifacts were housed, Library endowment matches, a Biomedical Research building, endowed chairs and professorships, and additional student scholarships. With an improving economy in mid-decade, and under the stewardship of new University President David Boren, all of these goals would be realized by the University prior to the millennium *[RM, 23048]*.

For fiscal year 1993, the Health Sciences Center E&G budget was increased by $1.5 million in state funds and $600,000 in tuition and fees. Of this sum, barely $100,000 was available for faculty promotions and equity increases. Only 10 percent of the faculty received increases, and one-half of these were increases of less than 6 percent. The outlook for salary increases in the immediate future was not much better, according to statements by the regents *[RM, 23050]*.

Provost Jay Stein initiated a series of personnel assignments and reassignments when, on September 10, he relieved Dr. Edward N. Brandt of his titles of executive dean, College of Medicine, Oklahoma City and Tulsa, as well as of the Lawrence N. Upjohn Chair of Medicine. Upon recommendation of Dr. Stein, Douglas Voth was named by the regents as interim executive dean August 1 for a term of three years (until November 11, 1995). Then, on November 10, Voth, former Veterans Hospital chief of staff and current acting dean, was made permanent executive dean of the College of Medicine, Oklahoma City and Tulsa. This was effected, at the urging of Provost Stein, without a formal search process involving the faculty *[RM, 23157]*. Finally, the appointment of Voth as executive dean was extended from three to five years, to end on March 31, 1997.

The new provost demonstrated that he was in full stride with personnel changes when, at the same September regents meeting, he relieved Gordon Deckert of his title of acting chair of Psychiatry and Behavioral Sciences. Later, Joseph Westermeyer, former chair of Psychiatry, "resigned." Joseph Kopta also "resigned" as chair of Orthopedic Surgery and Rehabilitation. Additionally, a new position—associate vice president for health sciences—was created by Stein, and Marcia Morris, previously assistant provost for academic affairs, was appointed to the position *[JR, 11–18–92]*.

In October the Samuel Roberts Noble Foundation of Ardmore announced the relocation of its biomedical research operations to the Oklahoma Medical Research Foundation in order to gain proximity of its investigators to an active research faculty *[DO, 10–2–92]*. This consolidation would directly benefit the Oklahoma Medical Research Foundation but not greatly affect the College of Medicine.

Malpractice Insurance

A significant cost of operation for the Health Sciences Center at year's end was, increasingly, that of malpractice insurance. In 1992, aggregate costs for this insurance were $2.3 million in Oklahoma City and $0.5 million in Tulsa. Of this total, Anesthesiology and Obstetrics accounted for nearly $1 million. Individual yearly malpractice insurance rates ranged from $2,900 for those not doing surgery to $14,000 for most surgical specialties and $21,000 for Neurological Surgery, Orthopedics, and Obstetrics. As charges escalated, there was increasing dissatisfaction at the Center with PLICO—the physician's liability company—which declined the Practice Plan's request to charge reduced premiums for faculty practicing only a few days a week.

1993

On January 27 the Family Medicine venture was revisited by the University president and Board of Regents, with the latter authorizing bids on construction as a single-phase project at $7.75 million, for which $3.25 million in state funds had previously been set aside. The increase in costs reflected mandated design changes due to the Americans with Disabilities Act and inflationary increases. Six months later, on 27 July, a bid was accepted from Lippert Brothers Construction Company in the amount of $4,556,193 *[RM, 23461]*. Ground breaking for the building occurred the same month.

The University of Oklahoma Health Sciences Center Publications and Printing Service, in existence since 1951, was privatized in January by decree of the regents, and Unique Printing, Inc. was selected from four firms responding to an "RFP" requesting bids for printing services. This action eliminated the jobs of ten University employees. The regents affirmed the action following a protest from the Oklahoma Public Employees' Association and a review of the sequence of events leading up to the change. At the same meeting, regents named Dr. Robin J. Elwood as chair of the Department of Anesthesiology.

On January 28 before more than 700 guests at the annual Oklahoma College of Medicine Alumni Association's Evening of Excellence, faculty leader and Dermatology chair Mark Allen Everett was honored with the Dean's Award for Distinguished Medical Service, while Norman business leader Paul H. Travis was cited for Distinguished Community Service *[DO, 2–6–92; 1–29–93]*. Travis' wife Dolly was the center of attention when, identified by the master of ceremonies as a ninety-year-old former Ziegfield Follies girl, she broke into the can-can! At the same time, the Stanton L. Young Master Teacher of the year award for 1993 was given to Leon Unger, Ph.D., from the Department of Biochemistry and Molecular Biology.

The Alumni Association's Evening of Excellence honorees over the years constituted a veritable who's-who of the College of Medicine and the local business community, as the following chart reveals:

TABLE 6.   EVENING OF EXCELLENCE HONOREES, 1985–1996

Year	College of Medicine	Business Community
1985	Don O'Donoghue, M.D.	Dean A. McGee
1986	George Garrison, M.D.	Stanton L. Young
1987	Gerald Rogers, M.D.	John Kirkpatrick
1988	George Bozalis, M.D.	Mrs. Fred Jones
1989	Tullos O. Coston, M.D.	Richard D. Harrison
1990	G. Rainey Williams, M.D.	Edward L. Gaylord
1991	Robert G. Tompkins, M.D.	Edward C. Joullian III
1992	Stewart Wolf, M.D.	John S. Gammill
1993	Mark Allen Everett, M.D.	Paul Travis & Presbyterian Foundation
1994	Thomas E. Acers, M.D.	Sarah C. Hogan & OCAST
1995	John R. Alexander, M.D.	Governor George Nigh
1996	Don F. Rhinehart, M.D.	James G. Harlow, Jr.
1997	Ronald C. Elkins, M.D.	James R. Tolbert III
1998	John R. Bozalis, M.D.	Jim and Christy Everett
1999	James L. Dennis, M.D.	Governor Henry Bellmon

In March 1993 the Board of Regents revised the Campus Master Plan for Capital Improvement Projects by classifying the Biomedical Research Center as a four-phase project, at a total cost of $45.1 million. This action was taken because regents decided that building the structure in one phase was not financially feasible.

The Declining Budget

In spite of the successful endowed chairs program, the bond issue for higher education construction, the constant growth in Professional Practice Plan revenue, and the increasing success in acquiring extramural grants, inadequate funding of higher education by the state legislature continued to exert a negative effect on all activities at the Health Sciences Center, as well as throughout higher education in Oklahoma. Early in 1993, the legislature proposed a five to seven percent cut in state funding. In April Regent Chair E. Murray Gullatt emphasized that "quality higher education is an absolute necessity to attract new industry and encourage industrial expansion within the State and also the key to attracting and retaining the brightest and best students. Oklahomans must understand that material reductions in State funding to higher education will have a very negative impact on the universities" *[RM, 22924–5]*. On May 28 the legislature voted an appropriation of nearly $20 million less than that of the previous year, while approving an increase in student tuition and fees. This necessitated a five percent overall cut in the budgets of the University in order to protect "core activities of degree-granting programs, research, libraries and computing" *[RM, 23411]*. Because the state's economy was not expected to improve significantly in the near future, competition from other state agencies—especially common education (which was now receiving 38.5 percent of all appropriated state funds), human services (24 percent), and corrections— was expected to place further pressure on higher education (which received only 15 percent of the appropriated budget) over the next few years. President Van Horn indicated that with appropriated funds and tuition being "far below the Big Eight and Big Ten average, to maintain a position as a significant institution of higher education, we have to behave like a private university" *[RM, 23416]*. This also necessitated a willingness to reallocate all appropriated state funds to the areas of greatest need.

The Board of Regents adopted a resolution commending former board member Ada Lois Sipuel for her courage and determination in the landmark Supreme Court case, "Sipuel v. Oklahoma," which changed state history by opening the doors of higher education to Black students in Oklahoma *[RM, 23295]*. Mrs. Sipuel had been admitted to the Law School at a time when institutions were still segregated, and she was provided with a seat isolated from that of fellow students. Following her pioneering enrollment, advanced degree programs would be open to all qualified students, regardless of race.

Dr. Donald B. Halverstadt, who completed his term on the State Regents for Higher Education on April 24, was appointed by Governor David Walters to a seven-year term as a University of Oklahoma regent, effective that same day. His appointment followed the governor's withdrawal of the nomination of Larry C. Brawner, a close friend, who had been charged with three felony counts of making illegal contributions to Walters' 1990 campaign. Brawner had been serving as a regent since his appointment the previous August, while awaiting confirmation by the state senate. Brawner and Walters had worked together at the Health Sciences Center during the second term of Governor George Nigh *[DO, 5–6–93]*.

Another Walters appointment was received with somewhat less public enthusiasm than that of Donald Halverstadt. Dr. Garth Splinter, a longtime friend of the governor, was named to a new $61,000 per year position with the State Health Department "at a time when agencies have been ordered to cut their budgets" *[DO, 4–4–93]*. Senator Bernest Cain questioned why a new position was being established at a time when, due to inadequate funding of the Health Department, there was a waiting list of patients needing medical care in local health clinics. Splinter was to retain his full-time position at the Health Sciences Center, at $65,000 per year, as well as the directorship of the Health Affairs' Rural Health Program at $8,700 annually. The total compensation of $134,700 per year was accompanied by a 20 percent benefits package, according to the April 4 *Daily Oklahoman*. Dr. Ron Elkins of the Department of Surgery felt that Garth Splinter tried, in his position as director of the Health Care Authority, to assist in the academic mission of the Center to the extent that he could. An example of this was: "his critical support for supplemental funding to forestall a reduction of hospital supplemental funding to the College of Medicine. Although it was sometimes difficult to follow the direction of his financial ideas, he performed exceedingly well in serving multiple masters: running his department, satisfying the legislature, and supporting the Health Sciences Center. He was considered very bright and worked honestly in the best interests of the Center."[2]

Also approved in April was a managed health care program for patients treated by physicians at the Health Sciences Center titled "Health Source," incorporating physician-staff of the University of Oklahoma professional practice, and the Oklahoma Health Center. According to Provost Stein, "The aim of the program is to allow faculty to gain experience in direct operation of a managed care program and to implement the cost cutting and risk management controls effective in reducing premium and operating expenses" *[JR, 4–6–93]*.

Appointments and reassignments occupied the University administration and board of regents in the spring of 1993. In April David Maloney, former vice president for development at Carnegie-Mellon University in Pittsburgh, Pennsylvania, was named executive director of development on the Health Sciences Center campus. He later would be appointed to the corresponding post for the entire University *[JR, 4–21–93]*. May saw Christian N. Ramsey Jr. relieved of the title of chair of Family Medicine and placed on administrative leave of absence with full pay effective July 1, 1993. This was due to the provost's lack of confidence that a comprehensive managed care environment would be rapidly developed in Family Medicine *[RM, 23421]*. Andrea U. Bircher, Ph.D., an outspoken campus leader and professor of nursing, who had been one of the principal designers of the Health Sciences Center Campus Senate, retired on May 7. Jerry B. Farley, vice president for administrative affairs at the Center, was made vice president for administrative affairs of the Norman campus. At the same time, Mark Lemons, associate vice president for administrative affairs, was made interim vice president for administrative affairs at the Health Sciences Center.

Also in May, the Oklahoma Medical Information Network Telemedicine Project was approved at a cost of $1.175 million and included in the Campus Master Plan of Capital Improvement projects. The project had been proposed for the purpose of tying six rural hospitals via computer to the center, and providing consultation by faculty specialists regarding X-rays, electrocardiograms, and clinical problems, as well as providing access to the College of Medicine Library *[RM, 23365–6]*. The previous November, the network had been expanded to include thirty-eight rural state hospitals *[JR, 11–04–93]*. The Departments of Family Medicine, Pediatrics, and Obstetrics and Gynecology were selected for audits in 1993–1994, as were the Tulsa branch departments of Obstetrics and Gynecology and Surgery.

For the current fiscal year, the University was allocated $9.4 million for matching endowed chairs and professorships, bringing the total number of campus chairs to seventy-seven since 1988. The total matching funds received to date was $34.7 million *[RM, 23448]*.

On May 28 a loan from the Tulsa Industrial Authority was paid from the state bond issue, passed in November 1992, retiring the mortgage on the University of Oklahoma College of Medicine in Tulsa. A formal ceremony was held early in June, when University of Oklahoma officials presented a check for $6.6 million to the Tulsa Industrial Authority, completing purchase of the 13.5 acre campus of the Tulsa medical branch. This freed about $600,000 annually (previously devoted to rent) for other uses by the College *[Tulsa World, 6–4–93]*.

Final payment of the Tulsa debt reminded observers of the controversial 1980 campaign to move the Tulsa branch of the College of Medicine to the former American Christian College campus, which came after then-assistant provost David Walters visited the campus incognito, disclaiming any association with the College's founder, the now discredited evangelist Billy James Hargis. Dr. Donald Halverstadt, current retiring chair of the State Regents and acting provost of the Health Sciences Center at the time, recalled that he was told three times by Chancellor E. T. Dunlap to "drop" the Tulsa project. "Dunlap said if I didn't desist, he would send me to McAlester [state prison] or some-place."[3] Walters, who was now governor, observed that the retirement of the $6.6 million debt, conferred "another level of permanancy (sic)" on the Tulsa college *[Tulsa World, 6–5–93]*. In 1980, when Walters was surreptitiously shopping the Tulsa real estate market, the Tulsa branch was under scrutiny by those who thought it was too expensive and had expanded far beyond its original mission. Even during the recent financing activity, the State Regents attempted to block it by asking the legislature to merge the eight-year-old school with the osteopathic school.

On July 1 as a result of Senate Bill 423, governance of Oklahoma's Teaching Hospitals was transferred from the Department of Human Services to a separate administrative authority. Under the umbrella of the University of Okla-homa until 1973, the Children's Hospital was transferred to the Department of Human Services in that year, primarily to enhance funding. University Hospital (Oklahoma Memorial) was transferred to the department in 1980. As Depart-ment of Human Services revenues declined (primarily due to loss of the dedi-cated state sales tax), the hospitals deteriorated, and funds were even transferred out of the hospital budget into other department programs. It was primarily due to the continuing funding crises that creation of the new, separate authority was decreed by the legislature *[DO, 5–28–93; JR, 6–24– 93]*.

In spite of continuing funding shortages, the Health Sciences Center admin-istration was often able to find money for important improvements or pet projects—sometimes at whopping costs. Throughout the decade of the 90s, millions of dollars were spent by the regents and the Center to update its telephone communication equipment, with purchases as large as $5 million for an AT&T switching device. In addition, the Center spent large sums on the purchase of computer systems for billing and collecting professional fees.

A legislative action of major significance in the summer of 1993 was passage of Senate Bill 76 and House Bill 1573, which restructured the state's Medicaid system by creating the Oklahoma Health Care Authority, the prin-cipal mission of which was to implement a managed care system for welfare clients *[JR, 7–14–93]*. These legislative bills were among several designed to bring about the "long discussed breakup of the sprawling DHS [which] is necessary to establish credibility with the public by improving oversight of DHS operations" *[Tulsa World, 3–11–93]*. The irony of this new push to break up the Department of Human Services lay in the fact that the legislature had only recently completed its decades–long effort to enlarge the gargantuan organization by placing under its umbrella every "welfare" service or institu-tion it could not otherwise adequately fund, or wished to "wash its hands of."

At its zenith (at the height of Director Lloyd Rader's power and influence), the Department of Human Services boasted a budget of a billion and a half dollars and more than 14,000 employees!

Provost Stein and Health Care Reform

Provost Jay Stein shared his vision regarding health care reform and the academic health center with the University of Oklahoma Board of Regents at their September 1993 meeting. His remarks were stimulated by a published report of Peat Marwick Management Consultants which stated that "30–40 percent of today's Academic Health Centers will not survive because of their inability to adapt to the new environment." These predictions stemmed from the Clinton administration's proposals for health care reform, which, although not enacted by Congress, were, except for the provisions for care of the indigent and those without insurance, largely implemented through pressure from the health care insurance industry. The chief factors which would adversely affect academic health centers were decentralization (point-of-service medical care delivery), imposition of primary care "gate-keepers," a shift from inpatient to outpatient care, and severe cost cutting measures, accompanied by development of a centralized bureaucracy of administrators with little or no interest in care of sick individuals *[JR, 11–6–93]*. Provost Stein stated that "It was clear that the traditional organizational relationships and structures within academic medical center entities—medical schools, practice plans, and hospitals—will no longer be effective, and it is imperative that the Health Sciences Center PPP become organized sufficiently to meet the demands of health care reform and managed care." To Stein, this meant total centralization of faculty physician practices—bringing all clinical departments under direct fiscal control of the central Practice Plan office and eliminating the independent billing activities of these departments *[RM, 23513]*. It also meant that all managers must share his dream and his goal. Under pressure from Provost Stein's "my way or the highway" mandate, Dr. Christian Ramsey "resigned" as chair of Family Practice in May and departed in July. Similarly, Dr. Alfred W. Brann Jr., was removed as chair of Pediatrics in July, presumably due to his lack of enthusiasm for implementing Stein's far-reaching managed program. Brann had also served as the Hobbs-Recknagel Professor of Pediatrics. Dr. John E. Grunow was named as acting chair in his place. Hospital administrator Andrew Lasser departed a few months later. The removal of Lasser would prompt a legislative leader to introduce a bill in the legislature which would prohibit the provost from being a voting member of University Hospital Authority *[DO, 2–2–94]*.

Dr. Joseph Kopta, former chair of Orthopedics, served for several years as president of the faculty's Practice Plan Advisory Council and Executive Committee. He recalls that Provost Stein "wanted to force changes in operational policy of this group to assure that control was vested in the dean rather than as originally set up, in the hands of the Executive Committee."[4] Dr. Kopta then described an incident relating to this issue:

Stein, like [former Provost] Thurman, was a master at imposing his views through the mechanism of passing them through the regents. He would come back from a regents meeting where he had advocated some policy he would like to see adopted, and to which the regents had assented, and he would say, 'The regents ordered so and so.' When I learned that Stein was going to take the reorganization of the PPP to the regents in this fashion, I met the night before with [Regent Don] Halverstadt to argue and plead that this action be delayed. The next day was the annual meeting of the PPP, and Stein presented the plan, 'approved by the regents,' to the group for their concurrence. On his way into the meeting, Stein commented to me, 'You just don't understand, Kopta.' It immediately became clear that Halverstadt had revealed everything I said to him in confidence. I shouted at Stein, 'I do now!'[5]

In November, Provost Stein restated his vision of a medical research park between the old Oklahoma Publishing Company (OPUBCO) building in downtown Oklahoma City and the Health Sciences Center campus. He indicated that the Oklahoma Medical Research Foundation was to utilize the OPUBCO building for research. The University Hospitals, newly under an independent Board of Governors (Senate Bill 423, May 1993), was the principal key to any campuswide health care plan. And Stein, as one of the trustees of the governing board of the hospital, was in position to promote this goal. When asked about his resignation as University administrator, Lasser, who had directed the hospitals since 1988, gracefully said, "The University Hospitals Authority is looking to move the hospitals in a new direction" *[DO, 9–8– 93]*. Lasser's chief detractor had been "Dr. Jay Stein, pivotal governing board member," according to the *Journal Record* of September 8. Representative James Hamilton, the powerful lawmaker, warned against any power shift at the Hospital: "There was very strong sentiment in both the House and Senate that we want to preserve the Hospitals as an independent body" *[JR, 9–8–93]*. He indicated that in shifting the hospitals from the University of Oklahoma to the Department of Human Services twenty years ago, and the removal from Department of Human Services to an independent authority recently, the legislature wanted to assure that hospital revenues would pay for patient care rather than being diverted to research, teaching, or support of Department of Human Services operating expenses. Stein said that the problem at Oklahoma Memorial Hospital was intensified by too great a reliance on Medicaid patients and a physical plant which "was allowed to deteriorate by the Department of Human Services" *[Tulsa World, 9–16–93]*. In December Stein stated that the "Executive Dean has worked to break down barriers between the various clinical departments in order to address the compelling issues facing the academic health center." He asked to be allowed to prepare a revision of the faculty practice bylaws. The regents approved the request *[RM, 23672–3]*.

Another vision entertained by Provost Stein—one that recalled the move for administrative independence by Dean James Dennis years earlier—was revealed by his proposal, discussed at the regents' November meeting, that the Health Sciences Center campus should report directly to the regents, and the provost would become president of an Oklahoma Health Sciences University. Regent Halverstadt said, "This is not an issue that we have been thinking about for a long time, but it is something that only comes into focus now that we will be getting a new [University] president" *[DO, 11–5–93]*.

On October 22 a special regents' meeting was held to consider the resignation of University of Oklahoma President Richard L. Van Horn. The resignation was accepted, and a search committee was organized to find his successor. Once Van Horn made his plans public, criticism of his policies and management techniques began to surface. Professor Mark Meo of the Norman campus commented on the "unhealthy communication among and between the faculty and the regents" during Van Horn's tenure *[RM, 23603]*. The *Daily Oklahoman* pointed out that President Van Horn: "downplayed probes of OU by the Oklahoma State Bureau of Investigation, the state auditor and inspector and the Cleveland County district attorney as reasons for his retirement, and he took full responsibility for not adequately presenting the university's case in the ongoing controversy over travel reimbursements and other alleged improprities involving former OU vice president Art Elbert . . . who has resigned but still draws a salary of more than $100,000 until the end of the calendar year *[DO, 10–15–93]*.

Professor Meo, commenting on the upcoming search for a replacement for the president, said, "In the last five years we have been subject to a number of . . . unfortunate surprises. I would encourage . . . you to thoroughly investigate ... each candidate. The University cannot afford to suffer any more individuals who treat the University as an opportunity for on-the-job training" *[RM, 23603]*. Meo also alluded to the unfortunate tendency of the University to select administrators—at both the Norman and Oklahoma City campuses—who were persona non grata at their originating institutions.

The Board of Regents approved another Site of Practice exception in October. Faculty of Neurology and Neurosurgery in the Department of Surgery were approved for practice in the independently incorporated Oklahoma Neurological Institute, located in the Presbyterian Hospital. This would possibly circumvent the planned centralization of billing and collecting of private fees for these faculty members. The action was concurrent with an announced deficit in the Health Sciences Center's Practice Plan account, due to lower Medicaid payments and increased competition for patients from managed health care systems that emphasized primary care—i.e., "gate-keepers"—to avoid specialist care *[Tulsa World, 11–16–93]*.

In November the search committee for a new University of Oklahoma president was named. No faculty members of the College of Medicine were proposed or selected for the committee by the Board of Regents. At this time, the College of Medicine was without strong faculty and administrative leadership, a problem recognized by the regents in a discussion at their November meeting. Five of the College of Medicine departments currently lacked chairs: Biochemistry; Psychiatry; Urology; Pediatrics, and Family Medicine *[RM, 23644]*.

In December the regents were informed by Provost Stein that the Oklahoma Health Center Foundation and the virtually unheard of "Medical Technology and Research Authority of Oklahoma" (MTRA)—created by the legislature in 1990 to build and maintain "improvement projects" at the Health Sciences Center—had developed plans for a child care center and parking facilities. These plans were proposed by consultants to the Oklahoma Health Center Foundation and Authority, in collaboration with the sixteen institutions on the campus. The project required conveyance of the block bounded by N.E. 13th, N.E. 14th, Phillips, and Lindsey Streets by the regents to the Authority. No regent action was taken on Provost Stein's proposal.

The MTRA's full-time personnel were employees of the University of Oklahoma Health Sciences Center, and Authority members were Dr. Stein, David Dunlap of Presbyterian Hospital, and Ron Yordi, described by the *Daily Oklahoman* as "one of Governor David Walters' so-called 'gang of five'" *[DO, 11–21–93]*. The thrust was to take over all parking on the Health Sciences Center campus (regardless of who had paid for the construction or who maintained it) and charge employees, students, patients, and visitors a parking fee in order to develop funds for future projects of the Authority. A spokesman said, "It's not something MTRA wants to shove down anybody's throat" *[RM, 23667]*. Subsequent efforts by the Authority would prove otherwise. Dr. Timothy Coussons commented years later that MTRA had been set up to help tax-supported institutions through its ability to issue bonds. "We didn't have the money to bring the garages up to standard; we needed more than $9 million. In some ways, DHS did the Center a disservice by building and paying for the garages, which gave employees the idea that parking should be free."[6] This leader also stated that Ron Yordi had been "most helpful to the hospitals," especially in urging that Presbyterian Foundation grants were consistently of benefit to the hospitals and to the strength of the Health Sciences Center overall.

The year ended with the a flurry of personnel actions, including promotion of Mark Lemons to the position of permanent vice president for administrative affairs at the Health Sciences Center. In addition, Dr. James R. Gavin III, the William K. Warren Professor of Medicine, resigned his position effective December 6. Finally, Dr. R. Timothy Coussons was named interim chief executive officer of the University Hospitals in December *[RM, 23812]*.

Richard Timothy Coussons

Dr. R. Timothy Coussons, a graduate of the University of Oklahoma in 1960 and its College of Medicine in 1963, served an internship and residency in Medicine at the Johns Hopkins Hospital in Maryland (1963–1965), was a staff associate at the National Institutes of Health in 1966–1967, and was resident and chief resident in Medicine at the University of Oklahoma from 1967 to 1969. He had served as director of the internship program at Oklahoma from 1969 to 1974, first as assistant and then as associate professor of Medicine. Named professor in 1974, he served as chief of the medical services at the Veterans Administration Hospital, the University Hospitals, and as acting head of the Department of Medicine on two occasions (1983, 1984–1985). In 1985 he was named medical director of the University Hospital and associate dean for clinical affairs of the College of Medicine. In December 1993, he became interim chief executive officer of the University Hospitals and permanent chief executive officer in 1994. Following amalgamation of the Presbyterian and University Hospitals in 1998, he was named chief medical officer for University Health Partners. "Tim" Coussons served with distinction in each of the positions to which he was named, and at the same time maintained a medical practice and his reputation as a consummate physician both with his patients and his professional colleagues. His friends believed that his reputation as a model train buff well qualified him to keep everything "on track."

The year 1993 was marked by several medical accomplishments at the University of Oklahoma Health Sciences Center. First, was the significant success of CytoDiagnostics (later UROCORP), the medical technology enterprise evolving from the work of Urology faculty member George Hemstreet, who developed quantitative fluorescence image analysis, and who, with others, founded CytoDiagnostics to market the technology. After several crises and infusions of new managerial talent and much-needed capital, the firm evolved into a vigorous, growing enterprise concerned with diagnosis of bladder, kidney, and prostate cancer, with two new buildings on the campus *[JR 3–31–93, 12–30–93]*. Second was the international success of the a technique of "catheter ablation" of severe cardiac arrhythmia carried out by the University of Oklahoma Health Sciences Center Cardiac Electrophysiology Group, led by Dr. Warren Jackman. From inception in 1987 through 1993, more than 551 patients with specific arrhythmias had undergone successful (99 percent) ablation *[DO, 4–25–93]*. At this time, Children's Hospital operated the state's only infant heart transplant program, was ranked third nationally in pediatric kidney transplants, and treated 75 percent of the pediatric cancer patients in Oklahoma *[DO, 4–25–93]*. Finally, an often vital role in bringing the needs of the Health Sciences Center to public attention, as well as to the legislature, was played by the in-depth, insightful, and positive reporting of two medical writers for the *Daily Oklahoman*, Jim Killackey and Karen Klinka. In previous decades, this unacknowledged but important function had been performed by Oklahoma medical writer Imogene Patrick.

On a smaller, more intimate scale, a member of the Health Sciences Center faculty, Dr. Mark Allen Everett, received the Governor's Award for Lifetime Contributions to the Arts, together with the University of Oklahoma Press's beloved emeritus director, Savoie Lottinville. The presentations were made on December 8 by Governor Walters in a ceremony in the state capitol rotunda *[DO 12–9–93]*.

1994

Nineteen ninety-four opened with the state media celebrating two successes of the Oklahoma Center for the Advancement of Science and Technology program: the previously mentioned catheter ablation technique developed by

Dr. Warren Jackman; and the use of living organisms to test quality of water and treat or detoxify hazardous wastes. Each of these brought international repute to the Center *[DO, 1–18–94; JR, 1–1–94]*. Also early in the new year, the Stanton L. Young Master Teacher Award for 1994 was presented to Dr. James Tomasek of the Department of Anatomical Sciences, while the honorees at the annual research award dinner were Dr. Thomas E . Acers, professor of Ophthalmology; Mrs. Sarah Hogan, former chair of the University of Oklahoma Regents; and the Oklahoma Center for the Advancement of Science and Technology.

In January the University of Oklahoma Board of Regents approved a revision of the Professional Practice Plan which clearly specified that the executive dean was ultimately responsible for operation of the plan. For years, the governing body for the plan had been the Advisory Council (consisting of the chairs of clinical departments and divisions, with a few elected members), and an Executive Committee which considered itself to be the ultimate authority, responsible only to the regents, on issues regarding private patient income. Traditionally, the paid director of the plan (in charge of billing, collecting, statistics, etc.) had been selected by, and reported to, the Advisory Council Executive Committee. Under the revised plan, it was clear that all Practice Plan employees reported to the dean, who in turn selected the plan director. This clarified (and further centralized) an administrative arrangement which had for a long time confused even some of its participating physicians *[RM, 23004]*.

Also at the January meeting, the regents sold a series of four lots on N.E. 14th Street in Oklahoma City for $50,400 to the "Medical Technology and Research Authority" (i.e., the Parking Authority) for the development of a child care center. At the same time, an interim report was received from Dr. George Kaludis regarding a study authorized by the regents on December 21 of the preceding year seeking recommendations for the University's executive structure. Regent Halverstadt expressed "his concerns about the direction this review is or is not going," saying that the project was initiated "by the desire to discuss the reporting relationship of the Health Sciences Center to the Board of Regents, given the need for a greater degree of flexibility, responsiveness, authority, and independence for Health Sciences Center" *[RM, 23714]*. On April 13, Kaludis presented his final report on executive structure. Of four alternatives, he strongly recommended a central University administration with two stand-alone campuses reporting through provosts/senior vice presidents. He also envisioned an office for the president on both campuses, shifting "the Board focus to planning and evaluation of plans", developing a new accord with the University of Oklahoma Foundation, opening a new dialogue with the state on relationships between the hospitals and the Center, and "developing a new concept for the commitment of regents' time and energy" *[RM, 23781–3; JR, 4–13–94]*. The principal structural changes suggested in the report were implemented during the subsequent year. To the surprise of almost no one, all talk of a separate "Health Sciences Center University," with its own president, was quickly stilled *[RM, 23780]*.

The Health Sciences Center administration itself grew considerably at this time, with two vice presidents, an assistant vice president (Thomas R. Godkins), two vice provosts, an associate vice provost (Marcia Morris), and directors of development, University relations, communications and media, and affirmative action, in addition to eight deans and their staffs *[RM, 24025; Regent Exhibit A, 4–1994]*. It is interesting to compare this bureaucracy, and the salaries paid to its members, with the administrative structure less than three decades earlier, when Mark R. Everett, then James Dennis, ran the entire establishment with the help of a business manager and a secretary.

In March the University braced itself for another austere financial year by endorsing a proposed five percent across-the-board budget cut to both campuses, which would require considerable reallocation of funds in Oklahoma City and in Norman *[RM, 23750]*. Also in March the Department of Human Services' interim director, former State Senator George Miller, was named permanent director, ending months of discussion and dissension within the governing Welfare Commission, after Steven Dow and Paula Hearn (favored by Governor Walters) withdrew from consideration for the post. Dow said, "I think it is important to have a harmonious decision" *[Tulsa World, 3–30–94]*. Dr. Timothy Coussons, interim CEO of the University Hospitals since December, was named permanent chief executive officer on March 8. Both Miller and Coussons would serve in their respective executive capacities until 1998.

At a special meeting of the Board of Regents on April 27, U.S. Senator David L. Boren was named president and chief executive officer of the University. Declaring that "public service is not about power but is about where one can do the most good," Boren accepted the position, saying, "This a great University which will become an engine of economic growth," a "flagship for education in our entire region," and "a national role model in American public higher education" *[DO 4–28–94]*. For a change, the University had selected a leader with the drive, the ability, and the people skills to carry out his promises.

At their next regular meeting in May, the regents appointed Dr. J. R. Morris, a retired former professor, provost, and interim University president (1982), as interim president effective June 6, two months earlier than President Van

Horn's announced retirement date of July 31. The *Tulsa World* stated that this action "effectively closes the books on [Van Horn's] administration" and noted that Senator Boren had called Morris several weeks prior to the regents' meeting, asking him to accept the position *[Tulsa World, 5–12–94]*.

At the Health Sciences Center in May, the programs in Cytotechnology and Medical Technology in the College of Health were discontinued in order to meet the legislatively imposed reduction in state funds for 1993–1994. These programs had been certificate programs of the University Hospital, but following creation of the College of Health, they became degree programs in the University. Their discontinuance would, in the future, work a hardship on all the hospitals in the state. The Health Sciences Center administration was directed to hold conversations with the hospitals to ascertain if they would resume these as certificate programs. Although the regents' minutes for May stated that "at the August meeting of University Hospitals Authority, the Board of directors 'approved the University Hospitals' assumption of the medical technology and cytotechnology programs,'" the hospitals never reinstated a certificate program *[RM, 23827]*. The "medtech" program was provided from existing resources of the Hospital for one year and then discontinued in 1995. The "cytotech" program was similarly supported for two years until 1996. A year later, there were no longer training programs in these most important areas of hospital laboratory operation, the Rose State College program in tissue technology having been discontinued several years previously.[7] This assured difficulty for all Oklahoma's hospitals in obtaining laboratory personnel from 1995 onward.

Although the regents predicted that upcoming state appropriations for the Health Sciences Center would be $2 million less than in FY 1993, they anticipated that Professional Practice Plan revenues would rise by a like amount. Once again the University was relying on faculty practice income to compensate for the shortcomings of the legislature. However, in September, practice revenues were $66.5 million as opposed to $68.7 million in the previous year. The regents attributed the decrease in practice income to Medicaid reimbursement rate adjustments, loss of contracted services, reduction of interest income, a decrease in patient volume, and the impact of the conversion to centralized billing. In actuality, it was the latter which most contributed to the decrease, with collection rates dropping from 85–90 percent to 60–70 percent in spite of increased charges *[RM, 24062]*.

Enabling legislation some months earlier had allowed the Medical Technology and Research Authority (MTRA) to "lease all existing lots within the Health Center, to impose user fees for parking, to manage, repair and maintain the lots, and to build additional parking facilities" *[RM, 23967]*. Naturally, the first action of the Authority was "to generate revenues by implementing user fees," effective August 1, 1994. The regents voted to lease all Health Sciences Center parking lots to MTRA for $1 per year, to collect fees from all users, and to remit such fees, "totaling about $360,000 annually," to MTRA *[RM, 23968]*. There was no obvious benefit to the University or to the Health Sciences Center from this action, and the proposal to collect fees drew the ire of the Oklahoma Public Employees Association, on whose behalf Senator Angela Monson authored a resolution requiring the authority to consult with the legislature before imposing fees *[DO, 5–25–94]*.

Managed Care

The Oklahoma Health Care Authority announced that by July 1, 1995, one-half of all Medicaid clients must be in managed care plans. All Medicaid programs would eventually be managed care programs, and several optional providers were to be selected within a year *[Tulsa World, 11–28–94]*. In Oklahoma, Medicaid was a $1.1 billion program. The change to managed care had been mandated by Senate Bill 76 in 1993, a bill which also removed the program from the Department of Human Services and placed it under the supervision of the newly created Oklahoma Health Care Authority (House Bill 1573, 1993). This was a profoundly significant change for the University Hospitals because the two institutions ranked first and second in the nation among hospitals dependent on Medicaid for 50 percent of their revenue—a total of about $100 million. Civic leader and Presbyterian Foundation president Jean Gumerson said, "Something needs to be done to safeguard those institutions where 75 percent of the state's doctors are trained" *[DO, 11–27–94]*. Senator Bernest Cain commented, "Our state has paid a lot of money to people at the teaching hospitals and the University to do things and make changes, but I don't know that we've gotten the leadership over there that we paid for" *[Tulsa World, 11–28–94]*. Admitted Provost Stein, "If the right things don't happen, we're in big trouble." Dean Luthey, chair of the Hospital Authority, stated that an increased appropriation from the legislature was unlikely, and that "another way to increase revenue is to grow the patient base,"—i.e., persuade people with private insurance that the University Hospitals offer advantages over private hospitals *[Tulsa World, 11–20–94]*.

On September 14 the Site of Practice policy was again revised by regents to include "all health care entities which comprise the Oklahoma Health Center in Oklahoma City, the Tulsa Medical Education foundation hospitals in Tulsa, and the University owned or operated practice sites." Thus, Presbyterian Hospital was included in the Site of Practice policy for the first time *[RM, 23998]*. At the same time, Provost Stein said, "I think we should have one Radiology department, one Anesthesia, one Pathology and so on and so forth and more and more use the resources of the group as a whole" *[RM, 24040]*. This seemed a reasonable vision, but one beset with insurmountable political complications that could not be effectively addressed until such time as the hospitals were combined under one administration. (This would occur in 1998 when Columbia-HCA took over the management of all the hospitals.)

At the same September regents' meeting, the Professional Practice Plan for the College of Medicine was revised to remove any distinction among full-time, part-time, and volunteer faculty if they participated in practice at the Health Sciences Center. The previous exclusion of part-time faculty was removed. "Certain specific arrangements that are exceptions" to the policy would be possible with approval of the department chair, the Management Committee, the executive dean, the senior vice president and provost, and with contractual approval of the University president and the Board of Regents *[RM, 24044]*. Inclusion of part-time faculty in Tulsa would be by recommendation of the chair, advisory board, and the dean.

On September 25, the *Daily Oklahoman* announced that a comprehensive pediatric cancer center was to be built at Children's Hospital. The center was to be named for Jimmy Everest, son of a prominent Oklahoma City family. Prior to his death, Everest had been a patient of Dr. Ruprecht Nitschke, director of the Children's Hospital Oncology Unit. Ultimately housed in a new third-floor addition to the hospital on 13th Street, the $2.1 million center was funded through a community effort spearheaded by the Everest family and Health Sciences Center physicians. Over $1.6 million in private funds, including major gifts from the Noble and Presbyterian Foundations, as well as more than $80,000 in memorial gifts in memory of Jimmy Everest, were combined with $500,000 in institutional funds to build this cooperative project between the hospital, the University, and a private architectural firm, the Benham Group.

The Presbyterian Health Foundation—Again

The Presbyterian Heath Foundation had recently awarded gifts and grants totaling more than $3 million to the Health Sciences Center, bringing the total since 1985 to nearly $24 million. Jean Gumerson, president of the Foundation, acknowledged her organization's focus on Biochemistry and Pediatrics, and emphasized the need to "make certain that Children's Hospital, unique and the only one of its kind in Oklahoma, survives and prospers" *[DO, 9–16–94]*. Stanton Young, chair of the board of the Presbyterian Foundation, pledged to continue to support the Health Sciences Center at the same or greater level, "as long as we stay with the long range plan" developed by the provost and approved by the regents. According to Young, "The Center faces turbulent times. Nineteen ninety-five and 1996 will be challenging; they will be the most difficult years you will be facing as far as the Health Sciences Center is concerned. I compare them to 1964 and 1965 when the regents made a decision that they wanted to keep a medical school for Oklahomans, as well as the difficult days of 1973 and 1974" *[RM, 24066–7]*. The new Phase I Biomedical Research Center building on the campus would be appropriately named for Stanton Young.

Another important private gift to the Center at this time was $500,000 from Mrs. Joy Ann Shideler of Grand Junction, Colorado, whose late husband Max had served as an assistant professor of Pathology from 1957–1959. The funds were matched by the Oklahoma State Regents Endowment Program, to create the Alfred M. Shideler Professorship in Pathology *[DO, 6–6–94]*.

As Medicaid converted to a managed care program, the virtual monopoly of University Hospital over this patient population was challenged by other health care providers which viewed the Medicaid millions as a source of new and profitable income. A leader in this search for new sources of revenue was the Oklahoma Health System (later Integris), parent company of the Baptist Medical Center and its sixteen affiliated hospitals *[JR, 8–31–94]*.

September saw the University hospitals join a network of nine hospitals in southwest Oklahoma called First Health West *[DO, 9–14–94]*. The sharing of resources and referral patterns stemming from the affiliation offered promise of much needed incremental support of University Hospital operation.

In October the Oklahoma Health Center Research Park was announced by Stanton L. Young, chair of the board of the Presbyterian Health Foundation. Situated between N.E. 4th and N.E. 8th Streets between the Centennial Expressway and the Health Center, the park was envisioned as ultimately including nine buildings and a parking garage. The first building, a $6.5 million, 110,000 square foot structure, would be completed in March 1995. The first tenant would be Cytodiagnositics, the firm started in the mid-1980s by Dr. George Hemstreet, that offered diagnostic services to urologists *[JR, 10–6–94; DO, 10–6–94]*.

Richard H. Fleischaker, longtime benefactor of the Health Sciences Center Dermatology and Radiology departments, died on October 4. A founder of Singer-Fleischaker Oil Co. and Chair of Jolen Operating Co., he was noted for his contributions to the Oklahoma City art community, especially American Indian art, as well as charitable organizations in Oklahoma City and in Santa Fe, New Mexico. A Jewish community leader, he had donated a chair in Plastic Surgery to the Hebrew University in Jerusalem and founded the Richard and Adeline Fleischaker Chair in Research Dermatology at the University of Oklahoma Health Sciences Center *[DO, 10–6–94]*.

In mid-October Ronald W. Stutes returned as administrator of University Hospital after serving eighteen months in hospitals in Louisiana. He had been chief executive officer of the Hermann Hospital in Houston and also an administrator at University Hospital from 1991 until 1993.

Dr. Mark Allen Everett, Regents Professor, was elected president of the American Board of Dermatology at its annual meeting in Chicago in late October. Founded in 1932, the board is one of the twenty-four member boards of the American Board of Medical Specialties which are responsible for establishing standards for training and certification in the medical specialties *[DO, 10–24–94]*.

In November University of Oklahoma President-designate David Boren attended the Board of Regents meeting where, because of the budget squeeze, one-time payments were made in lieu of raises to recognize dedicated faculty and staff and "temporarily address the highest funding priority: salary and wage increases" *[RM, 24131]*. At the Health Sciences Center, 2 percent of the E&G budget was distributed in one-time payments ($817,000), with 63 percent of faculty and 76 percent of staff receiving payments averaging 2.4 percent. Fortunately, Professional Practice Plan revenues were $16.7 million to date compared to $15.5 million in the previous year. Increases of 15 percent in tuition fees for students in Law, Medicine, and Dentistry—both in- and out-of-state—were voted by the regents.

The year ended with the Health Sciences Center hospitals expecting a $17 million shortfall, arousing fears that as many as 500 employees might have to be laid off. Governor Walters stated that the two hospitals have to "face up to reality" as they are "overstaffed and spend a lot of money." He said that they "would go under only if they have extraordinarily bad management and bad leadership. There is no reason that they cannot adjust, as every other private hospital has" *[DO, 12–14–94]*. Such statements reflected the sentiments of many politicians who had not familiarized themselves with the great burden of indigent patient care at the Center's hospitals—a burden experienced by no other medical institutions in the state.

On December 31, the dedication of the newly completed $7.7 million Family Medicine facility was held in a ceremony featuring both governor Walters and governor-elect Frank Keating, as well as new University President David Boren. Boren, while serving as governor years earlier, had been one of the original supporters of construction of such a building *[JR, 12–30–94]*.

1995–1996

Nineteen ninety-five dawned with the University of Oklahoma Board of Regents approving, at their January meeting, privatization of the Health Sciences Center dialysis services, which had for many years provided renal dialysis to patients needing long-term care, as well as to those with end-stage renal disease. A contract was awarded to the REN Corporation, a management company, which was to provide a cash payment of $1.5 million to the College of Medicine and an annual payment in excess of $250,000 to the Department of Medicine for physician and other services.

Also in January, the regents finally approved schematic design plans and a cost estimate of $4.8 million for the long-awaited Student Center to be located between the Colleges of Nursing and Pharmacy. The facility would be completed and dedicated in October 1996. The regents also announced the retirement of one of the College of Medicine's most senior professors, Sidney P. Traub, effective March 2, 1995. Dr. Traub, head of the Radiology department, was among that handful of department chairs appointed in the 1960s who had steered their departments effectively through the ebb and flow of several decades. Finally in January, regents reported that faculty practice income from 1995's final six months was $33.6 million, compared to $31.8 million in the same period the previous year.

Nineteen ninety-five was less than a month old when the University Hospital Authority announced the closure of the O'Donoghue Rehabilitation Institute, trimming staff at University and Children's Hospitals, relocating the Child Study Center within Children's Hospital, terminating 359 employees, and eliminating 265 "vacant" positions. Although the O'Donoghue Institute would close, political pressure from the legislature prevented the relocation of the Child Study Center away from its free-standing building across from the O'Donoghue Rehabilitation Institute and Children's Hospital. A portion of O'Donoghue would later be utilized for a community psychiatric "Crisis Center."

In March the Health Sciences Center announced the hiring of a private management company, at a cost of $1.67 million dollars, to develop and initiate a managed-care operation for Medicaid named "Heartland." On the Norman campus, G. T. Blankenship Jr. was elected president of the University of Oklahoma Board of Regents, and Governor Keating appointed Robin Siegfried of Tulsa to a nine-year term on the board *[Tulsa World, 3–17–95; DO, 3–22–95]*. For the first time in several years, the state experienced a significant growth in tax revenues according to reports issued in April, indicating that no budget cuts would be required in the coming fiscal year. Needless to say, this announcement from state officials was cause for rejoicing among cash-strapped educational institutions throughout the state, but especially at the Health Sciences Center, where administrators had been forced to look into a variety of new, painful cutbacks for the coming year.

A generous gift of $3,208,000 from the estate of Paul Jonas was announced by The Board of Regents in 1995. From this gift, three fully funded endowed chairs ($800,000 each plus state regent matches of $500,000) at the Health Sciences Center were created. These chairs would be named the Paul and Ruth Jonas Chairs in Cancer, Diabetes, and Mental Health. An additional new chair in Pathology, named the Presbyterian Health Foundation Chair, was authorized in May 1995, with fundraising to be completed in September 1996. Meanwhile, September 1995 saw three professorships authorized for the Tulsa campus. These were in Surgery (initial funds from St. John's Medical Center), Obstetrics, and Gynecology (the latter two funded by the Hillcrest Medical Center Foundation). This brought to 116 the number of endowed chairs at the University of Oklahoma.

The Bombing of the Murrah Building

On April 19, 1995, at two minutes past nine o'clock in the morning, Oklahoma City was devastated by the explosion of an enormous truck bomb at the downtown Alfred P. Murrah Federal Building, which resulted in 168 deaths. Community hospitals were well prepared for emergency care of the wounded, in part because only a few weeks earlier they fortunately had conducted a mock-disaster exercise to test city facilities and practices. In spite of the devastating death toll, only 153 patients were treated at St. Anthony Hospital, 70 at Presbyterian Hospital, and 41 at University and Children's Hospitals. By fortunate coincidence, all four major hospitals were within ten blocks of the bomb site—St. Anthony's close enough to suffer some glass damage in the blast. The small number of injuries brought to the hospitals (most of them pedestrians on the street hit by flying glass and explosive debris), was an ominous portent of the death count in the collapsed building, which would be slowly revealed as the days passed.

Personnel of the Health Sciences Center were heavily involved in post-bomb street triages, assisting in rescue operations at the blast sight, and providing care of the wounded. The Center also assisted with around-the-clock operation of the Medical Examiners office, which received and identified the dead. Scores of physicians from the Center—radiologists, pathologists, dentists, and other personnel—were mobilized for the identification effort. The Federal Emergency Management Agency would later commend the Medical Examiner's office and the Center's Pathology staff for handling swiftly and with precision the critical identification of the remains of the dead, as well as helping to identify—and reunite with loved ones—those brought out of the building alive *[DO, 5–26–95]*.

Although the Murrah bombing would occupy the minds and hearts of most residents of Oklahoma City for months—even years—to come, business continued as usual at the cash-strapped University hospitals. In May, the regents authorized, at the urging of Provost Stein, a discussion by a group of individuals from the University, the University Hospitals Authority, and the legislature to explore potential private-sector partners to participate in operation of the Center's two hospitals. This effort would culminate several years later (in January 1998) with a management merger between the University Hospitals and Presbyterian Hospital under the banner of Columbia/Presbyterian Hospital Corp.

Two significant departures by longtime faculty members occurred in May. Dr. Patrick A. McKee, the George Lynn Cross Professor of Medicine, resigned as chair of the Department of Medicine on May 5, while Dr. Carl R. Bogardus, head of the Radiation Therapy division of the Radiology department, retired early in May. Dean Douglas Voth proclaimed that Dr. McKee's resignation was "effective immediately," and he quickly named Dr. Douglas P. Fine as acting chair *[DO, 5–6–95]*. It was presumed by senior College of Medicine faculty that McKee's removal was attributable to dissatisfaction on the part of Provost Stein with the highly visible role played by McKee in the hospitals, with the legislature, at OCAST, at the School of Math and Science, and with the Warren Foundation, not to mention McKee's outspoken personal style.

In the view of many faculty members, Provost Jay Stein saw himself as both the morning and the evening star at the Health Sciences Center, and anyone who dared shine brightly enough to diminish his glow was destined to drift out of the firmament. Dr. McKee later recalled that the provost told him, "We're not getting along." Shortly thereafter, Dean Voth, who loyally carried out the dictates of his provost, suggested, "Maybe you need to try something else. Maybe you should give up the chair and go over there [to the Oklahoma Medical Research Foundation] and do research."[8]

The Provost Departs

Provost Jay Stein was mysteriously absent from the June meeting of the University Board of Regents, and then, on July 16, he announced his departure from the position of provost to become vice president and vice provost for health affairs at the University of Rochester (NY) Medical Center, effective August 1. Although when he arrived at Oklahoma in 1992, Stein had said that he wanted to finish his career in Oklahoma City, he stated in July that "even though it pains me to leave Oklahoma, there was just no way to say no." The *Daily Oklahoman* summarized Dr. Stein's years at the helm of the Health Sciences Center in these words:

> The Stein tenure was marked by achievement and controversy. Some at the medical campus and in the Oklahoma City power structure applauded the changes he instituted, while others expressed outrage over his tactics. One issue that also dogged the provost throughout his tenure involved the funding sources for his unprecedented $338,400 salary. Another was Stein's penchant for forcing out people who did not rubberstamp his policies. Finally, the trial balloon for separating the campus as a health sciences University, with Stein as president, was not warmly received by most of the regents, and certainly not by the president-designate, David L. Boren *[DO, 6–17–95]*.

The reaction of President Boren upon learning of Stein's intentions vis-a-vis Rochester was a terse, "I wish Dr. Stein well as he begins his new responsibilities" *[DO, 6–17–95]*.

Jay Stein was a dynamic, controversial provost. He vigorously sought the support of the local business community and championed the idea that the Health Sciences Center would invigorate the economy of Oklahoma City and its business sector. He wrote a weekly column in the *Journal Record* in which he discussed health care issues and publicized his view of the role of the Center. However, by no stretch of the imagination could he be called a "team player" with the faculty. Chairpersons were discarded if they did not play the provost's game. Furthermore, he sought to be the only visible figure from the faculty to the general public, local business leaders, and the legislature. His vision of faculty medical practice as a centrally controlled engine generating money for the Center, and not for the physicians who cared for the patients, led to an often adversarial relationship with the faculty.

As provost, Jay Stein managed to subordinate completely both the dean and the faculty of the College of Medicine to the office of the provost. However, he also strengthened the relationship of the administration of the Center with the Oklahoma City business community, and especially with the Presbyterian Health Foundation. Teaching and the education of medical students and health professionals were not the principal missions of a Health Sciences Center headed by Jay Stein. Business and economics were the chief goal. Many believed this to be an uncomfortable, and at best secondary, role for a University and its Medical Center. The *Tulsa World* said, "One might think the chief administrator of Oklahoma's largest medical school and research center would spend his days contemplating the shaping of young physicians or the pursuit of cures for deadly diseases. Instead, Dr. Jay Stein mostly is occupied with keeping the health-care movement from killing his hospital." Stein was quoted by the paper as saying, "There are going to be more changes around here in the next year or two than there have been in the last 50 years" *[Tulsa World, 6–29–94]*.

Jay Stein's chief administrative achievements were: (1) stimulating the removal of the Center's hospitals from control of the Department of Human Services; (2) initiating the search for a private "partner" for the Center's hospitals; (3) making the Professional Practice Plan examine, and transform, itself; and (4) forcing changes in the Center's health delivery system to develop a PPO organization. The result, a centralized faculty practice organization under one office and one set of rules, although hardly an academic advancement, prepared the center to function as a "player" in the new medical care environment. Stein's least endearing administrative "achievement" was his penchant for forcing out people who did not agree, publicly or privately, with his policies. Quality of work was never the primary concern of this provost in evaluating the performance of his employees. Several tenured faculty members reportedly were told by Stein to either "retire"or "make yourself scarce on campus." The *Daily Oklahoman*, in a summary article on Stein's stewardship, listed the men he forced out in his final three years, some of them the most brilliant chairs the University ever boasted: "Dr. Ed Brandt, former dean of the medical school; Dr. Al Brann, former chair of pediatrics; Dr. Gordon Deckert, former chair of psychiatry and behavioral sciences; Dr. Lee Holder, former dean of allied health; Dr. Pat McKee, former chair of medicine; Dr. Chris Ramsey, former chair of family practice; and Dr. Bailus Walker, former dean of public health" *[DO, 6–17– 95]*.

In addition to this group, the departures of Dr. Lenart Fagraeous (Anesthesiology), William Parry (Urology), and Sidney Traub (Radiology) were hastened by Provost Stein.

It was not only those chairs who failed to "rubberstamp" the provost's policies who came into disfavor with Jay Stein. Publicized, highly visible faculty members were tolerated with a decided lack of enthusiasm by the provost. Two chairpersons who fell into this category, but remained untouched by Stein, were G. Rainey Williams (Surgery) and Mark Allen Everett (Dermatology). The provost did not conceal his occasional dislike for the activities of these men, but he never attempted to remove them because, presumably, their long personal and family connections to the social and business structure of the community—connections not easily disrupted by a relative newcomer on the scene, regardless of his or her influence and strength—prevented it.

In response to Jay Stein's resignation, President Boren announced that Dr. Joseph Ferretti, chair of Microbiology and vice president for research administration, would be interim provost, and Dr. Jerry Vannatta, professor of Medicine and director of medical education at Presbyterian Hospital, would be interim associate provost for medical affairs, with a salary change from $69,696 to $170,000 for the year, effective July 1, 1996. A search committee to carry out "a national search" for a senior vice president and provost of the Health Sciences Center was appointed by the regents on November 1. Although several reports from this committee were scheduled for delivery over the next six months, that particular item was always stricken from the regents' agenda. Then on April 24, 1996, without recommendations from the search committee, the titles of both men were changed, following the recommendation of Regent Halverstadt: Ferretti to senior vice president and provost, Health Sciences Center, with a salary of $225,000 per year; and Vannatta to vice president for health affairs and associate provost, Health Sciences Center, at a salary of $200,000 per year. Later, following the departure of College of Medicine Dean Douglas Voth, Vannatta was additionally named interim dean, and the following year—on July 21, 1997—permanent executive dean of the College of Medicine. Douglas Voth was listed as "on leave of absence without pay" until July 1, 1999. Thus, the position of dean was effectively integrated into the provost's office, with an associate provost serving as dean. In a bizarre turn, things had come almost full circle from the '60s, when Deans Everett and Dennis were also the directors (nee provosts) of the Center.

In November 1993, Site of Practice exceptions had been voted for the faculty in Neurology and Neurosurgery, permitting offices in Presbyterian Hospital facilities. On April 24, 1996, the regents approved a $132,000 annual lease with Presbyterian for office space for these faculty members. Further diffusion of the Site-of-Practice rule occurred when, on June 19, the regents agreed to sell, for $268,000, just under two acres of land on the Oklahoma City campus to the Oklahoma Health Sciences Facilities, Inc. to develop a private renal dialysis operation called "Gambro Inc.," a joint venture with University faculty. (Later, in January 1997, a contract for $228.7,000 for 1.5 acres would be approved. The regents retained first refusal rights should Gambro sell the property.) Additionally, an annual rental fee of $225,000 to the Dean A. McGee Eye Institute was approved for office, clinical, and research space for the Department of Ophthalmology. Later, in March 1997, the regents would approve departmental purchase of a practice in Otorhinolaryngology located in the Presbyterian Office Building, as an "outreach" which would increase patient visits for faculty revenue and student education *[RM, 25288]*.

On May 31, 1996, Dr. G. Rainey Williams retired as chair of Surgery as well as from the faculty, due to a previously unsuspected illness which would prove fatal in 1997. During the intervening time, the South Pavilion of University Hospital was named in his honor. As previously stated, G. Rainey Williams had for thirty years played a central role as a member of the faculty and administration of the College of Medicine. He was a gentle, thoughtful, compassionate man of whom the Center and the state will always be proud.

In addition to Dr. Williams, several other prominent faculty left the Health Sciences Center in 1996. Long-term, dedicated faculty members Gordon Deckert, a David Ross Boyd Professor, and Regents Professor Mark Allen Everett retired from the University. Dr. Deckert was later granted professor emeritus status. Dr. Everett left following forty years of service that brought international repute in Dermatology to the Health Sciences Center and the University. Additionally, Dr. Dan Duffy, professor and chair of Medicine, Tulsa, resigned on November 15.

In other faculty changes, Dr. Joseph Kopta was changed from full-time faculty to "0.99% time," presumably another Site of Practice exception, and Dr. Lynn Drake was appointed professor and chair of Dermatology at a salary of $130,000 per year, effective September 16.

In other matters, a contract to build Phase I (four floors) of the Biomedical Research Center was let for $14.6 million, and the Student Center contract was let for $2.9 million. On September 26, 1995, the title of the Department of Family Medicine was changed to the Department of Family and Preventive Medicine, "to correspond to the changing role of medicine in society" (a title similar to that of the 1970s) [RM, 24580]. Also in September, the Presbyterian Health Foundation gave $500,000 to the University of Oklahoma Research Corporation, subject to acquisition of 501c3 status. And on December 8 Professional Practice Plan funds were authorized to purchase 0.3 acres adjacent to the Tulsa College of Medicine campus for expansion.

The never-ending problem of parking was addressed by the Board of Regents at their meeting on January 10, 1996. The legislature had, in 1991, created the Medical Technology and Research Authority (MTRA) "to construct and improve" support facilities at the Health Sciences Center. The first plan adopted by this organization's governing board was to "lease" the existing parking from the University (for a negligible fee) and "generate revenue through user fees"—i.e. to impose parking charges on faculty, staff, other employees, and visitors. The regents approved a $10 per month charge for faculty and $6.25 per month for staff for unassigned parking. Reserved parking was far more—$25 per month. The imposition of fees led to considerable dissatisfaction among employees, who regarded even the lower fees as unreasonable and granting them only a "hunting license" to roam around the campus looking for a parking place. Over the next five years, MTRA would attempt to gain control of all parking on campus. The only successful resistance to their plan came from facilities not built with state (University or Department of Human Services) appropriations or bond issues—e.g., lots at the Oklahoma Medical Research Foundation, the Dermatology Clinic, the Oklahoma Allergy and Asthma Clinic, and the Dean A. McGee Eye Institute. Even these were subject to recurrent pressures by the administration to "fork over" at least part of their revenues.

A review of the campus Affirmative Action Plan by regents on March 6, 1966, revealed that of twenty-seven faculty promotions at the Health Sciences Center in the preceding year, 52 percent went to women (14 positions) and 19 percent to minority faculty (5 positions). At the same regents meeting, the name of the faculty Professional Practice Plan in the College of Medicine was changed to "University Physicians Medical Group." In a related action, regents decided that any salary in excess of the approved University base would be tied to the "level of clinical income and support from grants and contracts."

On October 30 the long-anticipated and recently completed Student Center was accepted by the University from the builders. At the same meeting, regents provided a welcome but long overdue honor to former president

George Cross on December 11 when he was granted the title of Regents Professor Emeritus.

Nineteen ninety-five and 1996 were years of tremendous transformation on the Health Sciences Center campus, largely as a consequence of changes resulting from alterations in the health care reimbursement system nationally. G. Rainey Williams, professor of Surgery and frequent interim dean of the College of Medicine, commented on these alterations: "We have a generation of physicians who have seen the practice of medicine change very dramatically. They don't like it—and they are saying so."[9] He believed that the present generation of physicians will be followed by a group of young doctors who won't know what the previous medical situation was like, but will find the same satisfaction in caring for patients that has always been a key part of medicine *[DO, 8–27–90]*. Much of the change had been brought about because of the escalating cost of medical care, especially hospital costs. Williams recalled that in the 1920s, the cost of patient care in University Hospital was $15 a week. Mark Allen Everett remembered that a private room in the same hospital was $27 per day in 1949. The cost in 1996 was commonly in excess of $2,000 per day.

In 1995, the University of Oklahoma made history by securing more than $100 million in externally sponsored research and investigative programs. Of this sum, over $50 million went to Health Sciences Center faculty, with over $16 million from the National Institutes of Health (NIH). Over half of all NIH expenditures in the entire state of Oklahoma were on the Health Sciences Center campus.[10] In 1996 and 1997, fifteen additional endowed positions (eleven chairs, four professorships) would be added on the Oklahoma City Campus and eight in Tulsa (five chairs, three professorships). The total number of endowed University positions at the end of 1998 was sixty-one. Of these, forty-seven were fully funded chairs and one was partially funded. In addition, thirteen endowed professorships were established, twelve of which were fully funded. (*See Table, Appendix.*)

Additionally, there was finally a complicated solution to the political controversy over which higher education institution(s) would provide graduate education courses in Tulsa, without creating a new free-standing university. Oklahoma State University was to have an undergraduate branch in Tulsa (replacing "Rogers University," which would revert to a local operation); Oklahoma State University and the University of Oklahoma would jointly operate a Graduate Center; and the College of Medicine campus in Tulsa would undergo a $55 million expansion to offer recognized, accredited masters degree programs in Physical Therapy and Occupational Therapy.

Major changes were to occur under the Health Sciences Center administrative team of Dr. Ferretti and Dr. Vanatta in the early years of their administration. The teaching hospitals were to enter an operational agreement with Columbia HCA, which would manage and provide capital for improvement and expansion of facilities, including a new ambulatory care center and several peripheral primary care centers. The three hospitals (University, Presbyterian, and Children's) would operate under the rubric of University Health Partners, and the Center's focus would indeed be transformed from a primary concern with education and research to providing managed care delivery of health services.

In the view of many physicians, the first years under Columbia HCA saw many positive changes taking place at both Children's and University Hospitals. More than one doctor pointed out that "things seem once again to be looking up." Dr. Ron Elkins of the Department of Surgery noted some of these transformations as the Health Sciences Center prepared to enter the new millennium:

I see some very positive changes taking place at a very difficult time. I think the work force in the hospital is moving in the right direction, and is much better than it was. A major effort has been made to keep the hospitals clean and bright, and improvements are being made in the food service. For the first time since the Rader days, in the operating rooms it is not a question of 'Can you do this?' but 'We will do this and stay here until it's done!' Old equipment is being replaced, supplies are more readily available, and, most importantly, the personnel *want* to get the work done.[11]

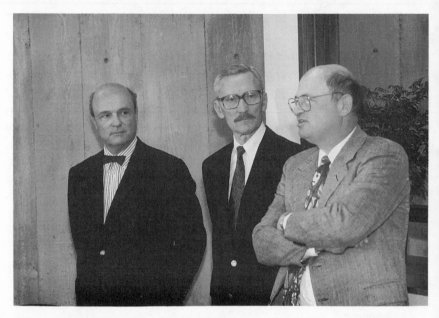

Left to right: Donald B. Halverstadt, M.D., University of Oklahoma Board of Regents; Douglas Voth, M.D., Executive Dean of the College of Medicine; and Jay Stein, M.D., Provost of the Health Sciences Center. (AAE)

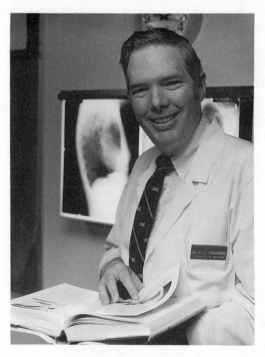

R. Timothy Coussons, M.D., Professor of Medicine, Medical Director and Chief Operating Officer of the University Hospitals. (OUHSC)

338

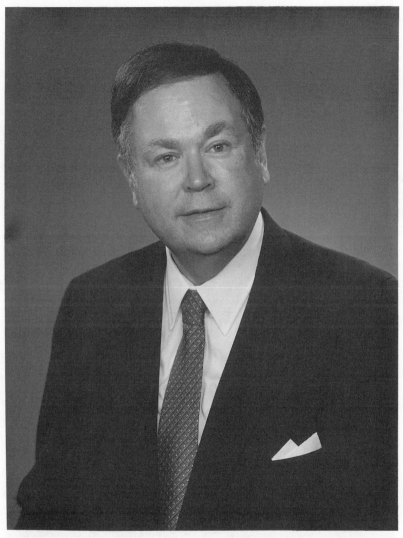

David Boren, J.D., President of the University of Oklahoma. (OUPA)

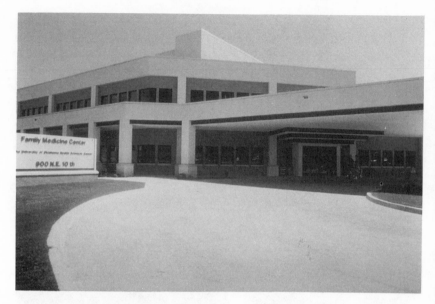

The Family Medicine building. (OUHSC)

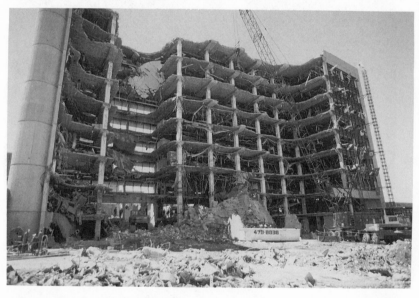

The Alfred P. Murrah Federal Building shortly after the April 19, 1995, bomb blast. (OUHSC)

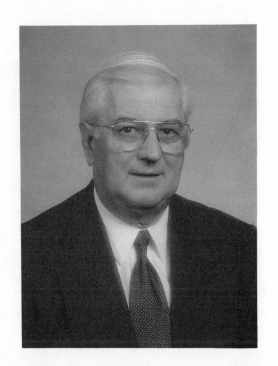

Joseph Ferretti, Ph.D., Provost
of the Health Sciences Center.
(OUHSC)

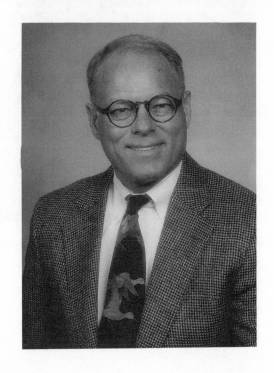

Jerry Vannatta, M.D.,
Associate Provost of the
Health Sciences Center and
Executive Dean of the College
of Medicine. (OUHSC)

341

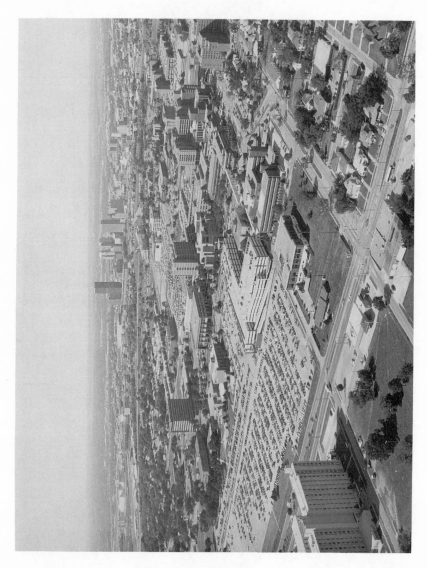

Aerial view of the
University of Oklahoma
Health Sciences Center
campus, 1998. (OUHSC)

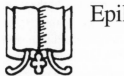

Epilogue

 The University of Oklahoma Health Sciences Center came full circle in the years between 1964 and 1996. In a distorted symmetry, Mark R. Everett, a Ph.D. scientist, was ultimately succeeded as director of the Health Sciences Center in 1995 by Joseph Ferretti, another Ph.D. scientist. It was unusual in the United States to find medical centers, hospitals, or colleges of medicine headed by Ph.D. scientists, and even more so to have two such leaders at one institution in thirty years. The style, commitment to medical education, and vision of what a Health Sciences Center should ultimately be, however, were dissimilar between the two regimes. The earlier leaders, dedicated to scholarship and clinical excellence in the College of Medicine, attracted strong, dynamic clinicians who taught medicine, accomplished internationally recognized scientific research, delivered quality care to Oklahoma's indigent and not-so-indigent citizens, and were mentors to a stream of talented medical specialists who achieved eminence in their own right. The Center's contemporary administrators, operating in a new age and under what they clearly view as a different mandate, are more oriented to managing a sprawling health care organization while competing in the arena of managed care.

More than anything else, the three-plus decades of this history were marked by the boom and bust financial cycle of the Oklahoma economy, and were characterized by inadequate funding and support by the state legislature, as well as by a chronic failure to address the provision of medical care to indigent Oklahoma citizens.

Mark R. Everett was succeeded in late 1964 by James Dennis, who pursued the dream of a multicollege Health Science Center that gradually replaced Everett's College of Medicine dominated by its faculty. Dennis set the stage for the vast health enterprise which subsequently evolved on the Oklahoma

City campus, as well as inadvertently subordinating the position of the dean of the College of Medicine to that of the provost/vice president of the Center.

An unexpected political and fiscal complication was the addition of a College of Medicine branch at Tulsa. A "Tulsa College of Medicine" was conceived by Tulsa hospital leaders, and brought to realization by powerful state senators from the area, at a time when the parent campus was suffering from inadequate funding. Opposition was fierce within the College of Medicine, since the creation of this additional institution could only further dilute legislative financial support for the Oklahoma City campus. Yet, as former University President Paul Sharp said, "Once the legislature had mandated the school, it became 'a good idea,' in spite of the failure of the legislature to provide adequate financing." Sharp believed that creation of the Tulsa medical branch increased statewide enthusiasm and support for the parent University in Norman. "I'm ready to defend it to this day. It did something we hadn't done before: it created teaching hospitals in Tulsa, and that was a great gain for them and for us. It brought to Tulsa an image of the University in the best possible light."

Between the administrations of Everett and Ferretti were two dynamic, decisive, at times even ruthless, provosts—Drs. William Thurman and Jay Stein—each of whom brought significant change and growth, as well as turmoil, to the institution they governed. Bridging these regimes was a twelve-year interregnum of relative calm, led by the well intentioned and socially suave Provost Clayton Rich.

Dr. Mark R. Everett and Dr. Merlin DuVal viewed themselves primarily as scholars, scientists, and leaders of their faculty; Dr. Ferretti and Dr. Vannatta, in the tangled new world of managed care and mergers, were more bureaucratic and process oriented, resembling CEOs of a vast business enterprise, ruling over an enormous complex of hospitals, colleges, health delivery and management groups, joint venture companies, office buildings, and research organizations. The dramatic shift between these models dredges up an inevitable sequence of questions: What was the purpose of establishing a College of Medicine within the University of Oklahoma almost a hundred years ago? Have we accomplished that goal? Are we at least headed in that direction? Has the intent of the founding fathers—to establish an institution to educate doctors for Oklahoma—been realized with today's vast medical complexes in Oklahoma City and Tulsa? Is our mission no longer the same?

A leading Health Sciences Center faculty member, Dr. Patrick McKee, in commenting on the changes during the 30-plus years of this history, observed recently that: "There has always been an impatience at this institution. There is a mind-set, based on the Oklahoma culture, which demands instant results. 'Successful' men just go out and punch a hole in the ground and suddenly you are a Phillips, a Warren, or a McGee. Some things take much longer than this to develop, and one has to stay with it. Because of the paucity of people with vision here, we have also had, in addition to impatience, an uncontrollable urge to declare excellence rather than achieve it."

A senior professor of Surgery believed that the increasing tendency to fill major administrative positions from within the Center would inevitably lead to "provincialism and mediocrity, rendering national prominence forever untenable." Only continual infusion of new ideas and administrative innovations from "larger and more imminent campuses" would reverse this trend.

Only time will tell whether the less complex, more idealistic, and far more academically oriented era of the post World War II period at the University of Oklahoma Health Sciences Center has given way to a more diverse golden age, or merely to a more bureaucratic and impersonal one with shifting emphases. A few weeks before his death, G. Rainey Williams asked the authors, perhaps rhetorically, "Why isn't Oklahoma on the A-list? Why didn't we quite get there?" One must examine closely the sea-changes charted in this history to find a definitive answer to his question. Perhaps the most optimistic response as the University begins the new millennium is, "The final chapter is yet to be written."

Appendix I.
Deans of the
College of Medicine,
1904–1996

1904–1910	Archa Kelly West, M.D. (Epworth College of Medicine)
1900–1904	Lawrence Northcote Upjohn, M.D. (Administrator, School of Medicine)
1904–1908	Roy Philson Stoops, M.D. (Director, Head, Acting Dean)
1908–1911	Charles Sharp Bobo, M.D.
1911–1913	Robert Findlater Williams, M.D.
1913–1914	William James Jolly, M.D.
1914–1915	Curtis Richard Day, M.D.
1915–1931	LeRoy Long, M.D.
1931–1935	Lewis Jefferson Moorman, M.D.
1935	Lewis Alvin Turley, Ph.D. (Acting)
1935–1942	Robert Urie Patterson, M.D.
1942–1943	Harold Adam Shoemaker, Ph.D. (Acting)
1943–1945	Thomas Claude Lowry, M.D.
1945–1946	Wann Langston, M.D.
1946–1947	Jacques Pierce Gray, M.D.
1947–1964	Mark Ruben Everett, Ph.D.
1964	Joseph M. White, M.D. (Acting)
1964–1970	James L. Dennis, M.D.
1970–1974	Robert Montgomery Bird, M.D.
1974–1980	Thomas N. Lynn, M.D.
1980–1982	George Rainey Williams, M.D. (Interim)
1982–1985	Charles McCall, M.D.
1984	William Knisley, Ph.D. (Acting)
1985–1986	George Rainey Williams, M.D. (Interim)
1986–1988	Donald G. Kassebaum, M.D.
1988–1989	George Rainey Williams, M.D. (Interim Executive Dean)
1989–1992	Edward N. Brandt, Jr., M.D. (Executive Dean)

1992–1995   Douglas W. Voth, M.D. (Executive Dean)
1995–1996   Jerry B. Vannatta, M.D. (Associate Provost & Interim Executive Dean)
1996–   Jerry B. Vannatta, M.D. (Associate Provost & Executive Dean)

Appendix II.
Chairs of the
Faculty Board,
1948–1998

1948–1972	Don O'Donoghue
1972–1974	John Schilling
1974–1990	Mark Allen Everett
1990–1994	G. Rainey Williams
1994–1996	Fred Silva
1996–1998	Jesus Medina
1998–2000	Douglas Fine

Appendix III.
Deans of the
College of Medicine,
Tulsa Branch, 1974–1992

1974–1975   Martin J. Fitzpatrick, M.D.
1975–1977   William G. Thurman, M.D.
1977–1978   James E. Lewis, Ph.D.
1978–1979   Daniel C. Plunket, M.D. (Interim)
1979–1991   Edward J. Tomsovic, M.D.
1991–1992   Daniel C. Plunket, M.D. (Interim)
1992–   Harold L. Brooks, M.D.

Appendix IV.
Chairs of the Department
of Anatomical Science,
1900–1998

1900–1904	Lawrence Northcote Upjohn, M.D.
1904–1908	Roy Philson Stoops, M.D.
1908–1915	Walter Leander Capshaw, M.D.
1915–1919	Reuben Morgan Hargrove, M.D.
(1918)	John Paine Torrey , M.D. (Acting)
1919–1931	Joseph Clark Stephenson, Ph.D., M.D.
1924–1925	Jacob Martin Essenberg, M.D. (Acting)
1931–1933	Carmen Russell Salsbury, M.D.
1933–1936	Lee Kenneth Emenhiser, M.D. (Acting)
1936–1945	Charles Francis DeGaris, Ph.D.
1945–1968	Ernst Lachman, M.D.
1968–1975	William J. L. Felts, Ph.D.
1975–1976	Kenneth K. Faulkner (Acting)
1976–1981	Joseph Ching-yuen Lee, M.D.
1981–1988	Kenneth Faulkner, Ph.D.
1988–1994	Joe G. Wood, Ph.D.
1994–1998	Raymond E. Papka, Ph.D.
1998–	Robert E. Anderson, Ph.D.
1998	(Name changed to Department of Cell Biology and combined with the Department of Pharmacology.)
1920–1950	Joseph Mario Thuringer (head of a separate Department of Histology and Embryology).

351

Appendix V.
Chairs of the
Department of Anesthesiology,
1936–1993

1936–1938	John Alfred Moffatt, M.D.
1938–1944	Hubert Eugene Doudna, M.D.
1945–1946	Albert D. Foster, M.D.
1946–1948	Hubert Eugene Doudna, M.D.
1948–1955	Howard A. Bennett, M.D.
1955–1956	Lawrence Stream, M.D. (acting)
1956–1965	Joseph A. White, M.D.
1965–1970	James A. Cutter, M.D.
1971–1982	Stanley Deutsch, M.D., Ph.D.
1983–1987	Lennert Fagraeous, M.D., Ph.D.
1987–1988	John Plewes, M.D. (Interim)
1988–1992	John Plewes, M.D.
1992–1993	Robin Elwood, M.D. (Interim)
1993–	Robin Elwood, M.D.

Appendix VI.
Chairs of the Department of
Biochemistry and Molecular
Biology, 1906–1994

1906–1923	Edwin C. DeBarr, Ph.D. (Chemistry Dept.)
1924–1965	Mark R. Everett, Ph.D.
1965	Arley Bever, Ph.D. (Term)
1965–1978	B. Connor Johnson, Ph.D.

(DEPARTMENT NAME CHANGED TO
BIOCHEMISTRY AND MOLECULAR BIOLOGY)

1978–1984	Peter Gray, Ph.D.
1984–1992	John Sokatch, Ph.D.
1992–1994	Albert Chandler, Ph.D. (Interim)
1994–	Paul Weigel, Ph.D.

Appendix VII.
Chairs of the
Department of Dermatology,
1916–1997

1916–1942	Everett S. Lain, M.D.
1942–1956	Charles Palmer Bondurant, M.D.
1956–1961	John H. Lamb, M.D.
1961–1963	Phyllis E. Jones, M.D.
1963–1997	Mark Allen Everett, M.D.
1997–2000	Lynn Drake, M.D.

Appendix VIII.
Chairs of the Department of
Family Medicine and Community
Health, 1912–1999

CHAIRS OF THE DEPARTMENT OF FAMILY
PRACTICE AND COMMUNITY MEDICINE

CHAIRS OF THE DEPARTMENT OF PREVENTIVE
MEDICINE AND PUBLIC HEALTH

1912–1932	Gayfree Ellison, M.D.
1934–1935	Hiram Dunlap Moor, M.D.
1936–1937	Onis George Hazel, M.D. (acting)
1938–1940	Egil Thorbjorn Olsen, M.D. (acting)
1940–1943	Donald Bard McMullen, D.S.C. (acting)
1943–1948	John Fielden Hackler, M.D.
1948–1951	Joseph Benjamin Goldsmith, Ph.D. (acting)
1951–1952	George M. Brother, M.D.
1952–1960	Kirk Thornton Mosley, M.D., D.P.H.
1960–1969	William W. Schottstaedt, M.D.
1965	Roger Lienke, M.D. (Division of Family Medicine, Department of Preventive Medicine and Community Health—Chair: 1966–72)
1969–1976	Thomas N. Lynn, M.D.
1970	(PMPH to Community Health, Colleges of Medicine and Dentistry)
1972	Division terminated: Department of Family Practice created
1973	Community Health changed to Family Practice and Community Norman L. Haug, Director of Family Practice Residency Program, 1973–1974
1977–1979	Dave Steen, Ph.D. (Interim)
1979–1980	Dave Steen, Ph.D.

355

1980   (Departments separated: Community Medicine now in College
                  of Health)

CHAIRS OF THE DEPARTMENT OF FAMILY PRACTICE

1979–1981   Jack Parrish, M.D. (Professor and Head of Family Practice in
             C/M)
1981–1982   Thomas Coniglione, M.D. (Interim Head)
1982–1994   Christian Ramsey, M.D.
1994–1999   Roy DeHart, M.D.
             (Department of Family Practice and Community Medicine)
1999–   Stephan Crawford, M.D. (Interim)

**Appendix IX.
Chairs of the
Department of Gynecology
and Obstetrics, 1924–1997**

CHAIRS OF THE DEPARTMENT OF GYNECOLOGY

1924–1939 John Frederick Kuhn, M.D.
1940–1950 Grider Penick, M.D.
1951–1961 Joseph Willard Kelso, M.D.

CHAIRS OF THE DEPARTMENT OF OBSTETRICS

1912–1933 John Archer Hatchett, M.D.
1933–1945 Walter William Wells, M.D.
1945–1946 Edward Pennington Allen, M.D.
1946–1954 James B. Eskridge Jr., M.D.
1954–1961 Milton John Serwer, M.D.

DEPARTMENT OF GYNECOLOGY AND OBSTETRICS

1961–1983 James A. Merrill, M.D.
1983–1997 John I. Fishburne Jr., M.D.
1997–   Robert S. Mannel, M.D.

Appendix X.
Chairs of the
Department of Medicine,
1912–1995

1912–1926   Archa Kelly West, M.D.
1926–1944   George Althouse LaMotte, M.D.
1944–1947   Wann Langston, M.D.
1947–1948   Robert H. Bayley, M.D. (Acting)
1948–1951   Rufus Quitman Goodwin, M.D.
1952–1967   Stewart G. Wolf, M.D.
1967–1977   James F. Hammersten, M.D.
1977–1984   Solomon Papper, M.D.
1983 (Oct–Dec) Richard T. Coussons, M.D. (Acting)
1984–1985   Richard T.Coussons, M.D. (Acting)
1985–1995   Patrick A. McKee, M.D.
1995–2000   Douglas Fine, M.D.

Appendix XI.
Chairs of the Department of
Microbiology and Immunology,
1912–1997

1912–1928	Gayafree Ellison, M.D.
1928–1929	William Alfred Buice, B.S. (Acting)
1929–1951	Hiram Dunlap Moor, M.D.
1951–1952	Homer F. Marsh, Ph.D.
1952–1958	Florene C. Kelly, Ph.D.
1959–1961	Martin M. Cummings, M.D.
1961–1982	L. Vernon Scott, D. Sc.
1982–1995	Joseph J. Ferretti, Ph.D.
1995–1997	Richard M. Hyde, Ph.D. (Interim)
1997–	John J. Iandolo, Ph.D.

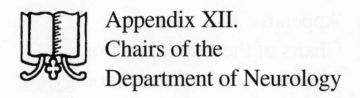

Appendix XII.
Chairs of the
Department of Neurology

(IN DEPARTMENT OF PSYCHIATRY PRIOR TO 1960)

1960–1964   Gunter R. Haase, M. D.
1970–1972   Ralph Druckman, M.D.
1972–1973   Richard Carpenter, M.D.
1973–1988   John D. Nelson, M.D.
1988–1990   Robert Schuman, M.D.
1990–1992   Douglas Voth, M.D.
1998–   James Couch, M.D.

Appendix XIII.
Chairs of the
Department of Ophthalmology,
1916–1992

1916–1938	Edmund S. Ferguson, M.D.
1938–1945	Leslie Marshall Westfall, M.D.
1945–1952	James Patton McGee, M.D.
1952–1962	James Robert Reed, M.D.
1962–1972	Tullos Oswell Coston, M.D.
1972–1992	Thomas E. Acers, M.D.
1992–	David W. Parkes II, M.D.

Appendix XIV.
Chairs of the
Department of Orthopedic
Surgery, 1927–1992

DEPARTMENT OF ORTHOPEDIC SURGERY

1927–1935   Samuel Robert Cunningham, M.D. (Elected)
1935–1938   Willis Kelly West, M.D. ("Acting") (Elected)
1938–1942   Paul Crenshaw Colonna, M.D. (First full-time)
1942–1948   Willis Kelly West, M.D. (Elected)
1948–1973   Don Horatio O'Donoghue, M.D. (Elected) (First resident 1927–30)
1973–1974   Marvin Margo, M.D.
1974–1992   Joseph Kopta, M.D.

DEPARTMENT OF ORTHOPEDIC SURGERY AND REHABILITATION

1992–   J. Andy Sullivan, M.D.

Appendix XV.
Chairs of the Department
of Otorhinolaryngology,
1912–1991

1912–1916	Edmund Shepard Ferguson, M.D. (Division of Surgery)
1916–1922	Lauren Haynes Buxton, M.D., L.L.D.
1922–1924	Edmund Shepard Ferguson, M.D.
1924–1936	H. Coulter Todd, M.D.
1936–1948	Theodore G. Wails, M.D.
1948–1951	Lawrence Chester McHenry, M.D.
1951–1959	O. Alton Watson, M.D.
1959–1962	Lee K. Emenhiser, M.D.
1962–1964	Ethan A. Walker Jr., M.D.
1964–1972	James Byron Snow Jr, M.D.
1972–1973	Willard Brown Moran Jr., M.D. (Acting)
1973–1978	Willard Brown Moran Jr., M.D. resigned 1978 (effect. 1 Jan 79))
1979	Robert Keim, M.D. (acting) resigned
1979–1981	Joseph E. Leonard, M.D. (Interim)
1981–1991	John Gail Neely, M.D.
1991–	Jesus Medina, M.D.

**Appendix XVI.
Chairs of the
Department of Pathology,
1906–1998**

1906–1908	Edward Marsh Williams, B.S. ("Instructor in charge of Pathology and Bacteriology")
1908–1944	Luis Alvin Turley, Ph.D. (Professor and Chair, 1909)
1944–1956	Howard C. Hopps, M.D.
1957–1966	William Jaques, M.D.
1966–1971	A. Lawrence Dee, M.D.
1971–1972	Clarke R. Stout, M.D. (Interim)
1972	Jaqueline Jones Coalson, Ph.D. (Administrator)
1972–1978	Robert M. O'Neal, M.D.
1978–1979	Jacqueline Jones Coalson, Ph.D. (Acting)
1979–1984	Mark Allen Everett, M.D. (Interim)
1984–1985	Jess Hensley, M.D. (Term)
1985–1989	Richard Leech, M.D. (Term)
1989–1998	Fred Silva, M.D.
1998–	Roger Brumback, M.D. (Interim)

Appendix XVII.
Chairs of the
Department of Laboratory
Medicine, 1964–1973

1964–1973 Ben I. Heller, M.D.
April 1973 Ben Heller departed; department dissolved and returned to
Department of Pathology

Appendix XVIII.
Chairs of the
Department of Pharmacology,
1924–1998

1924–1935	Mark Reuben Everett, Ph.D.
1935–1944	Harold Adam Shoemaker, Ph.C., Ph.D.
1944–1960	Arthur Alfred Hellbaum, Ph.D., M.D.
1945–1953	Department of Physiology and Pharmacology
1961–	Richard W. Payne, M.D.
1961–1969	Marion de Veaux Cotton, Ph.D.
1969–1998	Joanne Moore, Ph.D.
1998–	Combined with Anatomical Science into Department of Cell Biology

Appendix XIX.
Chairs of the
Department of Physiology,
1901–1984

1901–1903	Laurence N. Upjohn, M.D. (Head, Premedical Department)
1903–1906	Roy P. Stoops, M.D. (Head, Premedical Department)
1907–1911	John D. Maclaren, M.D. (Head)
1911–1912	Albert Clifford Hirshfield, M.D.
1912–1913	Richard L. Foster, M.D. (Acting Professor)
1913–1928	Leonard Blain Nice, Ph.D. (Chair of one faculty)
1928–1945	Edward C. Mason, M.D., Ph.D.
1945–1953	Arthur A. Hellbaum, MD, Ph.D.
1945–1961	Department of Physiology and Pharmacology
1953–1955	Ardell Nicholas Taylor, Ph.D. (Acting)
1955–1960	Ardell Nicholas Taylor, Ph.D. Chair
1960–1961	M. Jack Keyl, Ph.D. Acting Chair
1961–1966	Francis J. Haddy, M.D., Ph.D. Chair
1966–1971	Eugene D. Jacobson, M.D. Chair
1971–1977	M. Jack Keyl, Ph.D. Chair
1977–1984	H. Lowell Stone, Ph.D. (Head)

Appendix XX.
Chairs of the
Department of Physiology and
Biophysics (1978), 1984–1989

1984–1986   Robert D. Foreman, Ph.D.
1986–   Robert D. Foreman, Ph.D.

CHAIRS OF THE DEPARTMENT OF PHYSIOLOGY
(1989)

1989   Robert D. Foreman, Ph.D.

**Appendix XXI.
Chairs of the
Department of Pediatrics,
1930–1994**

1930–1938	William M. ("Baby") Taylor, M.D.
1938–1955	Clark Homer Hall, M.D.
1955–1957	Henry Bonheyo Strenge, M.D.
1957–1958	Theodore Pfundt, M.D. (acting)
1958–1976	Harris D. Riley Jr., M.D.
1976–1977	James Wenzl, M.D. (Acting)
1977–1988	Owen Rennert, M.D.
1990–1993	Alfred Brann, M.D.
1993–1994	John Grunow, M.D. (Acting)
1994	Terrence Stull, M.D.

**Appendix XXII.
Chairs of the
Department of Psychiatry,
1912–1996**

(PRIOR TO 1960: JOINT DEPARTMENT OF
PSYCHIATRY AND NEUROLOGY)

1912–1915	Antonio DeBord Young, M.D.
1916–1919	John Williams Duke, M.D.
1920–1940	David Wilson Griffin, M.D.
1940–1948	Charles Ralph Rayburn, M.D.
1948–1954	Coyne H. Campbell, M.D.
1954–1969	Louis Jolyon West, M.D.
1969–1986	Gordon H. Deckert, M.D.
1986–1989	Leroy Gathman, M.D. (Interim)
1989–1990	Ronald S. Krug, Ph.D. (Interim)
1990–1992	Joseph J. Westermeyer, M.D., Ph.D.
1992	Gordon H. Deckert, M.D. (Interim)
1992–1996	Ronald S. Krug, Ph.D. (Interim)
1996–	Betty Pfefferbaum, M.D., Ph.D.

Appendix XXIII.
Chairs of the
Department of Radiology,
1936–1996

1936–1948	John Evans Heatley, M.D.
1948–1957	Peter Ernest Russo, M.D.
1957–1962	Gus Ray Ridings, M.D.
1963	Gaylord S. Knox, M.D. (acting)
1963–1995	Sidney P. Traub, M.D.
1995	Bob Eaton, M.D. (Acting)
1996–	Bob Eaton, M.D.

CHAIRS OF THE DEPARTMENT OF RADIATION THERAPY, 1916–1948

1916–1942	Everett S. Lain, M.D.
1942–1948	William Eastland, M.D.
1948	Division of Radiology Department

Appendix XXIV.
Chairs of the
Department of Surgery,
1912–1997

1912–1913	William James Jolly, M.D.
1913–1915	John William Riley, M.D.
1915–1931	LeRoy Long, M.D.
1931–1943	Robert Mayburn Howard, M.D.
1943–1948	Cyril E. Clymer, M.D.
1948–1952	Leo Joseph Starry, M.D.
1952–1956	Forrest Merle Lingenfelter, M.D.
1956–1974	John A. Schilling, M.D.
1974–1996	George Rainey Williams, M.D.
1996–1997	Russell Postier, M.D. (Interim)
1997–	Russell Postier, M.D.

Appendix XXV. Chairs of the Department of Urology, 1913–1994

1913–1919	John W. Riley, M.D.
1919–1934	William Jones Wallace
1934–1936	Rex George Bolend, M.D. (Acting)
1936–1943	Rex George Bolend, M.D.
1943–1944	Charles B. Taylor, M.D. (Acting)
1945–1946	Basil Augustus Hayes, M.D. (Acting)
1946–1954	Basil Augustus Hayes, M.D.
1954–1962	Donald W. Branham, M.D.
1962–1994	William L. Parry, M.D.
1994–	Daniel J. Culkin, M.D.

Appendix XXVI.
Chairs of the
Department of Family Medicine—
Tulsa Branch, 1976–1999

1976–1977	Robert J. Capehart, M.D.
1977–1981	Roger C. Good, M.D.
1981–1982	Silvie L. Alfonso, M.D. (Interim)
1982–1988	Lesley L. Walls, M.D.
1988	Lester E. Krenning, M.D. (Interim)
1988–1991	Jon C. Calvert, M.D., Ph.D.
1991–1993	John W. Gastorf, Ph.D. (Interim)
1993–1999	Paul E. Tietze, M.D.
1999–	John W. Tipton, M.D. (Interim)

Appendix XXVII.
Chairs of the
Department of Internal Medicine—
Tulsa Branch, 1977–1999

1977	F. Daniel Duffy, M.D. (Interim)
1977–1996	F. Daniel Duffy, M.D.
1996–1999	Michel A. Weisz, M.D. (Interim)
1999–	Robert I. Wortmann, M.D.

Appendix XXVIII.
Chairs of the
Department of Obstetrics and
Gynecology—Tulsa Branch,
1975–1990

1975–1981	John B. Nettles, M.D.
1981–1982	Steven I. Saltzman, M.D. (Interim)
1982–1984	Donald R. Tredway, M.D.
1984–1985	Steven L. Saltzman, M.D. (Interim)
1985–1989	Steven L. Saltzman, M.D.
1989–1990	James H. Beeson, Ph.D., M.D. (Interim)
1990–	James H. Beeson, Ph.D., M.D.

Appendix XXIX.
Chairs of the
Department of Pediatrics—
Tulsa Branch, 1975–1996

1975–1996   Daniel C. Plunket, M.D.
1996–   Robert W. Block, M.D.

Appendix XXX.
Chairs of the
Department of Psychiatry—
Tulsa Branch, 1976–1997

1976–1985	James R. Allen, M.D.
1985–1986	Edward J. Tomsovic, M.D. (Interim)
1986–1988	Alan A. Lipton, M.D.
1988–1989	Edward J. Tomsovic, M.D. (Interim)
1989–1991	John T. (Tony) Brauchi, M.D. (Interim)
1991–1994	L. Blaine Shaffer, M.D. (Interim)
1994–1997	Milton C. Olsen, Ph.D. (Interim)
1997–	William R. Yeats, M.D.

Appendix XXXI.
Chairs of the
Department of Surgery—
Tulsa Branch, 1976–1997

1976–1981   James M. Guernsey, M.D.
1981–1984   Frank A. Clingan, M.D. (Interim)
1984–1996   Frank A. Clingan, M.D.
1997   J. Michael McGee, M.D. (Interim)
1997–   Thomas A. Broughan, M.D.

Appendix XXXII.
Chiefs of Staff of
University Hospital, 1963–2000

1963–1967	William A. Parry, M.D.
1967–1970	Ben Heller, M.D.
1970–1973	Gordon Deckert, M.D.
1973–1975	G. Rainey Williams, M.D.
1973	University Hospital Transferred to a Board of Trustees
1975–1977	Stanley Deutsch, M.D.
1977–1979	G. Rainey Williams, M.D.
1979–1980	James Merrill, M.D.
1980–1985	Mark Allen Everett, M.D. (Also CEO)
1980	University Hospital transferred to the Department of Human Services
1985–1990	D. Robert McCaffree, M.D. (Also CEO)
1990–1992	Russell G. Postier, M.D.
1992–1994	M. DeWayne Andrews, M.D.
1994–1996	M. Alex Jacocks, M.D.
1996	University Hospital transferred to University Hospitals Authority
1996–1998	Dwight W. Reynolds, M.D.
1998	University Hospital transferred to Columbia/HCA 1–1–98
1998–2000	Ronald Elkins, M.D.

Appendix XXXIII.
Administrators of the
"University Hospitals,"
1915–1979

SUPERINTENDENT (CEO)

1915–1931	LeRoy Long, M.D.
1931–1935	Wann Langston, M.D.
1935–1942	Robert Urie Patterson, M.D.
1942–1945	Thomas C. Lowry, M.D.
1945–1946	Wann Langston, M.D.
1946–1947	Jacques P. Gray, M.D.
1947–1957	Mark R. Everett, Ph.D.
1957	Dean becomes Director of Medical Center

MEDICAL DIRECTOR AND/OR ADMINISTRATOR

1946–1948	Robert C. Lowe
1948–1949	Vernon D. Cushing
1949–1958	Robert C. Lowe
1958–1965	Raymond Crews
1965–1973	Robert Terrill
1973	Transferred to University Hospital Authority
1973–1975	Jephtha Dalston
1975	Don Brown (interim)
1975–1979	Bruce M. Perry

Appendix XXXIV.
Administrators of
University Hospital since transfer
to DHS in 1980

1979	Donald L. Brown (Interim)
1980–1982	Donald L. Brown
1982–1983	James G. Borren
1984	Jimmie D. Scott (Interim)
1985–1986	Lyle Coit
1986–1988	Lowell Lenhart
1988	Robert McCaffree MD (Interim)
1989	Pam Troup (Interim)
1989–1990	Joel Hart
1991–1993	Ronald W. Stutes
1993–1994	M. DeWayne Andrews, M.D. (Interim)
1994–1999	Ronald W. Stutes

Appendix XXXV.
"CEO"s of Oklahoma Children's Memorial Hospital under the Department of Human Services, 1973–1998

1973–1983   Donald B. Halverstadt, M.D.
             (1980: Oklahoma Teaching Hospitals now includes University
             Hospital)
1983–1985   Owen R. Rennert, M.D. (Interim)
1985–1986   Antonio Padilla
1987   Bobby G. Thompson (Acting)
1988   Bobby G. Thompson
1988–1993   Andrew A. Lasser
             (1983: Transfer to Independent Hospital Authority in September)
1993–1998   R. Timothy Coussons, M.D.
1998–   Gerald J. Maier

Appendix XXXVI.
Hospital Administrators of Children's Hospital, 1974–1998

1974–1981	Ed Campbell
1980–1981	Lyle Coit
1982–1985	John Byrne
1985–1986	Don Doenitz
1986	Ed Finlay (Acting)
1987–1988	Andrew Lasser
1988	Robert Bonar (Acting)
1989–1991	Robert Bonar
1991–1998	Michael Noel
1998–	Sally Benn

Appendix XXXVII.
Chiefs of Staff of Children's Hospital, 1973–2001

1973–1980	Donald B. Halverstadt
1981–1987	Webb Thompson
1987–1989	Andy Sullivan
1989–1991	John Grunow
1991–1993	Joe C. Leonard
1993–1995	Tom Lera
1995–1997	Curtis Gruel
1997–1999	Morris Gessouroun
1999–2001	Andrew Walford

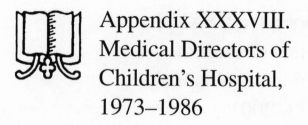 **Appendix XXXVIII.
Medical Directors of
Children's Hospital,
1973–1986**

1973–1975	Harris D. Riley
1975–1981	Webb Thompson
1981–1985	William Thurman
1986	Position discontinued.

Appendix XXXIX.
Chiefs of Staff of
O'Donoghue Rehabilitation
Center, 1980–1987

1980   Don H. O'Donoghue, M.D.
1980–1987   William G. Thurman, M.D.

Appendix XL.
Deans of the
College of Allied Health,
1970–1994

1970–1982   Philip E. Smith, Sc.D.
1982–1994   Lee Holder, Ph.D.
1994–   Carole A. Sullivan, Ph.D.

Appendix XLI.
Deans of the
College of Dentistry,
1969–1999

1969–1987	William E. Brown
1988–1999	Russell J. Stratton
1999	Stephen K. Young

Appendix XLII.
Deans and Directors of
the College of Nursing,
1911–1988

1911–1915	Annette Bourbon Cowles
1915–1916	Lucy Rennette Hill
1916	H. Mary Workman
1916–1919	Edna Holland
1919	Mary Ard McKenzie
1919–1924	Candice Monfort Lee
1924–1927	Ada Reitz Crocker
1928–1929	Mabel E. Smith
1929–1937	Candice Monfort Lee
1937–1941	Edythe Stith Triplett
1941–1943	Clara Marie Jackson Wangen
1943–1944	Kathlyn A. Krammes (LOA 1944–1945)
1944–1945	Clare Wolfe Jones (Acting)
1945–1947	Kathlyn A. Krammes
1947–1948	Ada Reitz Crocker (Acting)
1948–1951	Mary Rosch Caron
1951–1960	Ada Hawkins
1960–1969	Helen Patterson Chapman
1970–1973	Eleanor Knudson
1973–1975	Gloria R. Smith (Interim)
1975–1983	Gloria R. Smith
1984–1987	Lorraine Singer
1988	Constance Baker (Interim)
1988–	Patricia R. Forni

Appendix XLIII.
Deans of the
College of Pharmacy,
1893–1997

1893–1904	Edwin C. DeBarr
1904–1912	Homer Charles Washburn (LOA 1911–1912)
1911–1912	Edwin C. DeBarr (Acting)
1912–1917	Charles Howard Stocking
1917–1919	Howard Storm Browne
1919–1949	D. B. R. Johnson
1949–1962	Ralph William Clark
1962–1963	E. Blanche Sommers (Acting)
1963–1970	Loyd E. Harris
1970–1975	Charles W. Blissitt
1975–1976	John R. Sokatch (Interim)
1976–1983	Rodney D. Ice
1983–1985	H. Richard Shough (Interim)
1985–1996	Victor A. Yanchick
1997–	Carl K. Buckner

Appendix XLIV.
Deans of the
College of Public Health,
1967–1994

1967–1973   William Schottstaedt, M.D. (First Dean, School of Public
             Health)
1973–1981   Philip Smith, Sc.D. (With Allied Health in College of Health)
1978–1981   Paul Anderson, Ph.D. (Head, Division of Public Health)
1982–1984   Peter J. Levin, Sc.D. (College of Public Health)
1984–1989   Charles Cameron, Ph.D.
1990–1994   Bailus Walker, Ph.D.
1994–   Elisa T. Lee, Ph.D.

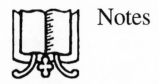 Notes

CHAPTER I. PASSING THE TORCH

1. At this point in history, the Oklahoma City campus of the University of Oklahoma consisted of the School of Medicine, the School of Nursing, the Crippled Children's Hospital, University Hospital ("Old Main"), and the Speech and Hearing Clinic. These were known collectively as the "Medical Center." The Dean of the School of Medicine served also as the Director of the Medical Center and its constituent institutions, and as such reported directly to the President of the University of Oklahoma. Also on the Oklahoma City campus were the Veterans Administration Hospital and the Oklahoma Medical Research Foundation, each an independent institution. In November 1971, the State Regents for Higher Education and the University of Oklahoma Board of Regents, reacting to the arrival of additional educational components on the Oklahoma City campus (e.g., the Dean A. McGee Eye Institute and Presbyterian Hospital), changed the designation of University components from "schools" to "colleges," and the name of the Medical Center itself to the "University of Oklahoma Health Sciences Center." In 1967, the title "Dean and Director" (created in 1957) was changed to "Dean, Director and Vice President." Later, in 1970, the title was changed to "Executive Vice President" and, later again, in 1973, to "Provost of the Health Sciences Center." In 1966, the "Oklahoma Health Center" had been incorporated by a group of interested Oklahoma City businessmen, the Oklahoma City Chamber of Commerce, and leaders of other institutions on the campus as an umbrella organization to coordinate activities of all institutions on the campus. The Board of Regents never formally acknowledged the primacy of the "Oklahoma Health Center" concept, however, and the official name continued to be the University of Oklahoma Health Sciences Center.

2. Mark R. Everett and Alice A. Everett, *Medical Education in Oklahoma, Vol. II, The University of Oklahoma School of Medicine and Medical Center, 1932–1964,* University of Oklahoma Press, Norman, OK, 1980, p. 313.

3. Ibid.

4. Ibid., p. 314.

5. Lloyd Rader, Comment to the authors, Oklahoma City, 1979.

6. Everett, op, cit., p. 314.

7. Rader, op. cit.

8. Rader, op. cit., 1981.

9. John Schilling, quoted by Robert Hardy in *HERO: An Oral History of the Oklahoma Health Center*, published by Robert Hardy, Oklahoma City, 1985, p. 17.

10. Everett, op. cit., p. 351.

11. Raymond Crews, quoted by Robert Hardy, p. 18.

12. John Schilling, quoted by Robert Hardy, ibid.

13. Stewart Wolf, Interview by author, Oklahoma City, 1997.

14. Harris "Pete" Riley, Interview by author, Oklahoma City, 1997.

15. Merlin DuVal, *Memorandum* to Rainey Williams, Oklahoma City, September 1994.

16. University of Oklahoma Medical Alumni Association, *Analysis*, Oklahoma City, March 26, 1963.

17. Everett, op. cit., p. 349.

18. Ibid., p. 347.

19. Ibid., p. 350.

20. Ibid., p. 348.

21. Ibid., p. 349.

22. Ibid., p. 348.

23. Ibid., p. 350.

CHAPTER II.

EXPANSION AND STRUGGLE

1. Stewart Wolf, Interview by author, Oklahoma City, 1997.

2. G. Rainey Williams, Interview by author, Oklahoma City, 1997.

3. William G. Thurman, Interview by author, Oklahoma City, 1998.

4. Stewart Wolf, op cit.

5. William G. Thurman, op. cit.

6. Ronald Elkins, Interview by author, Oklahoma City, 1999.

7. Boyd Gunning, *Minutes*, University of Oklahoma Foundation, Oklahoma City, May 1968.

8. Julian Rothbaum, Interview by author, Tulsa, OK, 1997.

9. John Kirkpatrick, Comment to the author, Oklahoma City, April 1998.

10. William G. Thurman, op. cit.

11. Julian Rothbaum, op. cit.

CHAPTER III. STRIFE IN THE EXECUTIVE SUITES

1. James Merrill, Interview by author, San Francisco, CA, 1998.
2. Thomas Lynn, Interview by author, Oklahoma City, 1999.
3. William Thurman, Interview by author, Oklahoma City, 1997.
4. Jeptha Dalston, "What Happened?", Paper delivered June 26, Oklahoma City, 1973.
5. Bruce Perry, Comment to the author, Oklahoma City, 1999.
6. Harris D. "Pete" Riley, Interview by author, Oklahoma City, 1997.
7. Ibid.
8. William Thurman, op. cit.
9. Gordon Deckert, Interview by author, Oklahoma City, 1997.
10. *Minutes*, Trust Fund Administrators, University of Oklahoma Health Sciences Center, Oklahoma City, November 17, 1972.
11. Bylaws, University of Oklahoma School of Medicine, Oklahoma City, 1971.
12. Baldwin G. Lamson, "Report on the University of Oklahoma College of Medicine," Oklahoma City, June 1, 1972.
13. James Merrill, op. cit.
14. Julian Rothbaum, Interview by author, Tulsa, OK, 1997.
15. William Thurman, op. cit.
16. Ibid.
17. Raymond Crews as told to William Thurman, op. cit.
18. Ron Elkins, Interview by author, Oklahoma City, 1999.
19. William Thurman, op. cit.
20. Vera Alder, Interview by author, Hugo, OK, 1996.
21. Ibid.
22. Harris D. "Pete" Riley, op. cit.
23. Donald B. Halverstadt, Interview by author, Oklahoma City, 1998.
24. Vera Alder, op. cit.
25. John Schilling, Letter to Paul Sharp, Oklahoma City, October 30, 1973.
26. John Schilling, Letter to Paul Sharp, Oklahoma City, April 12, 1974.
27. John Schilling, Letter to David Hall, Oklahoma City, October 30, 1974.
28. John Schilling, Letter to David Hall, Oklahoma City, March 14, 1973.
29. *Minutes*, Department of Surgery, University of Oklahoma Health Sciences Center, Oklahoma City, October 29, 1974.
30. Thomas Lynn, op. cit.
31. Ibid.
32. James Merrill, Interview, op. cit.
33. Harris D. "Pete" Riley, op. cit.
34. Thomas Lynn, op. cit.
35. Ronald Elkins, op. cit.

36. Donald B. Halverstadt, op. cit.

37. Ibid.

38. Lloyd Rader as quoted by Donald Halverstadt, op. cit.

39. Julian Rothbaum, op. cit.

40. Mark Allen Everett, Personal reminiscence, Oklahoma City, 1997.

41. James Merrill, op. cit.

CHAPTER IV. THE PROVOST GOVERNS

1. William G. Thurman, Interview by author, Oklahoma City, 1998.

2. Mark R. Everett, "By-Laws of the OMRF," *Pioneering for Research*, 1966, University of Oklahoma Medical Center, p. 34.

3. Ibid.

4. Ibid.

5. William G. Thurman, Letter to Dr. Mark A. Everett, Oklahoma City, March 19, 1976.

6. William G. Thurman, Letter to Dr. Mark A. Everett, Oklahoma City, September 9, 1975.

7. James Merrill, Letter to the University of Oklahoma Health Sciences Center Faculty Board, Oklahoma City, September 11, 1974.

8. William G. Thurman, Interview, op. cit.

9. Solomon Papper, Letter to Dr. Mark A. Everett, Oklahoma City, April 8, 1975.

10. Rainey Williams, Interview by author, Oklahoma City, 1998.

11. Oscar Parsons, Interview by author, Oklahoma City, 1998.

12. William G. Thurman, Interview, op. cit.

13. Oscar Parsons, op. cit.

14. William G. Thurman, Letter to Dr. Mark A. Everett, Oklahoma City, June 3, 1977.

15. Edgar B. Young, Letter to Dr. Mark A. Everett, Oklahoma City, July 26, 1978.

16. William G. Thurman, Letter to Dr. Mark A. Everett, Oklahoma City, April 1978.

17. Basic Science Department Chairs Meeting, *Minutes*, March-May 1977.

18. Thomas N. Lynn, Letter to College of Medicine Department Chairs, Oklahoma City, May 11, 1978.

19. Thomas N. Lynn, Interview by author, Oklahoma City, 1999.

20. Peggy Culver, Letter to Dean Thomas Lynn, Oklahoma City, August 19, 1977.

21. David Mock, Letter to Dr. Mark A. Everett, Oklahoma City, August 15, 1977.

22. Paul Sharp, Letter to Dr. William Thurman, Norman, OK, December 9, 1977.

23. Thomas Lynn, Interview, op. cit.

24. Liaison Committee on Medical Education, *Report of Survey of December 12–16, 1976*, Oklahoma City, February 28, 1978.

25. William G. Thurman, Letter to Dr. Mark A. Everett, Oklahoma City, April 20, 1977.

26. Third-Year Promotion Committee, *Minutes*, University of Oklahoma College of Medicine, June 6, 1977.

27. William G. Thurman, Letter to Dr. Mark A. Everett, Oklahoma City, June 1, 1978.

28. Mark A. Everett, *Memorandum* to Dr. William Thurman, Oklahoma City, June 3, 1978.

29. Thomas Lynn, Interview, op. cit.

30. William G. Thurman, Letter to Dr. Paul Sharp, Oklahoma City, June 19, 1978.

31. Paul Sharp, Letter to Dr. Mark Everett, Norman, OK, October 31, 1978.

32. Robert G. Mitchell, Letter to Dr. Mark Everett, Oklahoma City, October 31, 1978.

33. William G. Thurman, Letter to Dr. Mark Everett, Oklahoma City, October 31, 1978.

34. Mark A. Everett, Letter to Dr. William G. Thurman, Oklahoma City, November 7, 1978.

35. William G. Thurman, Letter to Dr. Mark A. Everett, Oklahoma City, February 23, 1979.

36. Thomas Lynn, Interview, op. cit.

37. Joseph Kopta, Interview by author, Oklahoma City, 1999.

38. *Minutes* of the General Faculty, University of Oklahoma Health Sciences Center, May 31, 1978.

39. Donald Halverstadt, Interview by author, Oklahoma City, October 1997.

40. William G. Thurman, Letter to Dr. Mark A. Everett, Oklahoma City, December 14, 1978.

41. William G. Thurman, Letter to Dr. Robert Keim, Oklahoma City, January 11, 1978.

42. Thomas Lynn, Interview, op. cit.

43. Ibid.

44. Julian Rothbaum, Interview by author, Tulsa, OK, 1998.

45. Ibid.

46. Nancy Hall, *Memorandum* to Dr. Mark A. Everett, Oklahoma City, December 1, 1977.

CHAPTER V. STORMS IN THE SEA OF TRANQUILITY

1. Donald Halverstadt, Interview by author, Oklahoma City, 1998.

2. Ibid.

3. Ibid.

4. Ibid.

5. Thomas Lynn, Interview by author, Oklahoma City, 1999.

6. Ibid.

7. University of Oklahoma Health Sciences Center Academic Program Council, *Memorandum* to Provost Clayton Rich, Oklahoma City, December 2, 1980.

8. University of Oklahoma Health Sciences Center Faculty Board, *Letter* to Dr. G. Rainey Williams, Oklahoma City, January 21, 1981.

9. Dean Harber, Reminiscence shared with the author, Oklahoma City, 1997.

10. Joseph Kopta, Interview by author, Oklahoma City, 1999.

11. Robert Fulton, Letter to Antonio Padilla, Oklahoma City, May 17, 1985.

12. Mark Allen Everett, Letter to Robert Fulton, May 18, 1985.

13. Joseph Kopta, Letter to Robert Fulton, Oklahoma City, May 20, 1985.

14. Bill Sylvester, Reminiscence shared with the author, Oklahoma City, 1997.

15. Joseph Kopta, Interview, op. cit.

16. Patrick McKee, Interview by author, Los Angeles, CA, 1998.

17. Ibid.

18. Joseph Kopta, Interview, op. cit.

19. Patrick McKee, op. cit.

20. Ibid.

21. Joseph Kopta, Interview, op. cit.

22. Ibid.

23. Thomas Lynn, Interview by author, Oklahoma City, 1999.

24. Donald Kassebaum, *Memorandum* to Dr. John Fishburne, Oklahoma City, January 4, 1988.

25. Patrick McKee, op. cit.

26. Dan Little, as reported by Patrick McKee, op. cit.

27. Patrick McKee, op. cit.

28. Ibid.

29. Joseph Kopta, Interview, op. cit.

CHAPTER VI. THE NEW CEOS

1. Mark Allen Everett, *Personal Recollection*, Oklahoma City, 1997.

2. Ron Elkins, Interview by author, Oklahoma City, 1999.

3. Donald B. Halverstadt, Interview by author, Oklahoma City, 1998.

4. Joseph Kopta, Interview by author, Oklahoma City, 1999.

5. Ibid.

6. R. Timothy Coussons, Interview by author, Oklahoma City, 1999.

7. Ron Gillum, *Reminiscence* with the author, Oklahoma City, 1997.

8. Douglas Voth, as reported by Patrick A. McKee, Interview by author, Oklahoma City, 1998.

9. G. Rainey Williams, Interview by author, Oklahoma City, 1998.

10. University of Oklahoma Health Sciences Center, *Notes*, Oklahoma City, Spring 1998.

11. Ron Elkins, op. cit.

Index of Persons

Acers, Thomas, 84, 247, 321
Albert, Carl, 106
Alder, Vera, 100, 106, *298*
Alexander, Leland, 114
Altmiller, Dale, 207
Altshuler, Geoffrey, 207, 217
Andrews, M. DeWayne, 218, 225
Anthony, Robert H., 226
Atkins, Hannah, 100, 157
Atkinson, Gordon, 151

Baggett, Bryce, 25, 31, 32
Bailey, Kenneth D., 144
Balyeat, Ray, 43
Banowsky, William, 43, 176–177, 178, 182, 185, 198, 205, 216, 220, 228, *298*
Barnes, Reginald, 227
Bartlett, Dewey, 32, 37, 46, 49
Bayley, Robert H., 37

Bell, Richard A., 144, 166, 183, 196, 199
Bell, William, 254
Bellmon, Henry, 17, 26, 28, 149, 214, 253, 260, 265, 270, 271
Bielstein, Charles, 23
Bircher, Andrea, 126, 313
Bird, Robert Montgomery, 21, 36, *56*, 62, 65, 91–93, 94, 103, 117, 127
Blacket, Piers, 207
Blankenship, G. T., 529
Bogardus, Carl, 287, 330
Boren, David, 12, 124, 151, 184, 265, 289, 308, 322, 327, 328, 331, *339*
Bozalis, George and John, 228
Braly, Mack, 103, 144, 153
Brandt, Edward N., 34, 36, 49, 43, 239, 269, 284, *304*, 305–306, 308
Brandt, Joseph A., 228
Brann, Alfred W. Jr., 315
Brawner, Donald, 121
Brawner, Larry, 311
Brett, Thomas R., 104, 110, 119, 144, 150
Brett, Tom, 104, 110, 119, 144, 150
Brisch, Hans, 208, 289, *304*
Brooks, Harold, 290
Brown, Charles R., 269
Brown, Don, 148
Brown, Irwin, 152

Brown, William, 39, 101, 260, *303*
Bruce, Thomas, 36, 116, 143
Bryan, Willie, 184
Bulmer, Glen S., 264
Burgdorf, Hans Conrad Walter, 207, 225
Byrne, John, 224

Cain, William Morgan, 23
Calhoon, Ed, 254, 272
Calvert, Horace K., 48
Cameron, Charles, 225
Campbell, J. Moore, 289
Cannon, Jay, 226
Chase, John D., 37
Clay, Richard A., 23, 35
Clingen, Frank, 157
Cloninger, C. Robert, 257
Coalson, Jackie, 110, 176, 182
Cohen, Wilbur J., 8ff
Colmore, John, 45, 49
Comp, Phillip, 284
Condit, Paul, 94
Cornelison, Raymond, 78
Counihan, Donald, 126, 180
Coussons, Harriett, 115
Coussons, Richard Timothy, 36, 110, 126, 148, 220, 224, 233, 238, 258, 265, 319–320, 312, *338*
Crews, Raymond, 3, 35, 91
Cross, George, 13, 17, 32, *58*, 62, 140, 156
Crowe, William, 28

Dalston, Jephtha, 4, 102, 147
Davies, Nancy J., 74, 192, 254
Dean, John, 84, 110
Deckert, Gordon, 39, 79, 82, *130*, 156, 159, 171, 205, 219, 258, 279, 305, 334
Dee, A. L., 34
Dennis, James L., 18, 21ff, 33, 35ff, 45ff, *56*, 64, 116, 143, 343

Deutsch, Stanley, 148, 212
Drake, Lynn, 334
Duffy, F. Daniel, 178, 183, 207, 272, 279, 334
Dumas, Jack, 88, 97
Dunlap, E. T., 11ff, 15, *53*, 88, 154, 166, 186, 200, 208, 313
DuVal, Merlin K., 14, 44, 77, 344

Edmundson, J. Howard, 75
Edwards, Archibald C., 127
Eliel, Leonard, 50, 60, 63, 67, 68, 78, 81, 91, 101, 111, 116
Elkins, Ronald, 27, 80, 85, 92, 108, 117, 312, 337
Ellis, Robert, 27, 43
Elwood, Robin, 309
Epstein, Robert, 235, 240
Everest, Harvey, 44
Everest, Jimmy, 325
Everett, Alice, 7, 17, 114, 218, 274
Everett, Mark Allen, 19, 37, 42, 51, 63ff, 67, 82, 94, 124, 126, *129*, 149, 159, 168, 170ff, 182, 207, 212, 224, 279, 309, 320, 327, 333, 334
Everett, Mark R., 7ff,17–20, 25, 51, *52*, 57, 58, 62, 140, 343ff

Fagraeus, Lennert, 212
Farley, Jerry B., 275, 284, 313
Felts, William J., 149
Ferretti, Joseph, 70, 333–334, 337, *341*, 343ff
Ferretti, Martha, 148, 183, 207
Fine, Douglas, 335
Fishburne, John, 225
Fitzpatrick, Martin, 114, 143, 151, 168
Fleischaker, Richard, 43, 277, 337
Foerster, Hervey, 278–279
Foreman, Robert, 229, 279
Forni, Patricia Brown, 268

Fulton, Robert, 219, 227, 229ff, 252, 258
Furman, Robert, 44

Gade, Nancy, 51
Gammill, John S., 289
Garrison, George, 149, 156, 218, 243, *302*
Gathman, LeRoy, 258
Gavin, James R., 273, 319
Gaylord, Edward K. II, 224
Gaylord, Edward L., 213
Gilmartin, Richard, 115
Godkins, Thomas, 307
Good, Robert A., 207, 220
Gorsline, Lester, 23, 27
Green, Jeanne, 35, 36
Greenfield, Lazar, 117
Gullatt, E. Murray, 311
Gumerson, Jean, 324, 326
Gunn, C. G., 36

Hall, David, 74, 78, 90, 92, 107
Hall, Nancy, 222, 225, 242, 265, 286
Halverstadt, Donald B., 36, 95, 101, 110, 118–119, 135, 177, 178, 185, 188, 196–197, 200ff, 211, 218, 220, 240, 254, 272, 311, 313, *338*
Hamilton, James, 88, 99,102, 106, 121, 255, 316
Hammarsten, James, 35, 163–164, 169; Award, 279
Hardy, Robert C., 91
Hartsuck, James, 117
Hazel, Onis, 140
Heller, Ben, 19, 67
Hemstreet, George, 320, 326
Henry, Jay, 111
Hensley, Jess, 222, 240
Hill, Anita, 291
Hobbs, Dan, 255, 259
Hogan, Sarah, 237, 321

Holliman, John, 235, 279
Holloman, Herbert, 33, 35, 37–38, 43, 45ff, 59
Horton, Frank, 236, 237, 244, 247, 252, 265–266
Howard, Gene, 121
Hudson, Katherine, 176
Huffman, Huston, 74, 84, 94
Hunter, David, 225
Hurst, Irvin, 29

Jackman, Warren 321
Jackson, Phil, 51
Jacobson, Eugene, 36, 67
Jacocks, M. Alex, 277
James, Frank, 243
Janike, Michael, 257
Jimerson, Gordon, 160
Jiske, Martin 229, 236
Joel, Walter, 37, 169
Johnson, B. Connor, 34, 207
Johnson, Mark R., 18, 187
Jonas, Pau,l 329
Jones, Dorothy, 100
Jones, Phyllis, 264
Joullian, Edward, 283

Kaplan, David, 224
Kassebaum, Donald G., 63, 113, 246–247, 252, 257–258, 265, 302
Keating, Frank, 328
Keim, Robert, 180–182
Kemp, Thomas Elwood, 237–238, 252, 254–256, 264, 266, 272
Kerr, Joffa, 272
Key, Janet, 183
Keys, John, 168
Killackey, Jim, 223, 225, 320
Kimmelstiel, Paul, 35–36
Kirkpatrick, John, 39
Klinka, Karen, 320
Knisley, William H., 275–276

Kopta, Joseph, 65, 174–175, 227, 231–232, 235, 251, *300*
Krug, Ronald, 258
Kurtz, Alton, 156

Lachman, Anya, 22
Lachman, Ernst, 22, 32–33, 183, 184
Lamb, John, 140
Lasser, Andrew, 258–259
Lazzara, Ralph, 273
Lee, Joseph, 205
Lee, Lela, 287
Lemons, Mark, 268
Leonard, Joseph, 181, 185
Leone, Joe, 208, 223, 252, 255
Lester, Boyd, 160
Levine, Norman, 218
Lewis, Sylvia, 272
Lienke, Roger, 72
Little, Dan, 281
Lockhard, Vernon M., 187
Love, F. C., 80
Lynn, Thomas N. Jr., 36, 111, 117, 124–125, 127, *135*, 138, 163, 168, 170, 184–185, 202–203, 204, 219, 252

Macer, Dan, 110, 152
Markland, Loy, 114–115
McCaffree, Robert, 226
McCall, Charles B., 179, 183, 210, 234, *297*
McCarter, "Pete," 35
McCreight, William George, 200
McGee, Dean A., 27, 228, 275
McGee, Reese, 50
McHale, Phi,l 279
McKee, Patrick, 63, 218, 224, 233–34, 240–241, 263, 264, 271, 279, 284, *301*, 330–331, 344
McLeod, Colin, 44
Medina, Jesus, 283, 287

Meo, Mark, 317–318
Merrill, James, 21, 63, 65, 80, 85, 94, 116, 121, 125, 143, 149, 165, 194, 205, 215–216
Metcoff, Jack, 45, 115
Middleton, Wiliam S., 23
Miller, Dorothy, 243
Miller, Ed, 266, 281
Miller, George, 93, 99, 322
Mitchell, Robert (Bob) G., 78, 109–110, 119, 144, 173, 182, 188
Mock, David, 45, 65
Monroe, Eph, 110, 138
Monson, Angela, 324
Moran, Willard, 179
Morris, J. R., 178, 217, 223, 322
Morrone, Jeanette, 30
Murray, Johnston, 75

Near, Harry, 156
Neely, J. Gail, 219
Neustadt, Walter Jr., 150, 156
Nichols, Michael, 122
Nicholson, Ben, 23, 63
Nigh, George, 196, 214, 219, 227, 243
Nitschke, Ruprecht, 325
Noble, Mary Jane, 254
Noble, Sam, 272
Nordby, Eugene, 39, 110, 126–127

O'Donoghue, Don H., 63, 125, 148, 175, *194*, 228, 290
Ockershauser, Kurt F., 168
Ordway, Nelson, 35

Padilla, Antonio, 226, 252, 258
Papper, Solomon, 164, 183, 185–186, 206, 224
Parke, David W. II, 288
Parrington, Vernon, 150
Parrish, Jack Walker, 183, 202
Parry, William, 288

Parsons, Oscar, 28, 125, 126, 156, 260, 288
Patnode, Robert, 149, 220
Patrick, Imogene, 320
Payne, Hugh, 50
Perry, Bruce, 75, 148, 156
Pfundt, Theodore, 115
Points, Thomas, 72
Porter, E. Melvin, 41, 122, 123, 242
Postier, Russell, 226, 230
Pumpian-Mindlin, Eugene, 39

Rader, Lloyd, 8ff, 23, 27, 75–76, 83, 89, 100, 106, 110, *130*, 178, 188, 197, 208–209, 213–214, 232, 251–252, 225, *300*, *303*
Ramsey, Christian, 207, 211, 227, 312, 315
Randel, Roger, 260
Reichlin, Morris, 287
Rennert, Owen, 115, 224, 226
Replogle, Dee A. Jr., 150, 154–155, 181, 185, *192*, 206, 211–212
Reynolds, Dwight, 240
Rhoades, Everett, 67
Rich, Clayton, 64, 186, *195*, 212, 238, 247, 248, 269, 276, 284, 292–293
Riley, Harris D. "Pete," 13, 21, 70, 76, 100, 115, 117, 225
Ritzhaupt, Louis, 15, 27, 70
Roberts, Alex, 264
Rogers, Gerald, 218
Rothbaum, Julian J., 24, 38, 87, 182, 185
Rucks, William, 23
Rumsey,Virginia Briscoe, 283

Santee, Jack H., 119, 138, 143
Sarratt, Charles F., 237–238, 266, 272
Saunders, John, 115
Schilling, John, 10, 13, 21, *54*, 63, 80, 82, 85, 105, 107, 111ff

Schmidt, James, 223
Schottstaedt, Mary Frances, 70
Schottstaedt, William, 35, 37, 117, 125
Scott, L. Vernon, 149, 218, 220
Sears, Bertram, 212
Seeley, Rodman, 183, 186
Serwer, Milton, 202
Sharp, Paul, 34, 66, 84, 95, 101, 108, 121, *129*, 151, 155
Sharp, Rose, 66, 68, 95
Shedrick, Bernice, 281
Shidler, Joy Ann, 326
Shurley, Jay T., 207
Siegfried, Robin, 329
Silva, Fred, 64, 259
Singer, Lorraine, 225, 253
Sipuel, Ada Lois, 310
Smalley, Phil, 88, 99, 102
Smith, Finis, 87–88
Smith, Gary, 71, 127, 200, 260, 268
Smith, Gloria, 148
Smith, Jerry, 148
Smith, Phillip E., 125, 212, 219
Smith, W. O., 148
Snow, James B. Jr., 19, 21, 83, 179
Sokatch, John R., 219, 225, 227
Sparks, Ruben, 40
Splinter, Garth, 312
Stansberry, Richard, 15, 27, 36, 37, 99
Steen, Wilson D., 91, 154
Stein, Jay, 258, 305ff, 325, 330–333, *338*, 344
Stone, S. N. "Newt," 17
Stratton, Russell Jr., 261
Stump, Ralph, 35
Stutes, Ronald W., 327
Sullivan, J. Andy, 290
Swank, David, 265

Tang, Jordan, 290
Terrill, Al, 147, 158
Terrill, Robert, 23, 35

Thomas, Ella, 115
Thompson, Bobby G., 258
Thompson, Webb M. Jr., 260, 264
Thurman, William, 26, 64, 79, 87,
　139ff, 148, 159, 164, 166, 168, 177,
　179ff, 184–185, *190*, *195*, 206, 344
Tillinghast, John, 231
Tomasek, James, 321
Tompkins, Robert G., 283
Tomsovic, Edward J., 181, 205, 282
Towle, William F., 222
Traub, Sidney, 19, 156, 328
Travis, Paul, 309
Tucker, Thomas, 110

Unger, Leon, 310

Van Horn, Richard L., 273, 305–307,
　317
Vannatta, Jerry B., 253, 333, 337, *341*,
　343ff
Voth, Douglas, 116, 308, 330–331, 333,
　338

Walters, David, 200, 212, 242, 282,
　311, 322, 327, 328
Warren, W. K., 254
Watson, Phil, 276
Weinberger, Casper, 106
Weiss, Kurt, 34, 156, 253
Wenzel, James, 269

West, Kelly M., 202
West, Louis Jolyon, 21, 31, 39, 152
Westermeyer, Joseph, 258
Whitcomb, Walter, 34, 186
White, Clayton S., 116
White, Joseph, 19, 36
White, Ronald H., 163, 188, 272, 286
Wiegand, Dennis Allen, 63, 279
Wilkinson, Carol, 228
Williams, G. Rainey, 26, 64, 68, 87–88,
　111–112, 117, *133*, 138, 146, 148,
　204, 225, 234, 243, 265, 266, 333,
　334, 336, 343
Williams, John Day, 90
Williams, Martha, 113–114, 228, 274
Williams, Victor, 188, 286
Willis, William P., 88, 99
Wizenberg, Morris J., 174
Wolf, Stewart, 13, 17, 21, 25, 26, 43,
　44, 57, 102, 289
Woodson, Fred, 140
Wright, Logan, 186

Yanchic, Victor, 225
Yordi, Ron, 318
Young, Stanton, 27, 39–40, *137*, 219,
　223, 236, 243, 286, 326
Young, Stephen, 207

Zahasky, Mary, 108–109
Zallen, Harold, 126–127

General Index

Italicized page numbers indicate illustrations.

Academic Council. *See* Faculty Board
Affirmative Action (desegregation), 161–162, 245–246, 265, 335
Agency Special Accounts, 256
Anatomical Science, Department of, chairs, 351
Anesthesiology, Department of, chairs, 352
Animal Research Facilities, 175, 205, 249
Anthony Foundation, 286

Basic Sciences Education Building, 30, 55
"Best Doctors in America," 290
Biochemistry Department, 36; chairs, 353
Biomedical Research Building (Stanton Young Building), 268, 277, 283, 306, 310, 326, 334–335
Biomedical Sciences Building, 65, 105, 149
Bird Library, 65, 142, 150, 178, 285–286, *296*, 313
Bizzell Library, 28
Bond Issues, 14ff, 21, 34, 38, 306; HERO, 34, 102

Bone Marrow Transplants, 235, 240, 253

Center for Molecular Medicine, 259, 284–285
Central Billing, 108
Central Oklahoma Parking and Transportation Authority (COPTA), 83
Chamber of Commerce, 109, 281
Child Study Center, 85, 114–115, 134, 328
Children's Hospital, 27–28, 55, 74, 77, 89, 94, 100, 106, 107, 131–132, 178, 196, 225, 235, *314*; Cancer Center-Jimmy Everest, 325; Chief Executive Officers, 383; Chiefs of Staff, 385; Medical Directors, 386;
Children's Medical Center, Tulsa, 147
Children's Medical Research, 218, 224, 225, 283, 286
Cogeneration Project, 244, 267
College of Allied Health, 105, 125, 151, 204, 212, *295*; deans, 388
College of Dentistry, 34, 66, 261, 270; deans, 389
College of Health, 29, 34, 35, 105, 125, 204, 220, 225, *295*, 323; deans, 392
College of Medicine, admissions, 69, 70, 166, 167, 273; admissions board, 96, 162; budget, 160–161, 165,

238–239, 244, 261; by-laws, 143;
class size, 69, 189; curriculum, 153,
162; dean(s), 4, 347–348; managed
care, 315, 324; Nichols Hills House,
36; "resignations," 308, 315; tuition,
153, 165, 208; Upjohn Gift, 286;
vacancies (Dept chairs), 318. *See
also* Faculty Board
College of Nursing, 29, 142, 169, 225,
268, *295*; deans, 390
College of Pharmacy, 50, 209, 220,
225, 264, *296*; deans, 391
Colleges, Schools to, 68
Columbia-Presbyterian merger with
University Hospitals, 330
Commencement, 33
Crippled Children's Commission, 75
Cytodiagnostics. *See* Urocorps

Daily Oklahoman, 177, 223, 226, 255,
320
Dean A. McGee Eye Institute, 27, 77,
86, 109, 126, 151, 158, 160, 193,
265, 278
Degree Granting Controversy
("Patterson Case"), 166, 169ff
Dermatology Building, 59, 208, 286,
307
Dermatology, Department, 41–42, 288;
chairs, 354
Dermatopathology, 276
Desegregation. *See* Affirmative Action
Dialysis, 328
Draper, Dan, 208

Emergency Medicine, 149
Endowed Chairs Program, 186, 241,
266, 268–269, 276, 277, 283, 289,
313, 326, 328
Enid, 157
"Evening of Excellence," 228, 243,
283, 289, 309–410

Eye Institute. *See* Dean A. McGee Eye
Institute

Faculty Board, 63, 110–111, 140ff,
157ff, 161, 280–281; Academic
Council, 143, 147, 156; chairs, 349;
vs. Provost, 164, 168, 170ff,
180–181
Faculty House, 29
Family Medicine, 31, 67, 70, 71ff, 102,
109, 157, 176, 183, 201–202, 207,
211, 224, 229, 246, 259, 264, 268,
277, 283, 288, 306, 309, 328, 335,
340; chairs, 355–356; laboratory, 282
Family Medicine, Tulsa, chairs, 374
Family Practice. *See* Family Medicine

"Gang of Five," 282, 318
Griffin Memorial Hospital, 85, 147,
229, 243
Gynecology and Obstetrics, chairs,
357

Hemstreet, George, 320
Herman Smith Study, 88, 97ff, 108;
Dumas Report, 97
Herzog Foundation and Chair, 269
Hillcrest Hospital, 147
House Bill 1017, 288–289
Hudgins-Tompkins-Ball, 70
Human Services, Department of
(DISRS, Welfare), 41, 107, 140, 187,
196–197, 201, 208, 214, 219, 227,
242, 276, 316–317; Master
Reimbursement Contract (Medicine),
242; "transfer" of funds from
University Hospital, 289. *See also*
Rader, Lloyd

Interim Building, 71
Internal Medicine, Tulsa, chairs, 375
Internal Revenue Service, 278

Kaludis Study, 321–322

Laboratory Medicine, chair, 365
Lamson Report, 82
Liaison Committee for Medical
    Education (LCME), 168, 204, 264

Magnetic Resonance Imaging (MRI),
    225
Malpractice Insurance, 309
"Managed Care," 315, 324
Master Teacher Award (Stanton
    Young), 219, 223, 235, 242, 272,
    277, 286, 310, 321
Medicaid, 324, 329
Medical Technology and Research
    Authority of Oklahoma (MTRA),
    318–319, 321, 323–324
Medicine, Department chairs, 358
Medi-Flight, 212–213, 297
Mercy Hospital, 30
M.D./Ph.D. Program, 285
Microbiology and Immunology,
    Department, chairs, 359
Moon School, 116, 126
Murrah Federal Building—Oklahoma
    City Bombing, 329–330, 340

National Board of Medical Examiners
    (NRMB Examination), 64ff,
    110–111, 138, 163, 165, 205, 207,
    257, 262
National Institutes of Health, 8, 65, 69,
    115, 285
Neurology Department, 37; chairs,
    360
Noble Foundation, 285, 308, 325

Obstetrics, 225; Tulsa department
    chairs, 376
O'Donoghue Rehabilitation Center,
    271, 328; Chiefs of Staff, 387

Oklahoma Academy of General
    Practice, 18
Oklahoma Asthma and Allergy Clinic,
    194, 201
Oklahoma Center for Advancement of
    Science and Technology (OCAST),
    262–263, 264, 272, 285, 287, 306,
    320–321
Oklahoma City Clinic, 23, *60*
Oklahoma City Urban Renewal
    Authority, 27, 28, 281
Oklahoma Health Care Authority,
    324
Oklahoma Health Center Foundation,
    26, 27, 31, 318
Oklahoma Health Sciences Facilities,
    Inc., 83, 178, 200, 220, 232, 334
Oklahoma Medical Alumni
    Association, 27, 38
Oklahoma Medical Research
    Foundation, 19, 50, 94, 140ff, 158,
    165, 200, 211, 284, 290, *294*;
    Physicians' Trust Fund, 80
Oklahoma Memorial Hospital. *See*
    University Hospital
Oklahoma Model for Medical
    Education (OMME-21),
    279–280
Oklahoma Museum of Natural History
    (Noble, Stoval), 276
Oklahoma Regional Medical Program,
    40–41
Oklahoma School of Science and
    Mathematics, 259, 281
Ophthalmology, Department, chairs,
    361; chairs, Tulsa, 376. *See also*
    Dean A. McGee Eye Institute
Oral Roberts School of Medicine, 166,
    275
Oral Surgery, 218
Orthopedic Department, 125, 182, 290,
    308; chairs 362

Osteopathic Medicine, 166, 219, 260, 270, 273
Otorhinolaryngology, 287; crisis, 180

Parking, 167, 169, 176, 199, 268, 318–319, 335
Pathology Department, 36, 149–150, 218, 222; chairs 354; Hartman Report, 261
Patterson Case. *See* Degree Granting Controversy
Pediatrics, Department, chairs, 369; chairs, Tulsa, 377
Penn Square Bank, 215

Pharmacology, Department, chairs, 366
Physician Associates Program, 184, 211
Physician Manpower Training Commission, 257
Physician Regents, 187–188
Physiology and Biophysics, Department, chairs, 367–368
Preceptorship, 71, 152
Presbyterian Foundation, 236, 240, 264, 266, 281, 283–284, 285, 286–287, 306, 325–326, 335
Presbyterian Hospital 23, 30, 86, 110, 119, 128, 136, 236, 278 , 288; Fitness Center, 184, 307; office building 153
Primary Care designation, 189
Professional Practice Plan (PPP), 80, 85, 108, 110, 118, 138, 167, 186, 189, 198, 229, 236, 242, 257, 262, 271, 274, 278, 283, 307, 318, 321, 324, 325, 327, 328, 335; billing services 274
Psychiatry and Behavioral Disorders, Department of, 150, 257, 261, 271, 290; chairs 370
Psychiatry, Department, Tulsa chairs, 378

Radiology, Department chairs, 371
Richardson Report, 91ff
Robert Wood Johnson Foundation, 70, 287
Rogers Building, 41

Sabbaticals, 291–292
St. Anthony Hospital, 67
St. Francis Hospital, Tulsa, 147, 271
Salaries, College of Medicine Faculty, 69, 100, 182, 199, 209–210, 218, 223–224, 241, 308
Sarkey's Foundation, 31
Senate, Faculty-Norman, 272
Senate, Oklahoma, bills ,111, 118, 314
"Sick-leave" policy, 239–240
Site of Practice Policy, 81, 278, 288, 318, 324–325, 334
Speech and Hearing Clinic, 158–159, 222–223. *See also* Otorhinolaryngology Crisis
Spina Bifida Controversy, 225
State Board of Medical Examiners, 170
State Board of Nursing, 45
State Health Department, 312
State of Oklahoma Preferred Provider Organization (PPO), 239, 312
State Regents for Higher Education, 25, 77, 95, 140, 145,161, 208, 272, 280
Steam and Chilled Water Plant, 41, 70, 79, 103, 128, 181–182, 199, 220, 282
Student Center, 277, 328, 335
Student Housing, 35
Summer Academy in Health Sciences, 287
Surgery, Department, chairs, 372; chairs, Tulsa, 379

Task Force on Hospital Governance (Bellmon), 254
Tenure, 200
Texas, 40, 269

TIAA/CREF, 157
Tulsa, deans, 390; medical education in, 36, 78, 86ff, 94, 96, 103, 110, 112–128, 138, 143–144, 152, 154, 158, 166–167, 169, 181, 198, 210, 219, 220, 236, 263–264, 265, 268, 270, 272– 273, 277, 290, 291, *294*, 313–314, 325, 336; Ungerman Trust 286

U.S. Dept. Health Education and Welfare, 41
University Hospital, 28, 34, 102, 109, 110, 121ff, *133*, 147, 182, 196, 225, 235, 314; administration, 381–382; Breast Institute, 291; "C" wing, 232; chiefs of staff, 380; Department of Corrections and, 229ff; Everett Tower, 34, 73, 77, 86, 99, 105, 107, 128, 157; nursing service, 222; "transfers" of funds to Human Services, 289
University Hospital Authority, 105, 328
University of Oklahoma Board of Regents, 21ff, 28, 53, 139, 152, 160;

Health Sciences Center Committee, 110, 140
University of Oklahoma Foundation, 36, 237, 254–256
University of Oklahoma Health Sciences (Medical) Center, 19, 27, 28, 138, 150–151, *191*, *301*; administration, 322; Faculty Senate, 126, 156; financial crisis, 40–41, 73, 152, 220, 226, 244–245, 248, 310–311, 314, 323, 327, 342; governance, 317, 393; publications and printing, 309; Research Park 306, 320, 321
Urocorp, 320
Urology, Department, chairs, 373

Vending Services, 273–274
Veterans Administration Hospital, 5, 37, 110, 178, 186, 248, 290

Wakita, 90
Walkways, 149, 165
Warren Foundation and Institute, 233, 257, 269, 273, 284–285